CW00952434

Plant Medicines, Healing and Psychedelic Science

Beatriz Caiuby Labate • Clancy Cavnar
Editors

Plant Medicines, Healing and Psychedelic Science

Cultural Perspectives

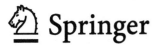 Springer

Editors
Beatriz Caiuby Labate
East-West Psychology Program
California Institute of Integral Studies (CIIS)
San Francisco, CA, USA

Center for Research and Post Graduate
Studies in Social Anthropology (CIESAS)
Guadalajara, Mexico

Clancy Cavnar
Psychiatric Alternatives
San Francisco, California, USA

ISBN 978-3-319-76719-2   ISBN 978-3-319-76720-8   (eBook)
https://doi.org/10.1007/978-3-319-76720-8

Library of Congress Control Number: 2018935154

Printed on acid-free paper

This Springer imprint is published by the registered company Springer International Publishing AG part of
Springer Nature.
The registered company address is: Gewerbestrasse 11, 6330 Cham, Switzerland

Acknowledgements

We thank all the authors of this book for their contributions and Rick Doblin and the Multidisciplinary Association for Psychedelic Studies (MAPS) for their support for this book.

Notes on Plant Medicines, Healing, and Scientists

Conferences are often boring affairs. Very serious people, often in ill-fitting suits, talk to one another about things they generally agree about. If you are an insider, you know what will happen, because it has happened before, the same conversations repeated again and again, the only difference being the color of the carpeting in an otherwise unremarkable conference room, in Atlanta, Chicago, Miami, wherever. Not so with Psychedelic Science 2017, promoted by MAPS and the Beckley Foundation, and held in April 2017 in Oakland, California, which provided the inspiration for this book.

There have been a series of Psychedelic Science conferences in the past that acted principally as forums in which researchers—who had either hewn very close to the cutting edge or gone over it into a sort of cloak and dagger, one step ahead of the law, mix of research and practice—came together to discuss their findings in what might be called a safe space, under the watchful eye of the law, but emboldened by their numbers and safe inasmuch as they were talking, only talking. This time, though, MAPS introduced new elements to the event: bigger and more diverse than before, the researchers, writers, activists, and enthusiasts who gathered for the conference had a whole new set of aspirations. They gathered in a state that had just voted to legalize marijuana, at a time when many of the participants could report on legally sanctioned trials of psychedelic drugs being used in experiments, exploring their use in palliative care, with depression, and with PTSD, among other things. And they met in a context where another difficult issue overlay the entire discussion. Just as some scientists and drug enthusiasts saw in these substances cures for physical and existential ills, a growing chorus of voices was crying foul about the transformed and profane place that many of these "medicines" seemed to occupy in contemporary society. Plant medicines, and particularly substances like ayahuasca, peyote, *Salvia divinorum*, iboga, and psilocybin mushrooms, have long played a central role in the spiritual lives and curing repertoires of a number of indigenous cultures in the Americas and in Africa, and for many of those in these communities, the current psychedelic vogue smacked of some form of appropriation.

This tension, which at times boiled over into open conflict in Psychedelic Science 2017, gave rise to this book. For the first time in the history of the Psychedelic Sciences conferences cosponsored by MAPS, the 2017 conference included a Plant Medicine track, organized by Beatriz Labate, and meant as a setting where fruitful dialogues might take place over the role of these plants in both indigenous and nonindigenous settings. The chapters in this volume represent the intellectual work that lay at the heart of that dialogue. They are the product of moments in which their authors opened themselves up to voices that applauded, critiqued, rejected, and, at times, simply misunderstood their intentions. These rich responses were possible because it was anything but the traditional staid academic conference. Instead, it often had a cacophonous feel, as scholars, activists, drug enthusiasts, and traditional users of these substances confronted the complexities of one another's views.

Through these dialogues, a few core issues emerged. First and foremost was the challenge of taxonomy. The plant medicines discussed at Psychedelic Science 2017 (principally, iboga, peyote, psilocybin mushrooms, *Salvia divinorum*, kratom, cannabis, ayahuasca, and toé) mean such profoundly different things in different settings that it is sometimes difficult to even agree that we are talking about common substances. Some will insist that these are gods, and sacred medicines, while others are much more interested in the chemical makeup of what they consider to be a plant drug. Uses also vary immensely from one setting to another, and these differences came up time and time again at Psychedelic Science 2017. These substances do not seem to have uniform impacts on the bodies of those who consume them, but instead become meaningful based on a complex set of factors that can include patterns of nutrition, living habits, traditions of exposure, and the cultural milieu within which these substances are consumed. In some contexts, they also seem to have profoundly different social meanings, either contributing to what we might call communal reproduction or being implicated in very individualized journeys of introspection. At Psychedelic Science 2017, we did not even see a common understanding of how to classify these substances as a whole. Whereas some participants used the term "drug" to describe these "hallucinogens," others chafed at the term and suggested that this did violence to a sacred plant: a deity, really. While some insisted that the appropriate term was "plant teacher," others suggested terms such as "sacraments" or "traditional medicine."

One might be inclined to categorize these conflicts through the concept of "appropriation," as indeed some attendees at Psychedelic Science 2017 suggested. In this way of seeing things, the plant medicines discussed at the conference were authentic to certain traditional indigenous settings, and those who sought to consume these substances outside of those settings (or who were themselves outsiders) had stolen Native patrimonies and were refashioning them in ways that were destructive of Native cultures. It is an argument that seems all the more salient given the ecological risk that the habitats for many of these plants face, and is one that has a long history in the Americas, where native plant medicines have faced prohibition largely because non-Natives have taken them up. Appropriation in this sense also relies on the claim that the meanings of these medicines have been transformed by consuming them out of context and that what was once a custom rooted in a communal healing process had become a dangerous drug in the hands of outsiders, placing everyone at risk.

And yet, even as these powerful arguments were being made, others at the conference were making similarly compelling arguments about the role that these plant medicines had played, and could potentially play, in healing processes outside of their traditional settings. These voices did not generally suggest that outsiders might replicate, or even understand, traditional Native uses, but relied on the claim—and on evidence that backed up that claim—that in certain carefully curated settings, psychedelic plant medicines could have a powerful healing effect that, while different in specific contexts, was nonetheless powerfully therapeutic. And all along, other advocates—especially the enthusiasts who simply believed that, in a free society, they should be entitled to consume substances that are not particularly dangerous and offer powerful mystical experiences—repeatedly made their voices heard. If they wanted to get high, whose business should that be?

This book makes an effort to capture the energy and tensions in that conversation by taking some of the presentations from Psychedelic Science 2017 and deepening the analysis in ways that are only possible in the aftermath of such an event. The chapters represent a series of conversations about sacred plants, modern medicine, communal healing, and journeys of self-discovery, as they were explored at Psychedelic Science 2017. They also reproduce some of the tensions in the conference through their strikingly different approaches to plant medicines. We have here some more standard social scientific efforts to understand the drug effect, as well as deeper concerns about reframing both the use of these plants and their conceptualizations away from a Western perspective. Nonnative communities of users are also closely and, at times, sympathetically interrogated. Some chapters approach the nonindigenous uses of these plants as interesting and important phenomena; others reflect the unease in the conference around the conflation of indigenous and nonindigenous use and the fear that the latter at times imperils the former. As a whole, then, these chapters offer a glimpse of a larger ongoing conversation about drugs, plant medicines, the sacred and the profane, science, and the law, a conversation that has yet to come to a conclusion and in which a great deal is at stake.

Organization of the Book

Considering the long history of these conflicts, we elected to begin our exploration of plant medicines with a chapter by the historian Erika Dyck, who reminds us that many of the challenges facing contemporary psychedelic research replay issues that arose decades ago. The field of "psychedelic science" has always been a sort of mix between culture and science; the psychedelic pioneers were certainly interested in the cultural aspects of plant medicines as well, and the tensions between clinical and nonclinical uses were always present. The author demonstrates how psychedelics fell from medical grace nearly half a century ago, but recent activity suggests that some researchers have "high hopes" for their return. Are we at risk, however, of facing the same historic challenges with a new generation of psychedelic enthusiasts, or have the circumstances changed sufficiently to allow for a new path forward? The twenty-first-century incarnation of psychedelic research resurrects some anticipated hypotheses and explores some of the same applications that clinicians experimented with 50 years ago. On the surface, then, the psychedelic renaissance might be dismissed for retreading familiar ground. A deeper look at the context that gave rise to these questions, though, suggests that, while some of the questions are common, the culture of neuroscience and the business of drug regulation have changed sufficiently to warrant a retrial. Dyck argues that, historically, LSD and its psychedelic cousins were not simply victims of unsophisticated science; drug regulators also clouded their legitimacy based on assumptions about their perceived effects, dangers, and potential for problematic use. The author examines the historical clinical uses of LSD in Canada, including the facility that led to the coining of the term "psychedelic," and the "infamous Hollywood hospital that offered psychedelic treatments for addictions," to explore some of the lessons that LSD's past has to offer.

Following on Dyck's analysis, Alexander Dawson, also a historian, reminds us that questions surrounding the legality and use of psychedelics have also historically been interwoven with larger issues of race, especially in the USA and Mexico. In the years since peyote became a controlled substance in Mexico and the USA, a steady stream of advocates and activists have laid claim to two types of exemption, rooted in both US law (the First Amendment) and international law (the 1971 Vienna Convention on Psychotropic Drugs). Indigenous peyotists, in particular, have been largely successful in making a claim to a legal right to be exempt from national prohibitions on peyote possession and consumption. This has represented a significant advance in indigenous rights; yet, according to Dawson, in both contexts it has had the unpleasant effect of signaling that a drug that is otherwise so dangerous as to be prohibited should be permitted for Indians, because they are somehow essentially different from all other citizens. This, then, is in the author's perspective, "peyote's race problem." The ways in which we have created a legal framework that makes peyote use licit among indigenous peoples, claims Dawson, have hardened a certain notion of profound, unalterable difference to the point that Indian bodies are said to be incommensurably different from the bodies of others who might desire to consume peyote, but for whom it is deemed too dangerous. Dawson argues that the frameworks that now exist for licit peyote not only resonate in an uncomfortable way with the colonial past but also offer important insights into the way that racist thinking continues to inform legal systems on both sides of the US–Mexican border.

Ben Feinberg then takes us on a journey from Psychedelic Science 2017 itself, to Huautla, and back again. He asks questions such as: What can Mazatec shamanism add to the field of psychedelic science, and what does the discourse about drugs tell us about different rankings of categories of people? While the physiological effects of the consumption of psychedelic mushrooms probably have much in common across individuals in different cultural and historical settings, the ways in which they are perceived to work, the contexts in which they are taken, the meanings that are attributed to them, the problems they are perceived to address, and the degree to which their efficacy is assessed are discursively constructed and may vary greatly. The town of Huautla de Jimenez in the Sierra Mazateca of Oaxaca, Mexico, is well known as a space where mushrooms are traditionally used, and national and international visitors have come to the area to consume them since the 1950s, producing what Feinberg calls an "often-imbalanced cross-cultural dialogue about their effects." Based on 25 years of ethnographic research, the author presents an overview of the different expectations of the visitors and the local Mazatec population regarding mushrooms and the changes in Mazatec discourse about their use. He suggests that the Western discourse about the "therapeutic value" of mushroom use, with its emphasis on individual wellness, often assumes a universality that erases the specificities of the Mazatec context and their understanding of the value of the "child saints." At the same time, these differences do not prevent productive engagement between Mazatec speakers and outsiders.

In Chap. 4, Ana Elda Maqueda keeps our focus on the Mazatecs but shifts our attention to another plant medicine that has had a growing impact outside of its communities of traditional use. *Salvia divinorum* is a medicinal plant endemic to the Mazatec Sierra of Oaxaca, Mexico, that has been used by this indigenous people for centuries as a treatment for different ailments. The chapter combines a description of traditional use, a review of the scientific literature, and a more experiential and down-to-earth "how-to" section on finding the best ways to use salvia for "medicinal, psychotherapeutic, and inner exploration purposes." The Mazatec consider salvia to be a very powerful plant being that should be treated with supreme respect and ingested based on a strict preparation regimen. They chew the fresh leaves at night, followed by chanting and praying. Among Westerners, however, dry leaves are potentiated in extracts and smoked, often resulting in overwhelming experiences due to the high potency and fast onset of the substance. The author aims to create a bridge between the two perspectives and also questions whether scientific findings back up Mazatec claims of salvia's therapeutic potentials.

In the following chapter, O. Hayden Griffin, III, extends the analysis beyond Mexico in an exploration of the potential medical uses of kratom, which comes from the Korth tree (*Mitragyna speciosa*) and is native to Africa and Southeast Asia. Kratom is one of many traditional drugs that have recently gained attention in the West. People indigenous to Southeast Asia have used kratom for hundreds of years, at least, but the first scientific reference to the plant appeared in 1836. The author offers a description of the scientific research on kratom and its rare combination of both stimulant and narcotic properties. As in the case of *Salvia divinorum*, traditional kratom use includes the treatment for a variety of ailments. More recently, many Westerners have begun to use it for medicinal and recreational purposes. In the USA, the Drug Enforcement Administration (DEA) has expressed some intent to regulate it, and a few individual states have already done so. Activists have discussed the possibility of regulation of kratom via the rules pertaining to dietary supplements, indicating the challenges of classifying the use of these traditional substances in our biomedical and legal categories.

In Chap. 6, Kevin Feeney, Beatriz C. Labate, and J. Hamilton Hudson combine legal and anthropological knowledge to confront the legal challenges to the use of plant medicines by nonindigenous users. The research is based on analysis of legal documents that are rarely available. The use of ayahuasca has been spreading rapidly worldwide; in the USA, the expansion has included the appearance of the Brazilian ayahuasca religions Santo Daime and União do Vegetal (UDV), underground ceremonial circles, workshops with itinerant Amazonian shamans, and spiritual retreat centers. This trend has also included the recent emergence of groups and organizations that publicly advertise "legal" ayahuasca ceremonies and retreats. The chapter maps the existence of a series of organizations and actors who have controversially claimed legal protection through incorporation as "branches" of the Native American Church (NAC). The legality, religious character, and sincerity of these churches are reviewed in light of governing law. As is the case with other substances discussed in this book, the use of ayahuasca has generated legal contradictions that remain unsolved.

Jordan Sloshower considers nonindigenous users of plant medicines in a different context in Chap. 7. Combining literature from varied disciplines and clinical perspectives with his experience in building a scientific research proposal on psilocybin mushrooms, the author brings to the forefront topics that are normally in the backstage of psychedelic science. He contrasts current psychiatric practices and their reductionist focus on biological paradigms with what he calls a psychedelic healing paradigm that actively engages in addressing root causes of illness at multiple levels, including the spiritual and energetic domains. He speculates on theoretical, methodological, and ethical challenges to the integration of the psychedelic healing paradigm into psychiatric practice. A model clinic is proposed that would serve as proof of concept for a new model of conceptualizing and treating mental illness.

In Chap. 8, Sidarta Ribeiro further complicates these questions in an examination of the differences between the use of whole plants and pharmaceutical extracts. He examines the scientific, economic, and political implications of the "war," or controversy, between those who advocate the traditional consumption of whole organisms and those who defend exclusively the utilization of purified compounds, presumably more specific and safer. He argues that traditional medicine, based on whole organisms, is complex and can't be reduced to single active principles. He evokes the examples of ayahuasca and cannabis. The first is the result of at least two plant species containing multiple psychoactive substances having complex interactions, and the second contains dozens of psychoactive substances whose specific combinations in different strains, he argues, correspond to different types of therapeutic and cognitive effects. Evidence indicates that it is time to embrace the "entourage effect": the synergistic effects of the multiple compounds present in whole organisms that may enhance clinical efficacy and attenuate side effects.

We are reminded of the particular challenges associated with psychedelic medicines in Katherine Handy's contribution, Chap. 8. This chapter is a must-read for all researchers involved in current scientific investigation of plant medicines. The author offers anthropological insights into the array of new studies with drugs like LSD, MDMA, and psilocybin. She poses questions such as: How is the placebo effect framed and shaped by clinical trial methodologies, and how could it be framed differently? What kind of a "problem" is a placebo? Placebo-controlled randomized controlled studies (RCTs), she argues, have become the institutional standard for research with psychopharmaceuticals. Hendy focuses on the fascinating topic of the placebo as a tool in blinding these studies (both to the subjects of the research and to the researchers themselves). She argues that, while anthropologists have examined placebos as examples of the power of symbolic healing or as ethically problematic research components, she examines instead placebos as a research technique around which the scientific status of a study is negotiated. In sum, the "problem of placebo" is a privileged space to reflect on the political struggle for psychedelics to be included under the sign of science.

We shift to a different community of users in the subsequent chapter by Joanna Steinhardt. The author addresses the use of mushrooms, covering a fertile intersection between "drugs" and "foods." She studies contemporary do-it-yourself (DIY) mycology, a movement that has emerged in the last decade in North America, specializing in methods of mushroom cultivation and mycological experimentation, and mobilizing a discourse of "alliance with the fungal kingdom." Drawing on ethnographic fieldwork in the San Francisco Bay Area and the Pacific Northwest, the chapter identifies the intersection of the psychedelic movement and ecological concerns. The DIY mycology exemplifies how the dissemination of mycological interests extends far beyond psychedelics. The individuals investigated by Steinhardt, and their love for and practices around mushrooms, make the definitions of "culinary," "medicinal," and "psychoactive" blurry and more complex. They invite us to shift our focus from the psychoactive properties per se and bring us back to the larger context of plants as beings in their natural environment, as is the case with indigenous beliefs and cultures described in other contributions to this book.

In the following chapter, Laura Dev continues discussing an interspecies or cross-kingdom engagement deeper south, in the Amazon, in ayahuasca "plant teachers" settings. While reviewing some academic literature on ayahuasca, she makes an original contribution by asking how the concept of "plant intelligences" could adequately be accounted for by research practices. In other words, the chapter aims to examine the ontological and epistemological assumptions that underlie current research practices and how they are related to certain hierarchies of knowledge. The challenge would be to end the reproduction of racialized knowledge hierarchies that continue to place plant spirits in the realm of "less valid" "indigenous beliefs." She suggests that we humbly engage with indigenous epistemologies and ways of producing knowledge, which include collaborating with plant teachers and their agency. What would a collaborative research that includes indigenous standpoints and multispecies perspectives look like?

In Chap. 12, Graham St John returns us to the pharmacological, but in a way that suggests that DMT's (N,N-dimethyltryptamine) uses among contemporary underground circles offer certain profoundly important opportunities for personal insight. DMT, known for its short-term "breakthrough effect," has experienced a growing appeal in the last decade. The author harvests accounts from key figures in the psychonautic literature, such as Terence McKenna and Jonathan Ott, and online "trip reports." Users report contact with "entities," the transmission of visual language, and connection to another reality from which modern humanity is imagined to have become alienated. The chapter speculates on the significance of DMT in modern Western esotericism and, like other contributions in this book, suggests that the uses of these substances are not easy to classify and can occur in a continuum of therapy, gnosis, and recreation. However, here, the urban "natives" are the ones to consider problematic the presence of a shaman and rather advocate for the absence of "intermediaries." In any case, these autonomous travels in "hyperspace" seem to forge the need for a new vocabulary and conceptual classifications about the "medical value" of psychedelics and ways to better investigate them.

Graham, like each one of the other eleven chapters in the book, captures a small but critical part of the many debates and conversations that one could find in the halls and conference rooms in Oakland. In each of these conversations, we can see the intersections of scientific analysis, religious belief, law, and indigenous rights, sometimes aligned together with specific goals, and at other times in profound tension: alignments and tensions that can be read throughout this book. The role of plant medicines in our societies is far from a settled matter, and these chapters, if unlikely to produce a uniform set of laws and practices, at the very least introduce us in a serious fashion to the questions we confront as we situate these substances (sometimes read as teachers) in our twenty-first-century societies. We hope that this book helps to advance a dialogue between science, culture, and society as the field of psychedelic science continues to flourish.

East-West Psychology Program   Beatriz Caiuby Labate
California Institute of Integral Studies
(CIIS), San Francisco, CA, USA

Center for Research and Post Graduate
Studies in Social Anthropology
(CIESAS), Guadalajara, Mexico

Nucleus for Interdisciplinary Studies of   Clancy Cavnar
Psychoactives (NEIP), São Paulo, Brazil

Psychiatric Alternatives, San Francisco,
California, USA

Department of History   Alexander Dawson
SUNY Albany, Albany, NY, USA

Contents

Chapter 1
Who Is Keeping Tabs? LSD Lessons from the Past for the Future

Erika Dyck

Abstract Psychedelics fell from medical grace nearly half a century ago, but recent activity suggests that some researchers are optimistic about their return. Are they at risk, however, of facing the same historic challenges with a new generation of psychedelic enthusiasts, or have the circumstances changed sufficiently to allow for a new path forward? The twenty-first-century incarnation of psychedelic research resurrects some anticipated hypotheses and explores some of the same applications that clinicians experimented with 50 years ago. On the surface then, the psychedelic renaissance might be dismissed for retreading familiar ground. A deeper look at the context that gave rise to these questions, though, suggests that while some of the questions are common, the culture of neuroscience and the business of drug regulation have changed sufficiently to warrant a retrial. A close look at the history of psychedelics encourages us to think carefully about the roles of regulators, the enthusiasm of researchers, and our cultural fascination and/or repulsion with mind-altering molecules.

In February 2014, *Scientific American* shocked readers with an editorial that called for an end to the ban on psychedelic drug research (End the Ban, 2014). The article criticized the mental health treatment industry for failing to advance therapies beyond the golden era of the 1950s and lambasted drug regulators for prohibiting psychedelic drugs, including LSD, ecstasy (MDMA), and psilocybin, drugs that had historically held clinical promise but were "designated as drugs of abuse" (End the Ban, p. 1). As the editors pointed out, the situation has created a paradox: "these drugs are banned because they have no accepted medical use, but researchers cannot explore their therapeutic potential because they are banned…The decades-long research hiatus has taken its toll" (End the Ban, 2014, pp. 1–2). Lest there be any confusion as to where the editors stood on the issue, they continued with explicit instructions: "This is a shame. The US government should move these drugs to the

---

E. Dyck (✉)
Department of History, University of Saskatchewan, Saskatoon, SK, Canada
e-mail: Erika.dyck@usask.ca

© Springer International Publishing AG, part of Springer Nature 2018
B. C. Labate, C. Cavnar (eds.), *Plant Medicines, Healing and Psychedelic Science*,
https://doi.org/10.1007/978-3-319-76720-8_1

1

less strict Schedule II classification…it would make it much easier for clinical researchers to study their effects" (End the Ban, 2014, p. 2). The article brought public and scientific attention to a growing contention among researchers and even some regulators that the clinical potential among psychedelic drugs had been dismissed in the past due to a moral panic about drug abuse.

But this article was just the tip of the proverbial iceberg. In the past decade, psychedelics have returned to the clinical arena with renewed optimism for their positive role in therapeutics, across a range of areas. Hundreds of published papers have looked back and criticized regulators, researchers, and consumers for distorting the truth about psychedelics. Several contemporary scientists have joined the chorus of support for renewed investigations into the therapeutic potential for psychedelics. Their criticisms of the current state of prohibition point to historical misconceptions about the dangers, as well as the benefits, of applying psychedelics in a healing context. The renewed interest, however, also reinforces some older trends in psychedelic science. In particular, the so-called renaissance criticizes the previous generation for applying sloppy scientific controls. Others blamed overzealous regulators for establishing demanding protocols that were considered unsuitable for the contours of psychedelic research. Journalists have also been the subjects of scorn, for fueling the moral panic about drug abuse, risky behavior, and even more conspiratorial claims about cultural changes inspired through psychedelic experiences. Nearly 70 years later, have we entered in a new social contract that allows us to mitigate these external challenges leveled at psychedelic science, or has the science advanced sufficiently to fend off these cultural and political challenges?

Historians are poorly equipped to make predictions about the future, but we are well trained to look back and situate events within a broader context. To do so requires sifting through elements of cause and effect and critically analyzing memories of events against evidence describing such events in real time. These skills are essential for altering the narrative or cultural assumptions about the past that, in turn, affects our reception of new ideas for the future. Historians do not simply tell stories about the past; we interpret the past, creating narratives that form part of our cultural memory. Those memories or legacies help to anchor our collective consciousness and allow us to gauge our future progress. In the case of a psychedelic renaissance, historical interpretations may be significant for carefully analyzing some of the long-held assumptions about why psychedelic science failed in the first place. This chapter examines the historical uses of LSD, as well as some of the shortcuts that may have hampered its more widespread reception or acceptance as a clinical tool. It reflects on the current reawakening by drawing contextual lessons from the past.

Tune In, Turn On, Step Back

Plant medicines have been used for thousands of years; Western scientific fascination has generated different ways of thinking about these substances. Regardless of the chemical structure of the substance used, the concepts that come to define the experiences also reveal different approaches to use. The category of entheogens describes plant teachers that generate the divine within, while hallucinogens are simply substances that cause hallucinations, regardless of any deeper subjective meaning; and psychedelics, the mind-manifesting molecules, have a comparatively shorter history and are associated with psychotherapy and clinical therapy. German psychiatrists, beginning in the 1920s, seized upon peyote for its healing capacity, not in the form of indigenous ritualized healing but instead as a distinctive chemical response to the isolated molecule, mescaline (Rouhier, 1927). Peyote had been used for hundreds of years in indigenous ceremonies to communicate with a spiritual world, as a healing agent and as a sacrament. Its first uses occurred in Mexico, and since at least the fifteenth century, it spread northward into the United States and southward through Mesoamerica (Maroukis, 2010). Peyote, the cactus, and peyotism, the practice of worship with the cactus, have attracted scholars, politicians, chemists, biologists, and indigenous and non-indigenous people who are captivated, and at times repulsed, by the connection between peyote and colonialism, settler-colonial relations, and science and religion (Labate and Cavnar, 2016).

In the twentieth century, as the peyote religion came under threat from colonial authorities eager to prohibit indigenous practices of religion and healing that were deemed backward or unmodern, Western scientists maintained their fascination with the peyote ritual and the potential science behind its culturally mysterious chemistry. Keen to distinguish the chemical reaction from the ritualistic context, early pharmacologists isolated mescaline, purifying the substance and opening the proverbial doors to a new era of scientific exploration with these substances that had long been revered in a different context for their capacity to inspire new insights or to generate spiritual encounters of a divine nature. While these elements were not altogether erased from the clinical encounters, the role of tradition, ritual, and spirituality were further muted, as deference to the molecule was pushed aside in exchange for deference to the researcher and scientific objectivity.

Mescaline attracted attention, but by the 1950s, its story was quickly overshadowed by LSD. D-lysergic acid diethylamide (LSD), on the surface, represented a triumph in modern science. This molecule originated in the laboratory setting, created and designed by the accouterments of modern science. It did not initially carry the trappings of a cultural discourse. Although it shared some experiential features with mescaline, it did not owe its history or future to a religious or cultural context and could readily appeal to Western scientists as a secular technology: a product of dedicated science. But, the history of LSD suggests that the molecule was not a typical pharmaceutical product but rather belonged, at least chemically and experientially, to a family of plant medicines that held both cultural and scientific fascination.

Albert Hofmann, the discoverer of LSD, famously reflected on the drug his book *LSD: My Problem Child*. His book captured the frustrating mixture of his excitement and joy with the new discovery and his hopes and dreams for the potential held within this tiny molecule. Hoffman was a Swiss biochemist working at Sandoz pharmaceutical laboratories when he began working with synthetic substances of the ergot family. In 1938, he first synthesized lysergic acid diethylamide-25, an internal name applied to the 25th compound in the lysergic acid series, which remained undisturbed for 5 years until he experienced its powerful effects in 1943 (Hofmann, 2013).

On Friday, April 16, 1943, Hofmann had his first LSD experience, though he had not realized that he had come into contact with the chemical, and the response took him by surprise. While disoriented, he "perceived an uninterrupted stream of fantastic pictures, extraordinary shapes and an intense, kaleidoscopic play of colors" (Hofmann, 2013, p. 18). His now infamous voyage into a gripping hallucination captured attention at the time and has since been a part of the psychedelic lore. His depiction expressed wonderment at the fantastical effects of a drug that disoriented his senses and disrupted his sense of reality. In the 2013 edition of his book, Amanda Fielding, editor, philanthropist, and LSD enthusiast, described Hofmann as "scientist who, through his most famous discovery, crossed the bridge from the world of science into the spiritual realm, transforming social and political culture in his wake. He was both rationalist and mystic, chemist and visionary..." (Hofmann, 2013, p. v). LSD had captured the attention of clinical, biomedical, spiritual, and political thinkers across the disciplinary spectrum; its unconventional status meant that it quickly became both revered and reviled.

Sandoz Pharmaceuticals began experiments with LSD first in animal models and eventually within the field of psychiatry. The drug's powerful psychological effects attracted people working in fields of psychiatry, psychotherapy, and psychoanalysis, in particular, due to its rather consistent capacity to affect cognition and to induce a period of reflection among users (Hofmann, 2013). By the early 1960s, over a thousand scientific articles had appeared with investigators using LSD in a wide variety of settings, applying diverse methods and instruments and drawing a number of different conclusions. The research community did not reach a consensus on a specific direction for LSD studies, but several promising avenues emerged throughout the 1950s. Chief among these was the use of LSD for treating alcoholism, but it was also tested in clinical settings on a range of behaviors, including homosexuality, depression, couples' therapy, aggression, and as a model psychosis (Abramson, 1960).

While researchers subscribed to different methods for testing LSD, its appeal widened to include non-clinical investigations, and it soon gained attention for being a catalyst for spiritual and creative thinking (Ellwood, 1994; Miller, 1991; Fuller, 2000). Some people tried to harness these reactions and put them to productive use in clinical settings, but others recognized the power of this substance to move beyond the confines of medicine and perhaps to better serve us by enriching human thinking along evolutionary terms. Yet others recognized a longer tradition of hallucinogens that connected with traditional healing practices among Aboriginal people or linked with non-Christian religions (Hoffer & Osmond, 1967). For instance, North American investigators looked to the use of peyote among members of the Native American Church, a religious organization that was first established in Oklahoma. Comparing religious interactions with hallucinogenic substances encouraged scientists to consider a longer tradition of combining spiritual healing into psychological treatments (Dyck & Bradford, 2012). Others looked to ololiuqui use among the

Aztecs who similarly derived meaning from drug-induced visions or hallucinations (Hoffer & Osmond, 1967).

In 1957, psychiatrist Humphry Osmond, then working in a mental hospital in western Canada, coined the term "psychedelic" to tap into its mind-manifesting properties and to describe how the drug brought psychological material to light (Osmond, 1957, p. 429). His introduction of the term came through his correspondence with British writer and philosopher, Aldous Huxley, and was a testament to the fundamentally interdisciplinary nature of the concept. After sharing a mescaline experience in Aldous Huxley's home in Hollywood, California, in 1953, these two men engaged in a decade-long relationship that produced over 700 pages of letters, countless visits, and kinship ties. Together they established a growing network of people committed to generating what Huxley would come to call "outsight": not simply the opposite of insight but a deep state of reflection that embraced both internal thoughts and the context in which we live in modern civilization. Humphry Osmond and Aldous Huxley attempted to create an organization dedicated to this cause. Outsight, in their words, would: "advance human consciousness and draw attention to a chemically induced way of accessing some higher dimension" (Symons, 2015, p. 136). Or, put more simply, they wanted to establish a psychedelic think tank: a group of expansive thinkers, intellectual elites even, who would come together under the influence of mescaline or LSD to tackle big problems.

Osmond and Huxley were uniquely positioned to create new language to describe the mescalinized responses, not because they were necessarily scientifically connected but because they drew from a rich and diverse set of experiences, ways of knowing, or ontologies, in their attempts to capture the concept of psychedelic science. Osmond was a British-trained psychiatrist with a side interest in being a playwright. Huxley was already a well-known literary figure from a famous family of writers and evolutionary biologists. By the time they met in 1953, Huxley was already a famous author and had a growing reputation for his personal interests in "fringe science" (Bisbee et al., 2018).

In their discussions leading up to developing the concept "psychedelic," they drew from diverse ideas—indigenous peyote rituals, biochemistry, evolutionary biology, musical performances, ancient Greek poetry, philosophy, history, neuroscience—with a heavy dose of Jungian psychology and spirituality. Not only were their discussions a veritable treasure trove of ideas about the power of the human mind to perceive or the capacity for chemicals to induce empathy, but they developed the language of psychedelics using concepts and approaches that were infused with an expansive set of possibilities that drew deeply from the past in an effort to imagine a different set of futures.

These psychedelic pioneers were interested in the clinical applications of psychedelics but were also deeply curious about the cultural uses of plant medicines and the ritualistic elements of ceremonial chemistry that was often ignored by Western science. Osmond, along with his colleagues in Saskatchewan, believed that LSD, along with other psychedelic drugs, including peyote (mescaline), ololiuqui, ibogaine, and others, provided Western medicine with a critical tool for linking biomedical approaches with spiritual and psychological healing: a feature that

Osmond believed had been leached away by modern biomedical interventions that tended to favor body over spirit.

The use of LSD in treating alcoholism gathered significant attention and showed tremendous promise throughout the 1950s, even within more conventional treatment modalities (Mangini, 1998). The concept behind its therapeutic approach involved single, albeit megadoses, of LSD. Patients were required to sit with a counselor, psychologist, psychiatrist, nurse, or social worker, throughout the experience, which usually lasted an entire day. Patients were encouraged to talk about themselves, often prompted by looking at family photographs or while listening to classical music or by looking at artwork. Results of follow-up studies indicated a long-term sobriety following these sessions. Individuals claimed that they had generated a new level of self-awareness and psychological fortitude to end their problem drinking (Krebs and Johansen, 2012). The results stymied contemporary addiction researchers, some of whom were less comfortable with a drug trial that did not conform to the emerging standards of randomized controlled testing, and debates over the value of psychedelics in therapy continued to engage mental health professionals (Dyck, 2006).

By the beginning of the 1960s, LSD had become a well-known substance within clinical research circles, but it had yet to reach mainstream society in any significant way. Ken Kesey was then a creative writing student at Stanford University who had volunteered to take LSD as part of a clinical trial before he burst onto the psychedelic scene as an apostle of LSD-induced mind freedom (Dodgson, 2013). Timothy Leary had explored a variety of drugs—both professionally and personally—before landing in trouble with Harvard University for his "unscientific" use of psilocybin mushrooms and drug experiments with prisoners (Greenfield, 2006).

These two figures became firmly associated with a different side of LSD's character by the mid-1960s. During that colorful decade, LSD's reputation changed dramatically. Leary had catapulted from Harvard University to Millbrook, an elite upstate New York getaway for acid gatherings, where he set himself up as an acid guru and an evangelical purveyor of a burgeoning psychedelic movement. Ken Kesey, meanwhile, had published his expose of American mental hospitals in *One Flew Over the Cuckoo's Nest* and quickly became associated with a rising tide of countercultural antics that included a rather flamboyant consumption of drugs (Kesey, 1962). Throughout North America, psychedelics coursed through the 1960s culture, inciting new genres of music, literature, hedonism, and anti-authority attitudes. While many of these connections were overblown, the presumed connection between LSD and immorality overwhelmed a more logical or clinical assessment of the situation (Dyck, 2012).

In the media, LSD became implicated with murder, suicide, and a slough of health problems, alongside a more generalized set of antipathies toward the American state (Osmond, 1967). Young people high on acid and caught in terrifying hallucinations were allegedly driven to madness and violence. Charles Manson's serial murders were in part attributed to LSD; elsewhere, a former medical student reportedly murdered his mother; LSD-soaked youths contracted venereal diseases at concerts; others went blind after taking LSD and believing they could stare at the sun (Dyck, 2008).

While sociologists have since pointed out that these claims were hyperbolic, medical researchers found themselves caught in a moral panic over the value of LSD. Sandoz Pharmaceuticals, undoubtedly worried about its reputation, temporarily suspended production of its LSD supplies in 1963. It became clear, however, that other substances had leaked into the black market and masqueraded as LSD, when in fact they bore no chemical similarities (Osmond, 1967). The rise of drug use in general, and psychedelics in particular, created challenges for medical researchers who were faced with the growing reputation that these substances were merely agents of abuse. By the same token, medical staff had difficulty treating patients who claimed to have taken LSD when the drugs in circulation were often not bona fide LSD and were often consumed in combination with other substances that further stymied medical staff in their ability to fully comprehend the LSD reaction or its management.

As public concerns heightened over the dangers associated with LSD use, drug regulators at first worked closely with scientists to chart a course of development for how best to regulate this drug. In the early 1960s, clinical optimism had tipped the scales in favor of a regulatory scheme that allowed for continued investigations along rather liberal lines (Oram, 2018). Some researchers maintained that LSD was on the cusp of making significant breakthroughs in addiction treatments and that further sustained study was necessary to see through the haze of misinformation surrounding the recreational abuse of the drug.

Meanwhile, acid on the streets wreaked havoc and induced psychotic breakdowns in otherwise sane people, according to news, police, and health reports. Bellevue Hospital in New York City claimed that it had never before received so many patients into its psychiatric division and had admitted 65 people in 1965 alone with LSD-induced psychoses. Fully nine of those cases involved "uncontrolled violent urges including homicide attempts by 2 individuals. Four others were found running or sitting nude in the streets" (Jonnes, 1996, p. 232).

The states of New York and California convened senate hearings in 1966 to outlaw LSD. The Canadian government had responded 4 years earlier with a more tepid response, placing LSD alongside thalidomide on a special new drug schedule reserved for drugs that were still under medical investigation, but which were not otherwise controlled through the criminal system. Iconic leaders of the psychedelic movement, including former psychologist Timothy Leary, writer Ken Kesey, poet Allen Ginsberg, and others, had become the new face of the drug and spoke publicly about the conservatism of the state attempting to stamp out a form of cultural consciousness. These self-appointed champions of psychedelia forged a strong popular connection between LSD and counterculture hedonism that may have galvanized supporters but also cleaved them off from mainstream society. The resulting cultural division cut deeply across conventional authority figures, including psychedelic researchers, who risked being labeled as bad scientists or bad citizens by association.

Spilling outside the confines of laboratory studies, LSD on the street posed a number of problems and inspired a more outspoken reaction to a drug that appeared to be spiraling out of control. In 1968, pressure came from all directions to regulate

LSD out of legal territory altogether. The scientific community could not come to an agreement on whether LSD's potential could truly be realized. While some researchers balked at its inability to perform consistently in controlled trials, others chided the spiritual dimension that had been attached to its healing potential. Either way, it had not found its way into a specific disease category or marketable psychopharmaceutical niche to warrant further sustained evaluation in this context. Furthermore, volunteers for trials increasingly came from a less desirable segment of society: those seeking thrills over legitimate, or even objective, test subjects. The capacity, therefore, of researchers to establish quantifiable and verifiable results became ever more difficult (Dyck, 2011). Despite these problems, some researchers remained dedicated to finding a credible scientific pathway through the cultural malaise, to demonstrate with clear evidence the efficacy of these molecules in psychotherapy (Oram, 2018). In spite of these efforts, it became increasingly difficult to justify continued studies of LSD while the substance appeared to produce violent and sustained health problems, primarily within psychiatric categories. Results, whether in clinical trials or on the streets, seemed to generate incredibly unpredictable and highly dangerous outcomes, compelling politicians and regulators to step in and restore public confidence in their ability to decrease public health risks (Oram, 2016).

By the 1970s, the psychedelic scene was dramatically different. Funded, legitimate scientific research directly using LSD ground almost entirely to a halt, while committed enthusiasts continued to manufacture the drug illegally and fuel an underground network of research. Spring Grove Hospital and its director Charles Savage were an exception (Oram, 2014, p. 241). Recreationally, LSD continued to be a force and was now readily joined by a host of other narcotics: psychedelics from peyote and mushrooms and others and from the comparably benign marijuana to a range of contraband amphetamines, to injectable heroin. The drug cornucopia, which had always been present but highly regulated, exploded onto the street with renewed enthusiasm as it comingled with ideas about consciousness-raising philosophies, anti-authoritarian attitudes, and risk-averse liberties (Elcock, 2015; Schneider, 2008; Henderson, 2011). Not without some irony, this was also the burgeoning era of psychopharmacology, when more pharmaceuticals moved into circulation than ever before. One of the key differences in their fates lay in the regulations that determined their classification as substances of medicine or those of abuse.

The tone of psychedelic research shifted from studies within the realm of pharmaceutical trials to ones exploring spiritual, philosophical, and cultural dimensions of the relationship of reality and consciousness. These kinds of questions moved beyond the comfort zone of modern Western medicine and developed small enclaves outside of university campuses (Aaronson & Osmond, 1970). Serious psychedelic research largely moved underground, while its more social persona took on a life of its own, seeping into cultural products, music, literature, and the visual arts as it became woven into the fabric of the 1960s, making public appearances only in times of desperation, whether in emergency rooms or in jail cells (Stevens, 1987). By the 1980s, it did not seem likely for LSD to resurface in legitimate scientific arenas.

The Psychedelic Renaissance: Lessons from the Past

Almost exactly 50 years after California banned the use of LSD, psychedelic researchers gathered for the largest meeting on psychedelic science yet. In April 2017, the Multidisciplinary Association for Psychedelic Studies, together with the Beckley Foundation, hosted over 3000 participants in Oakland, California, for a meeting to discuss the future of psychedelics. This time, they boldly married psychedelics of the past with the science of the future. The meeting featured several key figures in this community who have been collecting laboratory data, neuroscience imaging, and pharmacological information aimed at revising the historical record. This revision is based on assumptions that earlier attempts at accruing data were misled or unsophisticated. And, while it is true that researchers in the 1950s did not use the same techniques as the ones working in the 2010s, much of the research conducted in the past operated on the highest standards of research at the time. Unless our methods today fail to evolve, it is possible that the same fate will befall today's research teams.

The California gathering also included social scientists, filmmakers, and speakers whose experiences came directly from plant medicines. This acknowledgment of interdisciplinarity and cultural inclusion was an important gesture and could be a significant bridge between the past and future, as well as the science and culture of psychedelics. Psychedelics, past and present, straddle philosophical divides: mind and body, rational and irrational, and spiritualist and materialist. Collectively, we have not developed logic or methods for peaceful coexistence that have reached mainstream consensus. Indeed, these differences in how we interpret experience have penetrated deeply into our academic disciplines and are reinforced in our cultural attitudes about who qualifies as a legitimate psychedelic expert. These tensions remained on display at the 2017 meeting. *The New York Times* reported on the meeting, citing an attendee who accused Gabor Maté, a Canadian-based medical doctor who works with shamans and plant healers, of cultural appropriation and insensitivity toward this issue (Schwartz, 2017). The contests over indigenous rites and biomedical appropriation of plant medicines continue to incite controversy, which has yet to be resolved by past or present investigators. While figures such as Maté have attempted to bridge that divide by crossing from Western to non-Western approaches and by developing relationships with non-Western healers, the historical legacy of uneven power between colonizer and colonized deeply affects this relationship and continues to create unease within the context of psychedelics (Maté, 2009).

Race and indigeneity are not the only categories of identity that invoke tensions within the psychedelic community: men continue to dominate the discussions of psychedelic science, while women remain the handmaidens in this research enterprise. In both historical and current studies, women have been intrinsically involved in carrying out the research, particularly as therapeutic guides and empathic observers but rarely as principal investigators.[1] Historically, women played a vital role, most frequently as nurses and therapeutic guides, but they are rarely described in publications as central to the experiment or experience. Subjects, however, more readily refer to the empathetic women who guided them through their experiences or helped to ensure a safe environment for the experiment.

The new phase of psychedelic science seems to mirror this gender dimension rather than fostering a more inclusive atmosphere, either in terms of equity or in terms of prioritizing the empathic elements of qualitative and emotionally sensitive responses. This is not to say that women are exclusively capable of empathy, but they remain more on the sidelines in this rather male-dominated research arena, which may produce the combined effect that these empathic features are "less scientific" or less valued in the overall encounter. Scientists and policy makers alike have pointed to the systemic gender biases that exist within highly competitive research arenas and have begun pointing to its effects on innovation, collaboration, and scientific impact (Zippel, 2017; Kingston, 2017). *Nature* reported on gender discrimination in scientific research, indicating that less than 15% of full professors are women, which has a dramatic impact on who is setting scientific research agendas and policy (Loder, 1999). While most of these reports underscore the gender disparities, examining the history of psychedelic research provides a compelling case for why gender matters.

The new face of psychedelic enthusiasm is in fact not all together new. The male-dominated field today sounds unreflectively similar in some cases to the bravado of the last generation of researchers who felt that they were on the cusp of transforming our ideas about human consciousness and healing contexts. The kind of enthusiasm and stereotypically macho-style confidence that *this time* we have it right because we (a) have published more papers, (b) have better technology, and (c) understand regulations better is not the science of self-reflection. This is not exclusively a gender issue, but the process of gender inclusion would be a good starting point for developing strategies for scientific diplomacy, consensus building, and meaningful integration of qualitative and quantitative methods. This is not to suggest that including more women would dampen the enthusiasm, but the debates would be enriched by their presence and experiences and their allegedly increased capacity for self-reflection. Indeed, it is these qualities that appear to hold women back from succeeding in scientific careers; but what if those qualities were admired in a field that sought to bring rigor and self-reflection into harmony?

---

[1]One exception is Neilofar family, Director of Clinical Research at Eleusis. See also Mary Cosimano's role as guide at Johns Hopkins University.

Labyrinths of Regulation

In the twenty-first century, both researchers and consumers collectively have more experience with psychopharmaceuticals than ever before. Indeed, in the 1950s, the marketplace was only beginning to embrace psychopharmacology with real intensity. As Nikolas Rose suggests, this period also witnessed the dawn of the "psyences": a term that he uses to describe the pervasiveness of psychiatry, psychology, and social work in the everyday lives of citizens (Rose, 2003, p. 46). The return of psychedelics is, perhaps for the modern generation of consumers, neither off-putting nor obscene but rather a response to the culmination of a cultural shift toward chemically altering our consciousness as a natural response to modern living.

Yet, the issue of control or authority looms large. If we were to fast-forward to a time and place where LSD circulates on palliative care wards, where soldiers suffering from PTSD can apply for a psychedelic session, where addicts can qualify for an intense single-session consciousness-changing treatment, or where we might review an REB for a well-funded lab where neuroscientists unproblematically ask where spirituality activates the brain, who will keep tabs? Who will take responsibility for reevaluating safety or for establishing criteria for distribution, regulation, and prohibition? While there is compelling evidence for a place in medicine for psychedelics, we have yet to reconcile the question of control. If—and this is a big if—we overhaul the state drug regulators and impose an evidence-based policy approach, is the medical community prepared to take ownership of the psychedelic dilemmas? Investigators in the 1950s believed they could. They also produced libertarians like Timothy Leary, who believed that everyone should take LSD, and conservatives, like Abram Hoffer, who instead suggested that LSD should only be used in tightly controlled clinical settings. Others straddled these perspectives and handed it out to their friends, under the guise of research, to generate elite networks of psychedelic voyeurs who explored the expansive boundaries of consciousness but preferred to keep those experiences for themselves to probe the inner workings of their minds rather than to develop therapeutic options.

Psychedelic investigators in the so-called golden era had not yet articulated a coherent plan for regulating these substances in a manner that balanced the appetite for non-clinical use with the desire to retain psychedelics within the clinic. Famously, ex-Harvard University psychologist Timothy Leary proselytized the use of LSD, exclaiming that everyone should take it, and in fact he is rumored to have recommended its use even more indiscriminately—by putting it in water supplies—but no specific thought was given to how much or whether such a move should only be done on public holidays, whether they should use microdoses or combine it with "car-free" days. Others were more elitist, suggesting that understanding psychedelics required experimentation but that experimentation should involve intellectuals, physicians, theologians, neuroscientists, etc., a particular strand of highly educated individuals who might then harness the powers of psychedelics to improve society. These discussions over how to best regulate and control the use of psychedelics fell moot by the end of the 1960s, as black market versions circulated freely and the political climate of the Cold War gave rise to the damaging association between psychedelics and subversive behavior.

Historically, scientists were keen to separate the drugs from their cultural, spiritual, and healing contexts, even when they later compensated for this isolation by designing careful guidelines for establishing set and setting. Our accumulated knowledge about psychedelics has demonstrated that the experiences readily invoke reactions that are not necessarily reducible to scientific categorization. Perhaps it is time for psychedelic science to emphasize the *psychedelic* elements of this approach and to embrace a more holistic framework of understanding, interpreting, measuring, and ultimately treating modern human experiences.

Neuroscience was in its infancy in the 1950s, when LSD researchers first postulated that neuroreceptors were involved in regulating psychotic symptoms, among other things. Reactions to LSD seemed to suggest that brain areas could be turned on and off or that different levels of consciousness could be activated through the use of chemicals. These hypotheses were rather crude by today's standards but pointed scientists in the general direction. Today, neuroscience has exploded into a mega-discipline, with thousands of brain studies, more sophisticated instruments, expensive laboratories, and a pace of knowledge building that would be unrecognizable to the brain researchers of a generation ago.

Psychedelics have penetrated neuroscience in remarkable ways. Nicolas Langlitz has published a stunning ethnographic encounter of psychedelics in the brain lab and shows compelling evidence suggesting that the context of research has changed. He goes inside the lab of University of California, San Diego, neuroscientist Mark Geyer, who established one of the most prolific labs for investigating the effects of hallucinogens on animal behavior. The famous local escapades of Ken Kesey, Haight-Ashbury's reputation for fusing psychedelics with alternative living, music festivals, and countercultural activities, continue to loom large in the psychedelic folklore that still pulses through the California scene. Consequently, Geyer explained the historical reputation shaped his research approaches and meant that his work has focused exclusively on animal models to satisfy regulators and ethicists. Geyer's research program is therefore less motivated by these classical questions of mysticism or philosophy and instead more focused on the detailed, incremental accrual of data that can be gleaned from behavioral neuroscience (Langlitz, 2013).

Taking time to ponder the intersections of spirituality, consciousness, and brain science seems to be beyond the grasp of even the most successful researchers, whose time is increasingly devoted to securing grants, filling out ethics forms, and logging hours in the lab accumulating data. In other words, the context of modern science has refocused attention on data accrual and away from larger questions of ontology or impact. This shift away from the ideological connotations of psychedelic research might help to shield it from certain criticisms, but it might also restrict it from asking meaningful questions. Geyer's experiences are instructive; today's biomedical science necessitates large, financially secure labs and occupies principal investigators in grant writing and team management. The data production is impressive, but it may come at the cost of diminishing the political power of researchers to ask big questions.

The bureaucracy of drug regulation has grown exponentially over the past half century and has recently come under criticism for making political rather than evidence-based decisions. In 2007, British pharmacologist David Nutt published a harm scale in *The Lancet*, where he argued that psychedelic drugs were much less harmful than the regulated substances of nicotine and alcohol (Nutt, King, Saulsbury, & Blakemore, 2007). He was since fired from his position on the Advisory Council on the Misuse of Drugs, which catapulted him into the debates over renewing medical research on psychedelics. He subsequently pointed to the gulf that has grown between clinical drug trials and government regulations, lamenting the "daunting bureaucratic labyrinth" that dissuades "even the most committed investigator" (End the Ban, 2014, p. 2). Liberal regulation may contribute to hyperbolic scientific claims and overzealous research agendas, but tight regulatory controls may quash potential therapies or the development of basic scientific information. Regulation has come to represent a degree of safety or reduced liability that facilitates getting a drug to market, rather than setting the research parameters for a novel substance or a novel application (Marks, 1997; Healy, 2004; DeGrandpre, 2006). The critical attention being paid to the mega-industrial pharmaceutical complex and its regulation may help to better equip clinical researchers to wrest authority back from a regulatory bureaucracy, if an evidence-based agenda prevails.

Digital Humanities and Future Collaborations

The reawakening of interest in psychedelics has created a methodological conundrum: the bulk of the most rigorous studies from the past are 50–70 years old, while the new studies have small cohorts producing limited clinical data for analysis. The historic trials were conducted at the very early stages of the pharmacological revolution that ushered in new methods for evaluating efficacy and safety, culminating in the randomized controlled trial. Prior to standardizing that approach, however, most pharmacological experiments relied on case reports and data accumulation that did not necessarily involve blinded or comparative techniques. The thousands of experiences conducted in laboratory or clinical contexts captured qualitative and quantitative information about doses, experiences, reactions, and insights: valuable information for understanding the nature of the experience, but not necessarily conducive to current experimental protocols. This information was also generated using handwritten documents, not computer-generated datasets, nor readily comparable outcomes using databases, nor even simple statistical analyses.

Scientific methods have evolved, but so too have historical ones. Historians have embraced digital humanities and developed methods for evaluating large datasets that were produced before computers allowed for systematized, comparative analysis. Using these new ways of collecting and interpreting, historians can revisit the old clinical data to draw out more meaningful and comprehensive data from the case files created in the 1950s and 1960s. These methods allow us to move beyond anecdotal or case-based reports, to combine qualitative and quantitative methods to better appreciate how people experienced psychedelics in a systematic way with thousands of cases to draw from. Such studies are underway now and provide opportunities to bridge disciplines, methods, and, perhaps most importantly, clinical results with psychedelics that may help to illustrate the core features of the experiences.

Conclusion: Death and the Future

In 1963, Aldous Huxley received LSD on his deathbed: he died hours before John F. Kennedy was assassinated, and both deaths signaled losses for America. Huxley suggested that the effects of the drug bathed him in a vision of warmth and spiritual belonging, such that he could face death without fear. Palliative care has been an area identified for its potential use of psychedelics, for precisely this reason: not as a treatment but as a psychological therapy that helps people face the anxiety of dying or the experience of trauma (Mithoefer et al. 2011; Ross, 2012; Wolfson, 2011). Huxley also had direct experience as a caregiver a few years earlier; he had nursed his wife Maria through her final days as she succumbed to cancer. His care for her was aided in part by their mescaline experiences. He spoke candidly and compassionately about how their shared experiences in the Mojave desert had produced "genuine mystical experiences"; he suggested that it was "an abiding sense of divine immanence, of Reality totally present, moment by moment of every object, person and event... For her [Maria], it was not merely a geographical region; it was also a state of mind, a metaphysical reality, an unequivocal manifestation of God" (Bisbee et al. 2018).

He later wrote to his close friend and colleague, Humphry Osmond, explaining that psychedelics might have real potential in the art of dying care: to bring science and spirituality together in the act of caring. He was personally committed to this idea based on his own experiences. His intellectual articulation of psychedelic dying care is indicative of some of the tensions that existed in the context of Cold War science and its hyper-rational and secularized approaches to therapeutics and clinical care. Some observers at the time questioned whether Western methods confined to scientific environments necessarily provided a better or more efficient format to understand the value or benefits of psychedelics, while others, Huxley and Osmond included, were more wary of the consequences of isolation; they worried that the accompanying rituals imbued a kind of deference for psychedelics by treating them as sacred objects to be revered. Although that attitude did not necessarily fit in a 1950s laboratory, the notion of reverence they felt should be respected regardless of the context.

As new research units continue to explore the relationship between palliative care and psychedelics, these historical encounters may offer poignant reminders of how to remarry the science and humanities in a caring context. Will the growing demand for palliation change the context sufficiently to warrant a second look at LSD in the clinic? It would be the ultimate historical irony if the baby boomers, who have been at least superficially blamed for abusing drugs and giving rise to a moral panic about LSD, are the very same actors whose collective agitation for end-of-life care reinvents acid as a humanitarian, medically sanctioned palliative intervention. In doing so, they might also force us to reconcile bigger questions about how we consume drugs, what pain we are willing to endure, and the meaning of life.

References

Aaronson, B., & Osmond, H. (Eds.). (1970). *Psychedelics: The uses and implications of hallucinogenic drugs*. Garden City, NY: Anchor.

Abramson, H. (1960). *The use of LSD in psychotherapy: Transactions of a conference on d-Lysergic Acid Diethylamide (LSD-25)*. Princeton, NJ: Josiah Macy Foundation.

DeGrandpre, R. (2006). *The cult of pharmacology: How America became the world's most troubled drug culture*. Durham, NC: Duke University Press.

Dodgson, R. (2013). *It's all a kind of magic: The young Ken Kesey*. Madison: University of Wisconsin Press.

Dyck, E. (2006). Hitting highs at rock bottom: LSD treatment for alcoholism, 1950–1970. *Social History of Medicine, 19*(2), 313–330.

Dyck, E. (2008). *Psychedelic psychiatry: LSD from clinic to campus*. Baltimore, MD: Johns Hopkins University Press.

Dyck, E. (2011). "Just Say Know": Criminalizing LSD and the politics of psychedelic expertise, 1961–8. In E. Montigny (Ed.), *The real dope: Social, legal, and historical perspectives on the regulation of drugs in Canada* (pp. 169–196). Toronto: University of Toronto Press.

Dyck, E., & Bradford, T. (2012). Peyote on the prairies: Religion, scientists and Native-newcomer relations in western Canada. *Journal of Canadian Studies, 46*(1), 2852.

Dyck, E. (2012). The psychedelic sixties in North America: Drugs and identity. In L. Campbell, D. Clément, & G. S. Kealey (Eds.), *Debating dissent: Canada and the sixties* (pp. 47–66). Toronto: University of Toronto Press.

Elcock, C. (2015). High New York: The birth of a psychedelic subculture in the American City (Doctoral dissertation). Saskatchewan, University of Saskatchewan.

Ellwood, R. S. (1994). *The sixties spiritual awakening: American religion moving from modern to postmodern*. New Brunswick, N.J: Rutgers University Press.

End the Ban on Psychoactive Drug Research [Editorial]. (2014). *Scientific American, 310*(2), 33. Retrieved from: http://www.scientificamerican.com/article/end-the-ban-on-psychoactive-drug-research/.

Fuller, R. C. (2000). *Stairways to heaven: Drugs in American religious history*. Boulder, CO: Westview.

Greenfield, R. (2006). *Timothy Leary: A biography*. Orlando, FL: Harcourt.

Healy, D. (2004). *Let them eat Prozac: The unhealthy relationship between the pharmaceutical industry and depression*. New York City, NY: New York University Press.

Henderson, S. (2011). *Making the scene: Yorkville and hip Toronto in the 1960s*. Toronto: University of Toronto Press.

Hoffer, A., & Osmond, H. (1967). *The hallucinogens*. New York City, NY: Academic.

Hofmann, A. (2013). *LSD: My problem child and insights/outlooks*. New York City, NY: Oxford University Press. (Original work published in 1980 as *LSD: My problem child*.)

Jonnes, J. (1996). *Hep-cats, narcs, and pipe dreams: A history of America's romance with illegal drugs*. Baltimore, MD: Johns Hopkins University Press.

Kesey, K. (1962). *One flew over the cuckoo's nest*. New York City, NY: Viking Press.

Kingston, A. (2017, April 28). Canada's science minister speaks out on women in STEM. *MacLean's*. Retrieved from http://www.macleans.ca/society/canadas-science-minister-speaks-out-on-women-in-stem/

Krebs, T., & Johansen, P. (2012). Lysergic acid diethylamide (LSD) for alcoholism: A meta-analysis of randomized controlled trials. *Journal of Psychopharmacology, 25*, 1–9.

Labate, B. C., & Cavnar, C. (2016). *Peyote: History, tradition, politics, and conservation*. Santa Barbara, CA: Praeger.

Langlitz, N. (2013). *Neuropsychedelia: The revival of hallucinogen research since the decade of the brain*. Berkley: University of California Press.

Loder, N. (1999, November 25). Gender discrimination "undermines science." *Nature: News, 402*. Retrieved from: https://www.nature.com/nature/journal/v402/n6760/full/402337a0.html

Mangini, M. (1998). Treatment of alcoholism using psychedelic drugs: A review of the program of research. *Journal of Psychoactive Drugs, 30*(4), 381–418.

Marks, H. M. (1997). *The progress of experiment: Science and therapeutic reform in the United States, 1900–1990*. Cambridge, UK: Cambridge University Press.

Maroukis, T. (2010). *The peyote road: Religious freedom and the Native American Church*. Norman, OK: University of Oklahoma Press.

Maté, G. (2009). *In the realm of hungry ghosts: Close encounters with addiction*. Berkeley, CA: North Atlantic Books.

Miller, T. (1991). *The hippies and American values*. Knoxville, TN: University of Tennessee.

Mithoefer, M. C., Wagner, M. T., Mithoefer, A. T., Jerome, L., & Doblin, R. (2011). The safety and efficacy of ±3, 4-methylenedioxymethamphetamine-assisted psychotherapy in subjects with chronic, treatment-resistant posttraumatic stress disorder: The first randomized controlled pilot study. *Journal of Psychopharmacology, 25*(4), 439–452.

Nutt, D., King, L. A., Saulsbury, W., & Blakemore, C. (2007). Development of a rational scale to assess the harm of drugs of potential misuse. *The Lancet, 369*, 1047–1053.

Oram, M. (2014). Efficacy and enlightenment: LSD psychotherapy and the drug amendments of 1962. *Journal for the History of Medicine and Allied Sciences, 69*(2), 221–250.

Oram, M. (2016). Prohibited or regulated? LSD psychotherapy and the United States Food and Drug Administration. *History of Psychiatry, 27*(3), 290–306.

Oram, M. (2018). *The trials of psychedelic therapy: LSD psychotherapy in the United States*. Baltimore, MD: Johns Hopkins University Press.

Osmond, H. (1957). A review of the clinical effects of psychotomimetic agents. *Annals of The New York Academy of Sciences, 66*(3), 418–434.

Osmond, H. (1967, February 9). Letter to Jonathan Cole, Chief, Psychopharmacology Service Centre, National Institute of Health. *Provincial Archives of Saskatchewan*. A207, XVIII, 20. B.

Rouhier, A. (1927). *Le Peyotl: La plante qui fait les yeux émerveillés* [Peyote: The plant that amazes the eyes]. Paris, G. Doin.

Rose, N. (2003). Neurochemical selves. *Society, 41*(1), 46–59.

Ross, S. (2012). Serotonergic hallucinogens and emerging targets for addiction pharmacotherapies. *Psychiatric Clinics, 35*(2), 357–374.

Schneider, E. (2008). *Smack: Heroin and the American city*. Philadelphia: University of Pennsylvania Press.

Schwartz. C. (2017, May 6). Molly at the Marriott: Inside America's premier psychedelics conference. *The New York Times*. Retrieved from https://www.nytimes.com/2017/05/06/style/psychedelic-drug-resurgence-daily-life.html?mcubz=1

Spisak, J., with Cynthia, Bisbee, P., Dyck, E., Farrell, P., & Sexton, J. (2018). *Psychedelic Prophets: The letters of Aldous Huxley and Humphry Osmond*. Montreal: McGill-Queen's University Press.

Stevens, J. (1987). *Storming Heaven: LSD and the American Dream*. New York City, NY: Grove Press.

Symons, A. (2015). *Aldous Huxley's hands: His quest for perception and the origin and return of psychedelic science.* Amherst: NY. Prometheus Books.

Wolfson, P. (2011). Psychedelics, spirituality, and transformation. *Tikkun, 26*(1), 10–88.

Zippel, K. (2017). *Women in global science: Advancing academic careers through international collaboration.* Palo Alto, CA: Stanford University Press.

Chapter 2
Peyote's Race Problem

Alexander Dawson

Abstract In the years since peyote became a controlled substance in Mexico and the US, a steady stream of advocates and activists have laid claim to two types of exemption, rooted in both US Law (the First Amendment) and International Law (the 1971 Vienna Convention on Psychotropic Drugs). Indigenous peyotists in particular have been largely successful in making a claim to a legal right to be exempt from national prohibitions on peyote possession and consumption. This has represented a significant advance in indigenous rights, yet in both contexts it has had the unpleasant effect of signaling that a drug that is otherwise so dangerous as to be prohibited should be permitted for Indians, because they are somehow essentially different from all other citizens. This, then, is Peyote's Race Problem. The ways in which we have created a legal framework that makes peyote use licit among indigenous peoples has hardened a certain notion of profound, an unalterable difference to the point that Indian bodies are said to be incommensurably different from the bodies of others who might desire to consume peyote, but for whom it is deemed too dangerous. This notion of difference has been exacerbated by the increasing scarcity of peyote in the US and Mexico, which as further racialized the spaces where peyote grows.

The history of indigenous self-determination in the USA and Mexico is also the history of peyote. Battles over the legal status of peyote "cults" in the USA date back to the early twentieth century and provided the backdrop to struggles for indigenous rights in that country. The peyote religions, which ultimately became the Native American Church of North America (NAC-NA), were the means through which indigenous peoples north of the border established what was first heralded as a religious right and later became more broadly framed as a cultural right to practice indigenous traditions free from the watchful eye of the state. In Mexico, peyote has an even longer history. Banned by the Inquisition in 1620, peyote lays at the heart of

A. Dawson (✉)
Department of History, SUNY Albany, Albany, NY, USA
e-mail: asdawson@albany.edu

© Springer International Publishing AG, part of Springer Nature 2018
B. C. Labate, C. Cavnar (eds.), *Plant Medicines, Healing and Psychedelic Science*,
https://doi.org/10.1007/978-3-319-76720-8_2

19

a series of colonial battles over the mixing of indigenous and European traditions. It was not banned because indigenous peoples were drawn to its power; the Inquisition had no power over indigenous peoples. It was banned because Europeans and *castas* (people of mixed race) were drawn to it. Inquisitional trials reveal stories of slaves grown preternaturally brave and strong under its influence, of mestizos turning to peyote in the hopes it would work as a love potion, of prospectors using it to find mines, and even of priests being administered peyote to cure their troubled minds.

Centuries later, one of the first sustained challenges to the incorporationist politics of Mexico's revolutionary state would come from indigenous peyotists seeking to defend their traditions. In a country where the indigenous past is an integral part of nationalist iconography, the claim that groups like the Wixárika (Mexico's principle peyotists) merited consideration and respect for their autonomous traditions offered a radical departure to past practice and upended government policy in the latter years of the twentieth century.

We should, then, think of the interlocking histories of indigenous rights and peyote as something of a success story, except that certain parts of this story feel a little troubling. Peyote, which research scientists long ago determined to be virtually harmless (it is not habit forming and does not cause deleterious health effects, and it is virtually impossible to overdose on peyote in its natural form), remains a prohibited drug in both the USA and Mexico, classified in both countries as without therapeutic use and subject to a high risk of abuse. It is prohibited for all of those who do not meet strict criteria, which includes both membership in a small number of indigenous communities and also, in the US case, a blood relationship to that community. North of the border, one must be one-quarter Indian by blood and a member of the NAC-NA to legally consume peyote (Feeney, 2014).

In effect, these regulations dictate that one must meet certain racial criteria to legally consume peyote. These racial criteria have been justified through various means over the years, sometimes through a claim that peyotism is an ancient indigenous religion and therefore should be treated differently from other cultural practices, sometimes through an insistence that indigenous peoples use peyote in profoundly different ways than nonindigenous peoples and more recently through a claim that nonindigenous use of peyote has placed the ecosystems in which the peyote grows at enormous risk. Indeed, over time, the logics around peyote prohibitions have shifted, but one thing has remained constant: White bodies are not allowed to consume peyote, and indigenous bodies may consume the cactus.

If peyote is so dangerous that it must be classified as a Schedule 1 drug, and yet the state has determined that indigenous peoples can be allowed to use the drug, the only logical conclusions one can draw are that either modern states do not care about the physical health of indigenous bodies, while they do care about non-Native bodies, or that when an indigenous person consumes peyote, what happens is so profoundly different than what happens when a non-Native person consumes in that the effects cannot be said to be commensurate. As for these explanations, I think we should stipulate that modern states have long histories of not caring about indigenous bodies but that, at present, it would not be acceptable for any state to make this lack of concern so explicit. This leaves us with the second possibility, which forces its own discomfiting conclusions. It may be that it is the value system of those who consume the peyote that makes the experience different, but this is a claim that assumes that the value system is so deeply embedded in the physical body that, when an indigenous person consumes peyote, the effect on the body is somehow different than it would be on non-Native body. It does not allow for the possibility that a nonindigenous person might consume peyote in a traditional indigenous setting (in an NAC-NA ceremony or among Wixárika) and not be somehow endangered by the experience (i.e., the setting can be controlled enough to eliminate the danger). It assumes that, because of culture, tradition, or custom, indigenous and non-Native bodies experience the peyote effect in profoundly different ways and that what is safe for the former is dangerous for the latter. Moreover, US law specially treats peyote as safe for any indigenous body, regardless of the traditions from which that person came. Any person who is one-quarter Native American by blood and who joins a branch of the NAC-NA, is exempted from the ban. This arrangement aligns comfortably with the environmentalist claim that, because peyote habitats are endangered, access to these areas should be restricted to indigenous peyotists, because the loss of peyote would endanger their cultures. Non-Native peyotists, in this reasoning, are inauthentic interlopers whose desire for peyote is endangering an ancient Native tradition. But the logics of these bans fall apart when we acknowledge that peyotism is both quite new in some indigenous communities and long-standing in some non-Native communities; indeed, it leads us to the possibility that peyote may have a race problem.

The Origins of Prohibition

Drug prohibitions are funny things. As a rule, they rely on a series of logics that tell us a great deal about the context of their creation and about the things that the authorities implementing those prohibitions fear. When peyote was prohibited by the Spanish Inquisition, the edict signaled a fear that those who consumed the flesh of this small cactus were treading too closely to heresy. Inquisitors believed that the cactus had either been put in the earth by the devil to tempt the weak of spirit, or that those who took the cactus erroneously believed that it allowed them to communicate with the devil. At the very least, the cactus was tied to superstitious behavior that, while not heretical, was nonetheless illicit. Prohibition, in this case, spoke both to a fear of contamination (of the Indian realm into the Christian realm) and to a need to maintain religious discipline (Aguirre Beltrán, 1963).

Discipline, indeed, has been a feature of drug prohibitions since that time. From the gin panics of the eighteenth century to the international conventions aimed at limiting the flow of opium and cocaine in the early twentieth century, modern states have repeatedly intervened to restrict the consumption of substances that scientific, religious, and educational authorities associated with sloth and disorder (Schivelbusch, 1992; Courtwright, 2001). And, for the most part, the anxieties expressed through these prohibitions followed a series of logics. The substance (opium, marijuana, cocaine, alcohol) was said to poison the body, causing that body to degenerate and be unsuitable for work, discipline, and other forms of social reproduction. That personal tragedy then became a social tragedy through various forms of contamination, as that body first contaminated other bodies, encouraging the same behavior, and then contaminated society as a whole. Naturally, it helped if the thing itself was of foreign provenance, allowing authority in all its forms to transform the battle against the thing into a battle to defend the nation from a foreign invasion (Gootenberg, 2008; Campos, 2014; Peréz Montfort, 1999).

Of course, this narrative relied very heavily on the word of scientific experts, who were called upon again and again to remind government officials and other gate-keepers of the specifically pernicious effect of the substance on the human body. The historical record is filled with the tales of "reefer madness," of bodies made incapable of functioning by opium, and of dependence, addiction, health, and cognitive skills permanently impaired. These stories interest me a great deal, in part, because I think we are still attempting to sort through which of them do have a basis in evidence and which were simply the product of elite anxiety, spread as cautionary tales. We seem to be still struggling to separate out an empirical basis for under-standing the difference between prohibitions rooted in actual harm from those that arise from social panics (Goode, 2008). For instance, while it does seem that long-term use of inhalants (industrial cements, paint thinner) causes brain damage, there is no evidence for the claims about cerebral lesions or insanity associated with LSD (Krebs and Johansen, 2012). And as far as peyote is concerned, a variety of studies (many of them decades old) established not only that it poses no health risks to those who use it in clinical or controlled settings, but that it might actually be tied to positive health outcomes.

By way of a brief primer, social scientists and scientists have been studying peyote since the late nineteenth century and have, since at least the 1930s, held fairly uniform views about this substance. They agree it is a hallucinogen. They agree that, given the nature of the cactus, it is impossible to overdose on the alkaloids (principally mescaline) within the peyote. They agree that it is not habit forming and that it has no adverse effect on the health of those who take it. Some go further, arguing that it is in fact healthful for those who use it and that its antibiotic properties and the way it is often integrated into religious rituals have a positive impact on the physical health and social well-being on most of those who consume it. They suggest that it has been critical in helping some people, most of whom have an indigenous background, fight alcoholism and other maladies. The set and setting of peyote use seem to be important, but as a rule, these researchers have not argued that the potential benefits and absence of harm apply only to indigenous communities. What they have argued instead is that, given peyote's power to produce mild hallucinations, it is best consumed in a controlled setting and that, when done so, many users report a significant psychological or psychic benefit. Even outside of these settings however, they have found no evidence of addiction, degeneration, or overdoses due to peyote (Bergman, 1971; Anderson, 1980; Csordas, 1999; Halpern et al., 2005; Calabrese, 2014).

This makes the legal prohibitions that continue to surround peyote all the more perplexing. In Mexico, peyote was of almost no interest to the modern state prior to the late 1960s, largely because it circulated mostly in herbal markets and among a small number of indigenous groups who were generally seen as terribly backward. In the USA, state and federal attempts to ban peyote dated back to the end of the nineteenth century but here again went nowhere for two particular reasons: First, prior to the 1960s, peyote use was largely confined to Indian reservations and spread mostly through the NAC-NA; second, members of the NAC-NA, working with a series of allies (anthropologists, botanists, and occasionally government officials who supported an indigenous right to religious self-determination), repeatedly fought off federal efforts to pass a peyote ban. Over the course of these battles, the US courts established a religious right that it assigned only to bona fide peyotists, which jurists generally defined as members of the NAC-NA and Indian by blood (Feeney, 2016).

It was only once young, largely White, middle-class kids started getting interested in peyote that successful pushes toward federal bans in Mexico and the USA started to take shape. In the USA, peyote was outlawed in 1965 (interestingly, 6 years before mescaline, the synthetic derivative of the peyote cactus was outlawed in the Controlled Substances Act). Peyote was outlawed in Mexico in 1971 (declared "without therapeutic value" in the Sanitary Code that year) amidst a growing concern among Mexican conservatives that young Mexican hippies (often seen as poor copies of their North American cousins) were falling victim to the drug culture. Social conservatives responded to the *jipitecas* (we owe the term to Marroquín, 1975) with disgust, seeing in their *desmadre* (the term connotes an embrace of chaos and social rebellion) an existential threat to the modern, industrial, orderly, postrevolutionary state and society their parents had worked so hard to create (Zolov 1999; Agustín, 1996). Bodies seemingly damaged by drugs (there were claims about cerebral lesions, permanent psychosis, schizophrenia, and other permanent damage) were also sites of more fuzzy pathologies: depression, sloth, "moral contamination," and "corruption" ("Batalla Contra las Drogas," 1970; "Llamado a los Padres," 1970; Cabildo, 1974).

Peyote, with its association with Mexico's most primitive peoples, drew particular ire from the critics. It was rendered in the press like the Indian: "exotic" and "repugnant" ("Graves Peligros," 1969) . Youths attracted to its spell were said to be worshipping false gods, to be regressing to a primitive state, and to be embracing "perversity, vice, and degeneration" ("Graves Peligros," 1969; Shortall, 2014). All of this was causing "terrible spiritual damage" ("Graves Peligros," 1969).

What is perhaps remarkable in this critique is the way it collapsed a complex landscape of peyote use in Mexico into a single phenomenon. True, peyote was most closely associated with the Wixárika, but peyote also circulated somewhat openly in Mexico's herbal markets and among traditional healers, at least until the 1960s, and was used for a variety of illnesses. Some were of a more spiritual nature, such as *mal de ojo* (evil eye), though many of the uses of peyote were quite mundane. It was used, for instance, to treat joint pain and various forms of rheumatism, as an antibiotic and in some cases as a purgative. Peyote had also recently captured the attention of the controversial psychiatrist Salvador Roquet, who used it in his work with patients (Dawson, 2015). And yet, the very way that Roquet embraced peyote and other psychoactive plants—suggesting that indigenous value systems might have a powerful role to play in contemporary life—deeply alarmed his conservative critics, who associated indigeneity with chaos.

In a society not terribly far removed from a violent revolution, a civil war that many urban Mexicans blamed on indigenous barbarity (Gamio, 1916), these were not idle concerns. Mexicans lacked the easy confidence in their own modernity that could be seen north of the border, where the descent into indigeneity signaled by the hippies may have represented a threat to normative bourgeois Christian values, but did not pose quite the same sort of existential threat. Indigeneity was much closer in a country where millions within the urban underclasses were relatively recent migrants from the countryside, and a nationalist mythology had recently come to celebrate the mestizo as the true Mexican type. Moreover, the model citizen of the postrevolutionary era was orderly, disciplined, and committed to taking part in the sort of project of national progress that is essential in a society where dissent and *desmadre* risk causing the collapse of the entire social artifice. Drug takers, especially those who opted for those drugs that evoked indigenous alterity, represented a "generation in degeneration" ("Llamado a los Padres," 1970), weakened by their drugs, susceptible not just to indigenous mysticism but also to other forms of perversion, such as homosexuality (a *bête noire* of the revolutionary state) (UNAM, 1971; Grosser, 1969; Maynez Puente, 1969). Much like backward Indians, they needed help (Pacheco Santos, 1976; Cabildo, 1974; Cardiff, 1977; "El Problema de la Drogadicción," 1978; Iñigo, 1970; "Farmacodependencia," 1975; "Las Drogas, Aventura Mortal," 1980; Perez Isaak, 1979).

These anxieties were repeated over and over again by advocates of the two most prominent public initiatives in addiction treatment undertaken in Mexico during these years: Mexico's Centros de Integracion Juvenil (Youth Integration Centers), founded under the direction of Ernesto Lammoglia, and the Centro Mexicano de Estudios en Farmacodependencia (Mexican Center for the Study of Drug Dependence or CEMEF), which was founded under the leadership of Guido Belsasso in 1972. Expanding traditional definitions, the new specialists classified addiction (or dependence) as both a physiological need for the substance and by a body's ability to develop tolerance, thus requiring an ever-increasing quantity of the drug. While psychedelics were not associated with physical dependence, these specialists could use rather fuzzy evidence to claim that they caused "psychic dependence" due to the "distortions in perception" (Alarcón Navarro et al., n.d.) that they produced.

The CEMEF regularly beat the drum over psychedelics (e.g., Berruecos, 1974), claiming that chronic use produced a need for the drug that, when unfulfilled, resulted in psychotic states. Addicts "have dramatically changed their value systems," shifting from being useful citizens to embracing "passivity, mysticism, and fantasies" (Carranza Acevedo, 1971; UNAM, 1971). At their very worst, these drugs led to murder and suicide. Mescaline was specifically held to produce psychic dependency, tolerance, psychosis, panic, and extreme emotions. Psilocybin was said to have similar effects but was not known to produce psychosis. LSD was the worst, linked to the inability to work or study, possible genetic damage, cerebral lesions, and damage to the central nervous system (Consejo Nacional de Problemas en Farmacodependencia; Carranza Acevedo, 1972; Programa Nacional de Combate a los Problemas de Drogas, 1976; Uso y abuso de drogas, 1974; Mayoral Pardo, 1973).

Hallucinogens were thus core threats in what was said to be the "crisis of our time" ("Farmacodependencia, Crisis de Nuestro Tiempo," 1976). One story in *El Universal* in April 1976 claimed that there were between 500,000 and 800,000 minors in the federal district alone who needed treatment for industrial adhesives and solvents, marijuana, and other drugs ("Llamado a los Padres de Familia" 1976). Untethered to their traditional values, these youths were turning to crime, experimenting with dangerous lifestyles, and undermining society ("No Hay Centros," 1976; Payan, 1980).

Indigenous Exemptions in the USA

It goes without saying that the numbers were way off—that this was a classic instance of anxiety and self-interest coming together seamlessly to produce a moral panic about the dangers of drugs to youths: a panic that in the Mexican case was exacerbated by the larger social crisis that accompanied the 1968 student movement and Tlatelolco massacre (Carey, 2005). More interesting for our purposes, however, is the fact that this panic aligns remarkably well with the anxieties that prompted the US Congress to outlaw peyote in that country. Missionaries and public health officials working on US Indian reservations had for decades tried to get the American public's attention about the dangers posed by peyote to indigenous peoples, but their campaign had come to naught in part because indigenous peyotism seemed remote from the day-to-day concerns of Euro-Americans and in part because their own rhetoric—highlighting the primitiveness of the ceremony and the widespread appeal that peyote had among Indians—reinforced the assumption that indigenous peyotism was a natural thing, even if it was a new thing. It was only when beatniks and hippies took to peyote and the counterculture increasingly seemed capable of disrupting mainstream America that Congress took action. And in the debates leading up to the ban, North Americans mobilized language that was remarkably similar to the language used by their southern neighbors. Peyote led to sloth, laziness, and genetic and cerebral damage. It was tied to the collapse of civilized behavior. And, even if they could never become Indians (this, within the context of American life, seemed absurd), they were copying Indians as closely as they could. The guardians of order looked on with disgust (Smith, 2012).

It was also in this moment that the racial divide would be most clearly delineated through the law. In passing the peyote and mescaline bans, the US Congress created specific exemptions with unmistakable origins in racial thinking. Members of the NAC-NA had long argued that they should be exempted from state-level laws criminalizing peyote and, by 1965, had won a series of important legal challenges in federal and state courts preserving their rights as peyotists under the First Amendment's Freedom of Religion clause. Supplemented by state laws designed to protect the rights of members of the NAC-NA, these rulings created a context in which a universal ban would have created a constitutional mess.

Among the more prominent court rulings that established an indigenous right to peyote was *People v. Woody*, decided by California's Supreme Court in August 1964. In *Woody*, the court overturned the drug convictions of three members of the NAC-NA who had been arrested several years earlier while holding a ceremony in Needles, California. The court found that this was an ancient tradition; that it was an organized, bona fide religion; and that, as practiced within the NAC-NA, there was no evidence that peyote represented a danger to public health or to the participants in the ceremonies. The court did, however, conclude that the state had a compelling interest in otherwise controlling peyote. They did not overturn the California's state-level peyote ban. Instead, they found that within a very particular setting—an institutionalized and ancient church—peyote did not pose a risk, and as such, the ban violated the peyotists' First Amendment rights.

Race played only a shadowy role in the ruling. Indeed, in another ruling that day *(In re Grady)*, the court did not find that a White "way shower" who gave peyote to his followers had broken the law. Instead, they returned the case to the lower courts with the request that a finding be made as to whether his peyotism met the standards of "bona fide" belief that they set in *Woody*. Still, the contours of their ruling made the racialization of peyotism impossible to miss. If indeed peyote could be legal only as an ancient tradition, formally institutionalized through something like the NAC-NA, and within a specific cultural context that excluded nonindigenous peoples, peyote had to be an Indian thing.

This became explicit in subsequent court rulings and federal legislation that, over time, shaped a very strict standard for licit peyote in the USA. Federal officials denied petitions for a religious exemption to all groups but the NAC-NA and began insisting that, beyond being a member of the church, one had to also be at least one-quarter Indian by blood. This particular interpretation of the law was rooted in Texas state law, and, though it had not been a part of the legalization of peyote in other states, it became the national standard. To this day, it remains the federal standard for licit peyote.

A couple of caveats are worth mentioning here. First, as peyote use expanded in the USA during the 1950s and 1960s, so too did the number of religious organizations that professed a belief that peyote was a sacrament. Some of those groups were offshoots of the NAC-NA, and some of those groups were exclusively indigenous; that is to say, members of those groups insisted that indigeneity be a prerequisite for group membership and that non-Indians were not welcome and could never fully understand what happened within these communities. We have every reason to understand these as moments of anticolonial renaissance, in which group solidarity and exclusivity played a critical role. Peyotism had the feel of being ancient, even if its connection to the ancient past was problematic (it was a relatively new practice in many of the communities where the NAC-NA was growing), and this produced important and meaningful connections among members.

And still, not every peyotist group functioned this way. In some contexts, nonindigenous members were welcomed in, even "adopted" as members of peyote groups. We know of some prominent figures that played this role, such as George Morgan and J. S. Slotkin, because they wrote about their experiences. Others, like Robert Lawrence Boyll, come to us through court cases in which the complex intermingling of traditions within the NAC-NA can be seen. Still others sought to create their own peyote churches—the Church of the Awakening, the Neo-American Church, and the Peyote Way Church of God—pushing for licit spaces for nonindigenous peyote use within the USA.

Legal developments after 1965 have tended to put these diverse practices at risk. Federal law effectively made a clear distinction between indigenous and nonindigenous peyote use and created clear lines of demarcation between Indian and non-Indian, by seeking to punish both nonindigenous peyotists and indigenous groups that welcomed nonindigenous peyotists. These laws also created a series of perverse incentives, encouraging the NAC-NA to expel non-Indians, to carefully police membership (all-race chapters of the NAC-NA would not get legal sanction), and adopt narratives that created clear distinctions where they had once been rather fuzzy. NAC-NA leaders who had once taken a Catholic view of nonindigenous membership in the Church were succeeded by generations who increasingly cast Church membership in stark racial terms. A new history emerged in which the non-Indians who had long sought to participate in the Church were rendered as outsiders, always unwelcome, and barely tolerated (Schaefer, 2015).

There is no way to make clear sense of these claims. The history of court challenges around peyote, and at least some of the testimonials we have from the period prior to the federal ban suggest a complex terrain in which racial identities were in some ways fluid within the NAC-NA. This would make sense, at least in part, because the NAC-NA was itself a twentieth-century creation and was pan-indigenous, rather than rooted in one specific indigenous tradition. This was, however, too much for the law. Racial identities had to be simplified. And to defend their rights, at least some in the NAC-NA willingly participated in this process.

The imperatives toward this arrangement grew stronger as peyote supplies in the gardens of South Texas dwindled. The ecological challenges faced by the peyote gardens of South Texas are undeniable and come from at least two clear threats. One comes in the form of efforts to convert more and more of the desert landscape to commercial agriculture, a Sisyphean task enabled by the supposed promises of improved desert agriculture technologies. The second comes from the fact that, over the course of the past century, peyote in the desert in an around the Texas-Mexico border has been overharvested. As the NAC-NA has grown (its members now number around a quarter of a million), demand for peyote from Church members has steadily risen. Non-Native consumption of peyote also puts pressure on the cactus, especially when novice pickers venture into the desert to collect their own. Peyote has a decade-long growth cycle and needs to be carefully harvested and cut midway down the root so that the cactus regenerates. Novices sometimes pick the entire cactus, leaving no chance for future regeneration. Some enthusiasts, including the Peyote Way and Leo Mercado, have tried to cultivate peyote in other regions or in greenhouses but have had relatively little luck. Peyote Way has had difficulty creating the right conditions on their property in the Aravaipa Valley in eastern Arizona, and Mercado had his entire collection of peyote plants confiscated in a police raid (Sterling, 1999; Labate & Cavnar, 2016; Trout & Terry, 2016).

Some in the NAC-NA do not object to these efforts to cultivate, while others firmly believe that it is not just peyote, but the landscape within which it grows, that is sacred. For those members of the Church, the only reasonable solution to the peyote crisis lies in restricting access to the peyote gardens of South Texas to members of the NAC-NA. This proposition is more complex than it may seem, for a variety of reasons. First, not all members of NAC-NA have a demonstrable historical or cultural connection to this region. Peyotism was an evangelistic, largely twentieth-century religion, and was often introduced in settings far removed from the peyote gardens of South Texas. Beyond this, such a claim to exclusivity would leave local populations, who have long lived in proximity to the gardens and made their livelihoods there, in a tenuous position. Still, it is a claim that carries weight at least in part because the loss of peyote habitats does represent an existential threat to the NAC-NA. In this proposition, because the NAC is an Indian Church and because White peyotists are either charlatans or Johnny-come-latelies, the indigenous claim to the peyote gardens should take precedence.

South of the Border

South of the border, a similar logic has taken hold, though, in this case, the historical precedence of the claim is much more easily demonstrated. It may simply have been a manner of convenience (after Mexico signed the 1971 Vienna Convention on Psychotropic Drugs, the country was formally committed to guaranteeing the traditional use of these drugs by indigenous peoples), but Mexico's anti-addiction establishment (mainly centered on the CEMEF in the 1970s) never sought to eradicate indigenous peyotism. This was curious, because the very images they used to relay their alarm at youthful dalliances with peyote trafficked very heavily in tropes of indigenous backwardness and degeneration in order to condemn youth drug use; yet, they made no case to restrict indigenous access to peyote. Instead, distinguishing "ceremonial" use in Wixárika communities from peyote use among non-Indians, Belsasso and others repeatedly argued that indigenous drug users were of a different kind than others. Non-Indian bodies became intoxicated, degenerate, and were placed in physical danger by these drugs. In traditional settings however, where peyote was integrated into long-standing rituals and the truths it produced channeled through carefully stage-managed rituals, indigenous bodies were not placed at risk. The new drug addiction specialists even argued that in these settings, peyote might have a therapeutic value that was not available to nonindigenous peyotists. And yet, they also fell very easily into a series of orientalist traps, at times suggesting that the Wixárika were in fact so damaged by their peyote use that it made little sense to attempt to help them. At one point, members of the CEMEF even suggested that they represented a good case study for the long-term deleterious effects of drug use (Belsasso & Kramer, 1972; Alarcón Navarro, Miranda, & Pérez Ramírez, n.d.; Gurza, 1976; Centro Mexicano de Estudios en Salud Mental, 1979; Belsasso, 1976; García Salazar, 1970).

The Wixárika have been collecting peyote in a desert region of the State of San Luis Potosí near the town of Real de Catorce since before Europeans arrived in the Americas. The region, which they called Wirikúta, has long been one of the most sacred sites in Wixárika cosmology, and pilgrimages to the region are one of the most important events in their cultural life. Prior to the 1960s, the Wixárika undertook those pilgrimages largely out of view of the state, as they could cross relatively undeveloped landscapes and enter the desert with a minimum of interaction with the state or curious onlookers. Since the 1960s, however, both the Wixárika and Wirikúta have come under significant pressure from the forces of economic development and environmental change. Fencing now blocks off many of their old routes. First hippies, and later New Agers, have made their own journeys to Wirikúta, at times, indiscriminately taking the peyote and reducing the available supply. Already, during the 1970s, alarmists had suggested that hippie enthusiasm for peyote was placing the Wixárika at risk (Matta Torres, 1976), and, given the ecological fragility of the northern desert, it is unsurprising that it should become a concern that those same hippies were overrunning the desert and putting the long-term survival of the cactus at risk (Labate & Feeney, 2016).

Responding to pressures to protect peyote ecosystems, federal and state officials transformed Wirikúta into an ecological reserve during the 1990s (Frid, Poliakoff, Rajsbaum, & Martínez, 1994–95; Instituto Nacional Indigenista [INI], 1996). Peyote was placed on the Mexican government's endangered species list at the end of 1991, and 3 years later state authorities in San Luis Potosí declared Wirikúta to be a "protected natural area." As a part of this arrangement, the Instituto Nacional Indigenista (INI) secured permission from the governor of San Luis Potosí to grant the Wixárika unrestricted preferential access to 182,108 acres in the state to conduct ceremonies and gather peyote. The accords that enabled this arrangement envisioned shared governance over Wirikúta between several levels of government and Wixárika elders, an arrangement that was meant to ensure that the pressure to develop the desert economically would not take precedence over the need to preserve it for Wixárika use. More than this, the legislation and agreements that created a legal basis for Wixárika to collect peyote in Wirikúta were specially intended to prohibit the collection of peyote by non-Wixárika and for non-ritual purposes. Under the terms of the agreements, the Mexican government appointed "ecological guards" to protect the desert and maintain it as a zone of indigenous exclusivity.

It never quite worked out that way. Since the region was declared protected, local police and ecological guards have consistently used their authority to harass and humiliate Wixárika pilgrims. More shockingly, within months of signing a pact between Wixárika authorities and the federal government guaranteeing that they would have some say in development in the zone in November 2008 (the *Pacto De Hauxa Manaka Para La Preservación y Desarrollo De La Cultura Wixárika* [Hauxa Manaka's pact for the preservation and development of the Wixárika culture]), the federal government issued concessions to two Canadian companies to open silver mines in the protected zone. Given the fragile nature of the desert ecosystem and mining's insatiable demand for water, environmentalists and indigenous rights activists rightly feared that these concessions would spell the end for Wirikúta.

Completely frozen out of the decision process, the Wixárika authorities organized to protest the concessions on the local, national, and international levels. Their protests were custom-made for early twenty-first-century activism, pitting what activists purported to be an innocent Stone Age people against multinational mining companies. Between 2010 and 2014, Wixárika activists traveled to New York, Vancouver (where they protested at board meetings of First Majestic), and elsewhere, repeatedly making the case against the concessions based on international and domestic laws.

That they succeeded (the concessions were canceled in 2012, though the government reserved the right to revisit the issue) was a testament to the power of coalitions that combine the twin forces of a claim to indigenous rights and environmental protection. Given the urgency of the issue, it might seem like nit-picking to point out the fact that in all of this, the winning argument in defending the desert was one that both located peyote firmly in the indigenous sphere and then used an argument about racial exclusivity to suggest that the spaces associated with peyote must remain exclusively indigenous. And yet, I think this is a critically important point to make.

It is not just that the campaign made the Wixárika out to be a Stone Age people, so trapped in their mystical alterity that they could not possibly survive in the modern world, and cast the destruction of Wirikúta as the destruction of their being as a people (they are, in fact, a dynamic, diasporic community, with a very strong sense of ethnic belonging that has, in some ways, grown stronger even as their worlds have proliferated and been transformed through technological, social, and economic change). It is also that this campaign so thoroughly participated in the racial re-inscription of peyote that it left no room for the fact that, for centuries, peyote has played a role as medicine and source of spiritual well-being and other things within a variety of nonindigenous Mexican communities.

It is, for instance, a campaign that has left Mexico's nonindigenous peyotists in an uncomfortable place. Nonindigenous allies and collaborators of the Wixárika have a long history of taking part in peyote ceremonies and of working with Wixárika communities to protect and preserve Wirikúta; yet, their close collaboration and participation were largely erased from a public campaign that relied on the exotic Indian to gain global attention. This practice oddly coincided with the Mexican state's own tendency to view non-Wixárika participants in these ceremonies with disdain and to pressure Wixárika elders to exclude these outsiders, lest they risk losing their own licit access to Wirikúta (Sánchez Azua, 2004).

More than this, Mexico has its own versions of groups like the Neo-American Church, some of them as distinctly non-Indian as their northern counterparts. And yet, the Mexican case is complicated by the fact that, according to the standards of racial indigeneity that satisfy the US government, many members of these groups would in fact qualify for licit peyote use (blood quotients are impossible to determine in a country like Mexico, where a majority of the population has some indigenous origin). Mexico's version of the NAC-NA, the Iglesia Nativa Americana de Mexico (INAM), has for years been struggling for legal status in the country, with little success to this point. Though the Mexican Supreme Court ruled that the Secretaría de Gobernación could not take the beliefs of members of a Church into account when granting it legal status in November 2016, the government has yet to grant the INAM a legal charter. In the Latin American context, where claims to indigenous origin are both murky and increasingly politically salient, one cannot fairly accuse the members of the INAM of being frauds or charlatans. They simply fail to meet Mexico's particular criteria for licit peyote.

Concluding Thoughts

This, then, is why it does matter that we have created legal apparatuses in Mexico and the USA that have reserved licit peyote use (and the spaces associated with that use) for indigenous peoples, defined according to very limited criteria. In failing to acknowledge what has historically been a significant community of non-Natives who are drawn to peyote for both corporeal and spiritual reasons (and that the very notion of who is and who is not indigenous has shifted over time) while, accepting indigenous use as somehow natural, we reinscribe a critical difference that peyote might make us want to question. Instead of attempting to understand how it is that some indigenous peoples and some nonindigenous peoples are drawn to peyote and wondering whether there are moments of commensurability here (if, in these phenomena, we see similar forms of searching, longing for belonging, and belief in a world that is unseen and unknowable to the senses under normal circumstances), we make a world in which our actions reinforce the idea that peyote belongs to the indigenous realm and that those who try to enter this realm from the outside are fools, interlopers, and frauds.

There are no simple answers to the environmental challenges faced by peyote ecosystems in the early twenty-first century. What I propose here is merely that we step back from the ways in which environmental scarcity has moved Mexicans and North Americans into a posture in which creating racially exclusive spaces seems like a solution to this problem. I remain troubled by the fact that what is now a claim to an environmentally based proscription was at one time based in much more clearly racial stereotypes. In the 1970s, the state stepped in to protect White bodies from the dangers of peyote. Now, it steps in to protect peyote from the dangers of White bodies. The result is the same.

It is that peyote, while an indigenous heritage, is also a human heritage: a small cactus that has and continues to play an important role in the lives of indigenous and nonindigenous peoples. It may be that we have more to gain in remembering what it is that unites indigenous and nonindigenous peyotists and finding a way to protect what is a sacred medicine to all, rather than continuing to demarcate the one so starkly from the other.

There is a tradition in the West of laying claims to the spaces, cultures, and bodies of the other, a tradition that has been openly challenged in recent decades (Comaroff & Comaroff, 2009; Brown, 2003). I hope that the reader understands that this is not my intention here. I do not wish to stake a claim for nonindigenous peyote use that somehow subsumes or erases the particularity of different traditions. What I instead sought to do here was suggest that a close interrogation of the historical record of licit and illicit peyote use reveals a past in which indigenous and nonindigenous histories were more intertwined and less distinct from one another than contemporary legal and political debates about peyote suggest. And I want to suggest that we produce racial difference in the ways we distinguish indigenous from nonindigenous peyote use. The production of race here becomes an ongoing process, one in which modern states and systems of knowledge create and enforce essential difference. Where peyote's complex history might help us to destabilize racial boundaries, we instead simplify that history to enforce those boundaries.

References

Aguirre Beltán, G. (1963). *Medicina y magia: El proceso de aculturación en la estructura colonial [Medicine and magic: The process of acculturation into the colonial structure]*. Mexico City: Instituto Nacional Indigenista.

Agustín, J. (1996). *La contracultura en México: La historia y el significado de los rebeldes sin causa, los jipitecas, los punks y las bandas* (The Mexican counterculture: The history and significance of the rebels without a cause, the jipitecas, and the bands]. Mexico City: Editorial Grijalbo.

Alarcón Navarro, F., Miranda, J., & Ramírez, N. P. (n.d., ca. 1971–1973). Drogadicción [Drug addiction]. Secretaría de Salud Pública-SP 245.1.

Anderson, E. F. (1980). *Peyote: The divine cactus*. Tucson: The University of Arizona Press.

Batalla Contra las Drogas [Battle against drugs]. (1970, February 27). *Novedades*.

Belsasso, G., & Kramer, J. C. (1972, September 5). Joint memorandum. *Secretaría de Salud Pública-SP, 259*, 2.

Belsasso, G. (1976, August) Estrategias de prevención en farmacodependencia. Modelos de Prevención y Alternativas al Consumo de Drogas [Strategies of prevention in drug dependence: Prevention models and alternatives to drug consumption]. *Trabajo presentado en el V Congreso Nacional de Higiene Escolar* [Work presented at the 5th National Congress on School Hygiene], Acapulco, Mexico.

Bergman, R. L. (1971). Navajo peyote use: Its apparent safety. *American Journal of Psychiatry, 128* (6), 695–699.

Berruecos, L. (1974, March 15). La Función de la Antropología en las investigaciones sobre farmacodependencia [The role of anthropology in investigations about drug dependence] In Consejo Nacional de Problemas en Farmacodependencia, Informe, [National Council for Problems in Drug Dependence report). Secretaría de Salud Pública-SP 293.2.

Brown, M. F. (2003). *Who owns Native culture?* Cambridge, MA: Harvard University Press.

Calabrese, J. (2014) *A different medicine: Postcolonial healing in the Native American Church*. Oxford: Oxford University Press.

Campos, I. (2014). *Home grown: Marijuana and the origins of Mexico's war on drugs*. Chapel Hill, NC: University of North Carolina Press.

Carey, E. (2005). *Plaza of sacrifices: Gender, power, and terror in 1968 Mexico*. Albuquerque, NM: University of New Mexico Press.

Carranza Acevedo, J. (1971). Informe para los Consejo Nacional de Problemas en Farmacodependencia [National Council for Problems in Drug Dependence report]. *Secretaría de Salud Pública SP, 244,* 2.

Carranza Acevedo, José. (1972). *Información a Jóvenes, Consejo Nacional de Problemas en Farmacodependencia* [Information for youths, National Council for Problems in Drug Dependence]. Secretaría de Salud Pública SP 263.3.

Centro Mexicano de Estudios en Salud Mental [Mexican Center for Studies in Mental Health]. (1979). *La familia ante el problema de las drogas, Una programa de la Familia para la Prevención de la Dependencia a Sustancias Químicas* [The family confronts the drug problem: A family program for the prevention of dependence on chemical substances]. Mexico City: Author.

Comaroff, J., & Comaroff, J. (2009). *Ethnicity, Inc*. Chicago, IL: University of Chicago Press.

Courtwright, D. T. (2001). *Forces of habit: Drugs and the making of the modern world*. Cambridge, MA: Harvard University Press.

Csordas, T. J. (1999). Ritual healing and the politics of identity in contemporary Navajo society. *American Ethnologist, 26*(1), 3–23.

Dawson, A. (2015). Salvador Roquet, María Sabina, and the trouble with Jipis. *Hispanic American Historical Review, 95*(1), 103–133.

Cabildo, H. M. (1974, February 27). Epidemiologia y Prevención de la Farmacodependencia [Epidemiology and the prevention of drug addiction]. *El Día*.

Cardiff, G. (1977, December 14). Incultura Sexual y Drogadicción [Sexual illiteracy and drug addiction]. *El Heraldo de Mexico*.

Departamento de Psicología Medica, Psiquiatría y Salud Mental, Facultad de Medicina, Universidad Nacional Autónoma de México. (1971). El Problema de Farmacodependencia [The problem of drug dependence]. *Mexico City: Archivo Historico de la Secretaría de Salud Pública, SP, 244,* 2.

El Problema de la Drogadicción Juvenil [The problem of youth drug addiction]. (1978, October .24). *El Heraldo de Mexico*.

Farmacodependencia, Crisis de Nuestro Tiempo [Drug dependence: The crisis of our time. (1975, April 15) *El Dia*.

Feeney, K. (2014). Peyote, race, and equal protection in the United States. In B. C. Labate & C. Cavnar (Eds.), *Prohibition, religious freedom, and human rights: Regulating traditional drug use* (pp. 65–88). Berlin: Springer.

Feeney, K. (2016). Peyote, conservation, and Indian rights in the United States. In B. C. Labate & C. Cavnar (Eds.), *Peyote: History, traditions, politics, and conservation* (pp. 105–128). Santa Barbara, CA: Praeger.

Frid, K., Poliakoff, D., Rajsbaum, A. & Ramón Martínez, R. (ca. 1994–95) Evaluación del Trabajo de Protección a lugares Sagrados [Evaluation of the work of protecting sacred places]. INI, Dirección de Procuración de Justicia, Subdirección de Antropológica Jurídica, Departamento de Lugares Sagrados [INI, Directorate of Justice, Sub-Directorate of Juridical Anthropology, Department of Sacred Places]. Mexico City: CDI Historical Archive (CDI) FD 09/2310.

Gamio, M. (1916). *Forjando patria (pro nacionalismo) [Forging a nation (pro-nationalism)]*. Mexico City: Librería de Porrúa Hermanos.

García Salazar, H. (1970). Drogadicción, Etnología, y Cambio Social a Vuelo de Pájaro [Drug addiction, ethnology, and social change to bird flight). *Annuario Antropológico Universidad Veracruzana, 1,* 65–70.

Goode, E. (2008). Moral panics and disproportionality: The case of LSD use in the sixties. *Deviant Behavior, 29*(6), 533–543.

Gootenberg, P. (2008). *Andean cocaine: The making of a global drug*. Chapel Hill, NC: University of North Carolina Press.

Graves Peligros [Grave Dangers]. (1969, July 11). *El Universal.*
Grosser, A. (1969, September 28). La Droga y el Vacío [The drug and the void]. *Excelsior.*
Gurza, T. (1976, April 8). Las Drogas, Recurso Terapéutico Pervertido en el uso Clandestino [Drugs: A therapeutic resource perverted by clandestine use]. *El Dia.*
Halpern, J. H., Sherwood, A. R., Hudson, J. I., Yurgelun-Todd, D., & Pope, H. G. Jr. (2005). Psychological and cognitive effects of long-term peyote use among Native Americans. *Biological Psychiatry, 58*(8), 624–631.
Instituto Nacional Indigenista, Coordinadora Estatal de Nayarit. (1996). Reunión de rescate cultural de la costumbres Wirraritari [Wirraritari customs cultural rescue meeting]. Mexico City: CDI Historical Archive, FD 18/048.
Iñigo, A. (1970, May 21). El Huichol, Hermanado con el Peyote Casi Desde que Nace [The Huichol: United with peyote practically since birth] *Excelsior.*
Krebs, T. S., & Johansen, P.-O. (2012). Lysergic acid diethylamide (LSD) for alcoholism: Meta-analysis of randomized controlled trials. *Journal of Psychopharmacology, 26*(7), 994–1002.
Labate, B. C., & Cavnar, C. (Eds.). (2016). *Peyote: History, traditions, politics, and conservation.* Santa Barbara, CA: Praeger.
Labate, B. C., & Feeney, K. (2016). Paradoxes of drug regulation in Mexico: Drug conventions and environmental laws. In B. C. Labate & C. Cavnar (Eds.), *Peyote: History, traditions, politics, and conservation* (pp. 211–238). Santa Barbara, CA: Praeger.
Las Drogas, Aventura Mortal [Drugs: A mortal adventure). (1980, July 4). *El Heraldo de Mexico.*
Llamado a los Padres de Familia [Calling the parents]. (1970, April 10). *El Universal.*
Marroquín, E. (1975). *La contracultura como protesta. análisis de un fenómeno juvenil* [The counterculture as protest: Analysis of a youth phenomenon]. Mexico City: Joaquin Mortiz (Cuadernos).
Matta Torres, R. (1976). *Los Peyoteros.* Guadalajara: Author.
Maynez Puente, S. (1969, April 26). Sucedáneos del Afecto [Substitutes for affection]. *Excelsior.*
Mayoral Pardo, D. (1973). Toxicomanía-Farmacodependencia [Drug addiction-drug dependence]. *CEMEF Informe, 1*(6). Secretaría de Salud Pública SP 266.1, 4.
No hay centros para rehabilitar a los niños farmacodependientes [There are no centers for rehabilitating drug dependent children]. (1976, April 19). *El Universal.*
Payan, V. (1980, April 24). 200,000 Llamadas Recibieron en 1979 en los Centros de Integración Juvenil [The youth integration centers received 200,000 calls in 1979). *Excelsior.*
Pacheco Santos, G. (1976, April 14). *Conocer el Lenguaje de los Farmacodependientes Ayuda a Ganar su Confianza* [Understanding the language of drug dependents helps win their trust]. El Día.
Pérez Isaak, A. (1979, February 11). Alerta la a Cívica Femenina Contra Drogas y Pornografía [The civic feminine association raises the alarm against drugs and pornography]. *Excelsior.*
Pérez Montfort, R. (1999). *Yerba, goma y polvo: drogas ambientales y policías en México, 1900–1940 [Herb, gum, and dust: Everyday drugs and police in Mexico, 1900–1940].* Mexico: Ediciones Era.
Programa Nacional de Combate a los Problemas de Drogas [National program to combat the problems of drugs]. (1976). *¿Como Identificar las drogas y sus usuarios?* [How to Identify drugs and their users?) Mexico City: CEMEF and SEP.
Sánchez Azua, A. (2004, June 7). Extranjeros se disfrazan y roban peyote mexicano [Foreigners in disguise steal Mexican peyote]. *El Siglo de Torreón.*
Sterling, T. G. (1999, February 18). A vision gone bust. *Phoenix New Times.*
Schaefer, S. (2015). *Amada's blessings from the Peyote Gardens of South Texas.* Albuquerque: University of New Mexico Press.
Schivelbusch, W. (1992). *The tastes of paradise.* New York City, NY: Vintage.
Shortall, S. (2014). Psychedelic drugs and the problem of experience. *Past and Present, 222*(Supp. 9), 187–206. https://doi.org/10.1093/pastj/gtt035
Smith, S. L. (2012). *Hippies, Indians, and the fight for Red Power.* New York City, NY: Oxford University Press.

Trout, K., & Terry, M. (2016). Decline of the genus *Lophophora* in Texas. In B. C. Labate & C. Cavnar (Eds.), *Peyote: History, traditions, politics, and conservation* (pp. 1–20). Santa Barbara, CA: Praeger.

Uso y abuso de drogas. Información para maestros [Use and abuse of drugs: Information for teachers]. (1974). Mexico City: SEP. Secretaría de Salud Pública SP 295.1.

Zolov, E. (1999). *Refried Elvis: The rise of the Mexican counterculture*. Berkeley: University of California Press.

Chapter 3
Undiscovering the Pueblo Mágico: Lessons from Huautla for the Psychedelic Renaissance

Ben Feinberg

Abstract The people of the Sierra Mazateca region of Mexico became internationally known in the 1950s for their ritual use of psilocybin mushrooms, and the Mazatec town of Huautla became a destination for mushroom seeking visitors. This chapter provides an overview of changing Mazatec and "outsider" discourses about mushrooms and the Sierra Mazateca over the last 60 years. It argues that "outsider" representations of the Sierra Mazateca and mushroom use—whether framed in terms of spiritual journeys or scientific research—tend to recapitulate some consistent patterns common to other forms of cultural tourism that owe more to the role of substances in marking distinctive cultural identities than to the effects of the substances themselves. It concludes by suggesting lessons from this history for the current moment, in which a discourse framing the use of psychedelic substances through universalizing narratives of science and individual health is becoming ascendant

Nothing signaled the triumphalist moment in the biomedical approach to psychedelics like the Psychedelic Science conference at the Marriott Hotel in Oakland in April 2017. *The New York Times* compared the event to the Coachella music festival taking place over the same weekend, only "rather than rock stars, scientists from schools like Johns Hopkins and N.Y.U. were the main attraction," bringing evidence for the effectiveness of psychedelic substances—once exclusively the territory of the counterculture—to treat a broad range of maladies, from PTSD to depression (Schwartz, 2017). While scientists dominated the conference rooms, an anthropologist wandering through the exhibition hall could marvel at the eclectic, and at times contradictory, mix of pro-psychedelic discourses and cultural domains, united only by a shared optimism.

Here, a section of the room was devoted to poster presentations overflowing with charts and graphs and margins of errors demonstrating, for example, the

---

B. Feinberg (✉)
Warren Wilson College, Asheville, NC, USA
e-mail: feinberg@warren-wilson.edu

© Springer International Publishing AG, part of Springer Nature 2018
B. C. Labate, C. Cavnar (eds.), *Plant Medicines, Healing and Psychedelic Science*,
https://doi.org/10.1007/978-3-319-76720-8_3

"characterization of mystical experiences occasioned by 5-MeO-DMT containing toad bufotoxin" or the success rates of "3,4-methylenedioxymethamphetamine (MDMA) on conditional fear extinction." There, a young man sold coloring books based on visions he experienced while taking ayahuasca. Here, a drug company, using a font and logo as alienating and disembodied as that of any other pharmaceutical product, marketed distinct cannabis-based treatments for pain relief, sleep disorders, and finding calm with the slogan "Targeted formulas. Precise dosages." There, brochures used classic psychedelic imagery to advertise an online university as "The Ultimate Learning Hub for All-things Ayahuasca," where you can "Go deep in powerful online courses taught by experts" and "learn how to maximize your ayahuasca journey." I watched one of the most renowned of the celebrity scientists, psychologist James Fadiman, on a screen in the overflow room as he spoke from the Grand Ballroom, breathlessly listing the infinite benefits of regular microdosing with LSD: from reducing procrastination and increasing productivity for Silicon Valley coders to enabling better relationships for lovers to guaranteeing more intense workouts and performance for elite athletes.

One could interpret this dizzying spectacle of reputability through the narrative of the inevitable conquest of reason over superstition, a kind of twenty-first-century Scopes Trial heralding the reemergence of scientific progress after a 50-year-long dark age of ignorance and repression. Or one could view it through a darker lens, as an extreme manifestation of the kind of dystopian cooptation imagined by the Bay Area punk band Dead Kennedys in their song, California Über Alles: "I am Governor Jerry Brown, my aura smiles and never frowns... You will jog for the master race, and always wear the happy face" (Biafra & Greenway, 1979). But if one steps back from the splendor of this scientific renaissance in psychedelic studies, where (almost entirely) White scientists hawk the benefits of psychedelic substances in treating mostly White patients in front of an overwhelmingly White audience in a convention center in the heart of a great city, one must encounter the story of a Mexican town called Huautla de Jiménez. In Huautla, even as science retreated from its earlier enthusiastic engagement with psychedelic research, the centrality of a particular psychedelic organism—the hallucinogenic mushroom—never went away. What does the story of Huautla, a Mazatec-speaking community that improbably achieved international fame in the 1950s, have to say to the current moment of excitement about psychedelic medicines?

In this chapter, based on my research over the last 25 years in the Sierra Mazateca, my goal is to go beyond the stereotype of "magical" Huautla, "city of the magic mushrooms," and provide an overview of Mazatec and "outsider" discourses about mushrooms and the Sierra Mazateca over the last 60 years. I highlight the ways that these representations are fluid and dynamic and involve forms of connection and misunderstanding within and between these two broad (and themselves heteroge-neous) groupings. I argue that "outsider" representations of the Sierra Mazateca and mushroom use—whether framed in terms of spiritual journeys or scientific research—tend to recapitulate some consistent patterns common to other forms of cultural tourism that owe more to the role of substances in marking distinctive cultural identities than to the effects of the substances themselves. I will conclude by suggesting lessons from this history for the current moment, in which a discourse framing the use of psychedelic substances through universalizing narratives of science and individual health is becoming ascendant.

Huautla: *Pueblo Mágico*

For outsiders, the history of the Sierra Mazateca area of Oaxaca began in 1955, when the American banker and mushroom enthusiast Gordon Wasson visited, participated in mushroom rituals, and then wrote about his experience for *Life* magazine (Wasson, 1957). Wasson had developed a theory that the different cultures of the world could be classified as mycophiliac (like that of his Russian wife) or mycophobic (like his own New England Protestant family). After the American missionary Eunice Pike tipped him off that there were Indians in Mexico who consumed a mushroom that they considered sacred and which gave them visions, he realized that this could confirm his theory and determined to experience the mushroom for himself. He spent the remaining 30 years of his life researching and promoting psychedelic mushrooms and making frequent visits back to Huautla.

Wasson's article in *Life* led to a fungus rush, as foreigners descended on Huautla, led at first by avant-garde intellectuals who rented rooms in the town's only hotel, but followed by thousands of countercultural pilgrims who ultimately set up a large camp by a river a few miles outside of town. After tiring of the scandal and disruption they caused, in 1969 the town president asked the military to intervene. Sixty-four Mexican *jipis* were arrested, and 22 foreigners were deported (Zolov, 1999). For years thereafter, a military checkpoint on the only road into town blocked foreigners from access. In the mid-1970s, the army checkpoint was removed, and mushroom tourism resumed on a smaller scale.

Today, the image of Huautla is intimately connected with the image of the mushroom, which has become an official symbol of town identity. Visitors to the town pass a statue of María Sabina, the curer Wasson made famous, with her arms outstretched, and then drive under a great stone arch, in which the word *Bienvenido* (welcome) is flanked by carved mushrooms. Public space in Huautla is decorated with murals depicting María Sabina, and local businesses—from pizza restaurants to the ubiquitous taxis that navigate the city's network of impossibly narrow and steep roads—use the mushroom image for marketing. Even school parades, in which children wear costumes to demonstrate their town pride, emphasize the psychedelic substances as indexes of identity. In the parade I witnessed in 2014, kindergartners waved from a truck festooned with images of the hallucinogenic plant *Salvia divinorum*, known locally as *pastora*; the bed of the truck, besides carrying the children, overflowed with samples of the plant. Older children stopped and performed a staged reenactment of a typical mushroom ceremony, with a huipil-clad girl playing the role of the shaman, blessing children playing the roles of her patients.

In 2015, Huautla's application to be officially designated as a *Pueblo Mágico* (Magical Town) was approved by the Ministry of Tourism, providing the town with an additional stream of revenue to be used to promote tourism. The Pueblo Mágico program aims "to revalue a set of populations in the country that have always been in the collective imagination of the nation as a whole and which represent fresh and different alternatives for national and foreign visitors" (Secretaría de Turismo, 2016, para. 1). While the program's web page for Huautla lists a few natural attractions, the focus is on "spirituality" and the "cosmovision and legacy of the Priestess of the Mushrooms, María Sabina" (Secretaría de Turismo, 2016, para. 2). After years of official ambivalence toward Huautla's reputation (preceded by a period of outright repression), this designation represented the government's official embrace of Huautla's mushroom-based commercial potential. Huautla was officially placed in the chronotope of the "magical"—a bounded place like Narnia or Oz, outside normal space and time and permeated by a permanent liminality and way of life and thought distinct from the everyday world.

Parts of the world that do not come to mind with great frequency except with regard to a particular trait or quality that has received broader recognition often become conflated with that trait, so that the people and the trait come to signify each other, and we imagine that the whole meaning or purpose of the people is to remind us, in case we have forgotten, of the importance of sensuality (for Micronesia, see Lutz & Collins, 1993), of the grand adventure of viewing big animals (for Africa, see Mathers & Hubbard, 2009), or of relaxation on deck chairs while swaying to reggae music (for anywhere on the "global beach," see Lofgren, 2004). A visitor viewing Huautla through the lens of the "magical," and seeing the mushroom images on walls and in parades, might be forgiven for assuming that Huautla means mushrooms and psychedelic spirituality, just as Cancún means sand, surf, and margaritas.

But the life of the people of the Sierra Mazateca is multifaceted, and if one lives there for any period, one realizes that the amount of time that most residents spend thinking and talking about hallucinogenic mushrooms is compared to time spent pondering questions such as work, migration, and navigating the intricacies of a complex and dangerous geography of kinship and social obligations, extraordinarily small, except for a very few. They are no more the "people of the mushrooms" than Texans are the "people of the chicken fried steaks."

Here I must offer a disclaimer: I am not an expert on the pharmacological "effects" of ingesting substances such as psilocybin, though I have consumed them a number of times in Huautla and elsewhere; nor, really, am I an expert on the intricacies of Mazatec shamanism, though I draw heavily in this chapter from the pioneering and comprehensive work of Edward Abse (2007). But I argue that any attempt to understand the meaning of substance use that relies only an individualist and medicalizing focus on their therapeutic "effects" will miss the point in understanding the social meaning of substances and their circulation. Similarly, a detailed analysis of the ritual meaning of "the mushroom ceremony," imagined as a private event meaningful only to the physically present participants, does not capture the broader role of mushrooms in reproducing social identities and groups. Pierre Bourdieu (1984, p. 2) wrote that, "To the socially recognized hierarchy of the arts, and within each of them, corresponds a social hierarchy of the consumers." He could have added as a corollary that, to the socially recognized hierarchy of "drugs," and within each of them, corresponds a social hierarchy of consumers. Much of my time over the last 30 years in the Sierra Mazateca has been spent studying the construction of identity and the politics of representation. It became abundantly clear to me that the discourses of mushrooms and mushroom shamanism, like those about *all* drugs in *all* contemporary societies, are largely about differentiating, defining, and ranking different categories of people.

Is It the Same for Us and Them?

First, I would like to address a basic anthropological question: is "their" experience on mushrooms the same as "ours?" Can we make broad assumptions about the effects of substances across cultural borders between peoples with different ontologies and social structures? Whether our answer is a firm "yes" or "no," with regard to the effects of mushrooms, there are implications that we should be aware of.

Individuals who consume psilocybin mushrooms may experience their effects as transcending the everyday barriers of language, culture, and the body and bringing them to a shared liminal space. As in Victor Turner's (1977, p. 138) description of communitas, they may discover "a transformative experience that goes to the root of each person's being and finds in that root something profoundly communal and shared." Alexander Dawson (2015, p. 105) argues that both María Sabina and the psychiatrist Salvador Roquet experienced mushrooms "as actants, or vibrant matter that produced bodily effects independent of language and other meaning-making practices" and "since many of these effects took place outside language, they undermined the sense of difference produced by linguistic and cultural barriers."

An answer of "yes" to the question of whether mushroom experience transcends difference allows us to see commonalities with others and recognized shared experiences but ignores the basic fact that, while substances may have common recognizable pharmacological effects on the human brain, these shared processes are interpreted in ways that are profoundly influenced and framed by culture, history, and social relationships. The assumption of similitude enables a leap of identification with others but also allows them, their social universe, and their interpretations to be ignored. By denying the possibility of the others with truly different experiences, it projects dominant metropolitan categories—such as the "individual self" and "spirituality"—onto them and elides the necessity of questioning Western cultural assumptions about what these mean. If indigenous experience of psychedelic substances does not offer anything genuinely different, then the role of indigenous people is reduced to their historical function as preservers of these practices until they can be "discovered" by more sophisticated people better able to understand and explain them. Local voices, such as shamans, are incorporated into the story only when they can be read (or modified) to corroborate Western biases; where they don't, they can be ignored or dismissed as "superstitious" or "inauthentic."

The goal of inquiry, then, becomes the documentation of a secret history of indigenous substance use rather than the interpretation of how substances acquire meaning in particular settings. This parallels the approaches of second-wave feminist and early LGBT scholars who assumed that categories like "female" and "homosexual" were universally experienced in the same way. Recognizing that, in order to build a social movement, it was vital to have knowledge of a shared history, these scholar/activists read their own experience backward and constructed a "myth of silence, invisibility, and isolation" in which people just like them always existed but were hidden (D'Emilio, 1983, p. 101). The meanings of others' experiences, in this framework, are already incorporated into the observer's perspective and experiences.

But if the answer of "yes" ignores the possibility of fundamentally different cultural understandings, the alternative "no" answer, emphasizing difference, when taken to extremes, also leads to problematic and ahistorical representations of the other. As Roger Lancaster (1997, p. 195) writes with regard to the scholarship that examines sexuality cross-culturally, it often generates "excesses of absolutist relativism" that "abstract human existences into posed and frozen daguerreotypes, arrayed like exhibits in a vast museum that suspiciously resembles a mausoleum." The "other" is seen as different, beyond any possibility of connection or dialogue, and also static and outside of history. From this perspective, people like the Mazatec may be seen as genuinely different, but only to the degree that they can be associated with labels such as "isolated," "traditional," and "ancient" that deny the reality that practices such as the use of mushrooms are dynamic and acquire meaning through constant interaction across cultural borders in evolving social structural contexts.

Popular understandings that individuals in different cultures experience drugs differently also have roots in the notion that people categorized in different races have different kinds of bodies. Spanish colonial drug laws banned non-Indians from using peyote because the drug, while appropriate for inherently irrational Indians, was believed to cause degeneracy for *gente de razón*, while the belief that cocaine drove Black people to rape White women justified mass incarceration in the United States (Dawson, 2018; Provine, 2007). In the 1990s, Jamaican folk beliefs categorized crack cocaine as a "White drug" for White bodies, while marijuana was a "Black drug" suitable for Black bodies (Broad & Feinberg, 1995). In each case, drug discourse functions to reify essentialized notions of biological difference in ways that tend to naturalize the effects of social inequality. Today, notions of essential "cultural" differences often replace biological explanations but serve the same function of mystifying exploitation while denying both the possibilities of connection across cultural borders and the diversity of experience within them.

In practice, many outsider representations of Mazatec mushroom pay lip service to the idea of cultural difference, but rarely examine their own perspectives as culturally specific, and generally ignore the ways in which cultural contact and difference are integral to Mazatec mushroom practice. The "cultural" (as a possession of indigenous people) is still bracketed out and recognized—but as something that affects "them," and not us. Only rarely do accounts of nonindigenous use of mushrooms seriously consider their own cultural specificity.

When taken in their purer forms, both the "yes" and "no" options, then, fail to recognize indigenous experience on its own terms. Hence, an assumption of universality erases others by locating them within the all-encompassing metropolitan self. Conversely, indigenous people like the Mazatec are often recognized as different but relegated to the space of the metropolitan other—as timeless, ahistorical objects of curiosity and charity and icons of authenticity, but not partners in dialogue.

Ceremony, Authority, and Travel: Changes in Mazatec Mushroom Shamanism

I will now briefly give an overview of some of elements of mushroom discourse in the Sierra Mazateca, highlighting how it has evolved, and some ways it contrasts with Western representations.

Abse (2007, p. 152) estimates that 1% of the people of the Sierra Mazateca are *Chjota chine*, or "people of knowledge" (referred to as *curanderos* in Spanish, although the use of the term *chaman* is increasing). These people typically serve a clientele that is based in their extended family groups. Curanderos provide mushrooms to their clients, and possibly other family members, during a ritual called a *velada*, or "stay awake," that takes place indoors and at night. In the nineteenth and early twentieth centuries, curanderos played important formal political roles in their communities: advising and serving as rulers, mediating between villages and kinship groups, and conducting community-wide rituals to deal with drought and in support of community projects. This formal role declined, but curanderos still often serve as informal leaders of their extended families.

While mushroom rituals may once have addressed community-wide concerns, today, most Mazatecos say that they should be taken to treat a particular health problem. These health problems may be psychological, such as *susto* (a condition caused by a sudden fright that forces the soul to leave the body) or postpartum depression, but they may also be conditions that foreigners consider biological, such as an injury or back pain. They may also be taken for other reasons, and Mazatec ritual practice has a strong streak of experimentation and very little dogma. In some lowland regions of the Sierra Mazateca, curers will use *Salvia divinorum* (*pastora*) as well as mushrooms, but Huautecos consider pastora a poor substitute for the real thing. People in the sierra view *Salvia* as similar to mushrooms, although the two substances are differentiated through the hot/cold Mesoamerican classification system: one woman told me that she does not like to use salvia as it is "cold," while mushrooms are "hot."

While Western visitors often emphasize visual and nonlinguistic experience, Mazatec shamanic practice highlights the importance of the curer as a speaker who uses a special charged and figurative form of language. Curers like Maria Sabina end each line with *tso*, or "says," highlighting how they convey speech coming directly from the "child saints" (a term often used for mushrooms) (Munn, 1973). Language, in Mazatec ceremonies, is the most important element of healing and often takes on material qualities; it evokes a purifying rain as participants may experience words, as Abse (2007, p. 171) writes, as "luminous objects or invisible textures coming down to them from the saints and Virgins."

The special language of the shaman seeks out and identifies the cause of the patient's malady, which is often couched in accordance with Mesoamerican container/contained models of the body and multiple souls. The curer may identify and remove intrusive substances by sucking or inducing vomiting or discover that a patient's soul has been lost in the wilds of the *monte* (uncultivated forest) or in a place of confinement. The idea that people may "become lost" is central to Mazatec discourse beyond shamanism, and I have heard many stories of individuals who vanished into hidden caves in the monte, only to reemerge with no recollection of how they got there but with fantastic stories of underground cities and magical wealth.

Like Westerners, Mazatecs speak of mushrooms as a vehicle of travel: they describe "trips" and say that the substances "take you far away." Shamanic language enacts and invokes travel, particularly between their home and spaces of power like oceans and cities. Like caves, mushrooms open up a pathway in which intermediaries, like the Mayan Hero Twins in the *Popol Vuh* (a pre-Hispanic book of Mayan myths), can enter spaces of symbolic and real power and intervene on behalf of their patients (Tedlock, 1985). The Hero Twins descended into the underground world to enter into a contest with powerful others—the Lords of Death—before returning to benefit their people, and Mazatec mythology is full of figures, like the light-skinned Mazatec Earth Lord named Chikon Tokoxho, who also personifies borders and transactions. A curer recorded by Henry Munn (1973, p. 106) in the 1970s used language to travel to Córdoba and Orizaba, the cities where *campesinos* would sell their coffee. He invoked the relevant symbols of power in his chants: "Where the Big Bank is, says. Where there is money of gold, says."

While outsiders refer to the Sierra Mazateca through the tropes of "isolation" and the maintenance of an ancient tradition, mushroom discourse, at its core, has always been one of cross-cultural exchange and mediation, focusing on crossing the magically charged borders of day and night, the sacred and profane, and us and them.

Wasson, in his prologue to María Sabina's autobiography, tried paternalistically to defend her against the charge that she was "illiterate" by comparing her to ancient oral poets, because she lived in a completely enclosed world: a fossilized, "protohistorical" version of our own Euro-American past, unlike the undeserving poor of our modern world who "lack the wit to learn to read and write" (Wasson, 1981, p. 15). This totally misses the point. María Sabina's shamanism did not represent an idealized distinct culture on the cusp of its inevitable degradation but told the story of a continually reproduced marginality within a transforming system of exploitation. And books, far from being foreign to this world, play a central role as symbols of power and domination that curers like María Sabina could access. In her ceremonies, this illiterate woman accessed and read a magical book as a symbol of her appropriation of a form of power she was very aware of. Most Mazatec curers, whether they can read or not, take possession of magical books through which they connect to sources of power (Feinberg, 1997, 2003).

The way Mazatec people view ritual has changed over the last 50 years (as it likely had in the 50 years before that), though this change should not be viewed, as a narcissistic tourist model would have it, simply an "effect" of visitors. Neither can we accurately describe this change as a "degradation" of tradition through loss of "isolation" and the presence of media and foreigners.

The main change probably involves a shift in attribution in the cause of the patient's suffering. While, for a previous generation, the victim's misfortune was usually caused by an accidental transgression of a sacred space, such as by crossing a stream connected to particular sprites at noon, today the cause is more sinister. Shamans more typically identify the problem as the conscious, malevolent action of a person in the community. This relates to a particularly resonant Mazatec word, *kjoaxintokon*, that signifies "a hideous malevolence often concealed behind the mask of friendship"—an amplified version of envy (Abse, 2007, p. 31). Fortunato, a *campesino* in a lowland village, told me that mushrooms were "good for seeing who is trying to harm you." Abse argues that this shift reflects the loss of trust following the transformation of community through the penetration of a capitalist cash economy and political parties. Mazatec curing, then, does not separate individual from social health; the two are always intertwined. Cures may require a patient to take certain actions. including, in some cases, the repeated ingestion of the substance every few days for a period of time.

The second main change is the decline of the authority of the curandero. In the mid-twentieth century, the curandero would take a large quantity of mushrooms, while the clients had smaller amounts, or sometimes none at all. The experience, language, and authority of the curandero, which corresponded to his or her social position within the community, were central. Today, individuals are more inclined to take mushrooms without a shaman and to usurp the shaman's authority to interpret their experiences. Juana, for example, took mushrooms alone every few nights, about five or six times, until her leg was healed from a nasty injury. And Julia, who had never taken mushrooms before, decided to take them by herself after her husband abandoned her. She discovered, through this unconventional episode, that she possessed a previously unrecognized shamanic power to see the true nature of her situation and realized that the envy of her husband's sisters had made him crazy. Through the ritual, she resolved the problem, and he returned shortly afterward to take his normal seat at the table, and she went on to regularly lead her family in mushroom ceremonies. My Mazatec informants frequently state that it is appropriate to "experiment" with mushrooms. "There are some problems that medicine doesn't cure," says Braulio, "and mushrooms may cure them. You experiment with them" to see if they can.

Mazatec mushroom practice and ideas about mushrooms are not static and have modified and adapted to changing circumstances. A famous quote from María Sabina attributes a general decline in the mushroom's power to the arrival of mushroom-seeking foreigners after Wasson. "From the moment the foreigners arrived to search for God," she told Alvaro Estrada (1981, p. 90), "the saint children lost their purity. They lost their force; the foreigners spoiled them." But, despite this claim, many of the historical changes in Mazatec curing, including the shift in attribution for sickness and the decline of the curandero's authority, are responding to other changes and should not be seen only as a "decline" caused by foreign "contamination." However, as I will discuss later, some curers have developed a non-Mazatec clientele, and this has led them to make more innovations in their practices.

Outsider Representations of Mazatec Culture and Curing

I will now discuss the key themes of outsiders' representations of Mazatec mushroom practice, which are similar to themes that anthropologists have identified in other sites of so-called spiritual tourism (Gomez-Barris, 2012).

The first is the overwhelming, repeated-to-oblivion claim that the people of the Sierra Mazateca represent the preserved past. From Wasson's description of María Sabina as a fossilized survivor of a lost world to the present, visitors describe Mazatecs as creatures of another time. In a recent television program on the Viceland Network, the young American protagonist Hamilton Morris (2016) could not help but frame his journey to Huautla in the same terms and to locate Mazatec ritual through the past tense. Morris first interviewed a scientist who had studied salvia in the Sierra Mazateca in the 1970s. The scientist explained "why the Mazatecs used this," and Morris added that "indigenous groups preserved religious traditions." He then journeyed to Huautla, falsely described as a "small" and "secluded mountain town," because "I hope to learn if the tradition he observed has remained the same." He consistently describes the Mazatec through the rhetoric of discovery, and the episode is framed as a rite of passage: a journey that begins and ends in a hypermodern, urban world, marked with the signifiers of scientific and avant-garde authority, and passes through a world of Mazatec shamanism framed as part of the past, whose function is to inscribe the first-world host with authenticity. The rhetoric of discovery reduces Mazatec history to the single dimension of continuity/change and produces a framework in which all change is interpreted as loss or contamination of an original purity.

These tales of the Mushroom People fix Mazatecs in a limited role as passive bearers of an unchanging tradition. Now that their historical function has been met, it's time to "pass on the torch" to the more "enlightened and sophisticated" foreigners who "discovered" them. María Sabina joined other commodified icons of "Latin American culture"—as a t-shirt next to Che Guevara and Frida Kahlo—or of "indigenous wisdom" that function as a source of inspiration for high culture. Like La Malinche of Mexican nationalist myth, the lover and translator of Hernán Cortés who revealed indigenous secrets, she is seen as passing ancient wisdom on to the bearers of the future. Once "discovered," the Mazatecs lose any right to agency. As the immensely popular Mexican rock band El Tri sang in their song dedicated to her, she functions only as a "symbol of wisdom and love": generic Western projections of spirituality (Lora, 1989). The song details how she "taught secrets" to journalists, philosophers, and poets, and "opened the eyes of the whole universe," achieving worldwide fame. Her role is to "show us the path" and then die—and it is clear who gets to be included in "us."

The representation of curers as women is a second theme. Visitors to Huautla who take mushrooms there usually do so with female curers, even though some 60% of Mazatec chjota chine are men (Abse, 2007, p. 152). Throughout Latin America, tourist discourses identify Indian women with the comforting, non-threatening aspects of the other, and as bearers of conservative cultural traits such as clothing and language. Indian women, unlike Black women, are desexualized (Weismantel, 2001, p. xl). The association of femininity with a form of indigeneity valued by tourists as the "principal signifiers of traditional culture, the indigenous, and the 'Other'" opens possibilities for indigenous women in the tourist economy to strategically turn these stereotypes into economic capital (Babb, 2012, p. 38). Visitors to Huautla highlight these gender differences by ignoring men or by describing them as sinister and suspicious while viewing women as more appropriate points of entry into an authentic cultural experience.

A third theme is the lack of interest in culture, history, or language beyond its role as an authenticating backdrop. Very few of the mushroom-seeking visitors to Huautla I have talked to (with some significant exceptions), including many who have participated in mushroom ceremonies, express much curiosity about Mazatec interpretations of healing, or the social and political landscape of the region. As in other forms of adventure travel, "there is minimal attempt to get to know strangers, to risk one's emotional and mental comfort zones and disturb any preconceived ideas" (Mathers & Hubbard, 2009, p. 202). The countercultural visitors of the 1960s whom I interviewed emphasized their own future-oriented utopian community, which was connected to other spaces of a globe-trotting drug culture. Huautla was the "poor man's Nepal," not a region in Oaxaca (Feinberg, 2009; Zolov, 1999). As in other locations of spiritual tourism, an "individualized spiritual journey replaces any broader social and cultural understanding of the local situation" beyond the "incorporation of native people as symbols of authentic purity" (Gomez-Barris, 2012, p. 73).

While most Mazatec healers who have attracted a small foreign clientele have remained poor and unable to transcend the unequal nature of this exchange, a few entrepreneurs have been able to position themselves as cultural mediators in ways that are very lucrative. One, in particular, has benefited greatly by the way that outsider discourse leads to uncritical celebration of a few culture brokers seen through a stereotypical lens. Julieta Casimiro is the most famous and wealthy living Mazatec curer. In an interview conducted by her daughter, Doña Julieta explained how her chjota chine mother-in-law taught her about mushrooms, commenting, "The truth is, I liked it" (Pineda Casmiro, 2007). In 1968, the hippie wave was cresting in Huautla. "At that time no one liked foreigners," she said, "whether from other countries or other parts of Mexico." Julieta was one of the first to sense the opportunity they provided while recognizing the risk. At first, she had to cultivate foreign clients in secret, "because it was frowned on to give niños santos to foreigners. That is, we worked against our culture and ran the risk that comes with opening your doors to those who don't belong to your culture." By 1993, when I

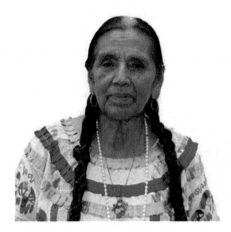

> **❝** *Our Mother Earth is hurting.*
> *They are destroying our*
> *Mother Earth. They are*
> *destroying our Mother. They*
> *need to have respect for Her.*
> – Grandmother Julieta Casimiro

Julieta is a Mazatec elder, from Huautla de Jimenez, and carries the tradition of healing and ceremonies with the use of sacred plants, the pre-hispanic Teonanactl, "Ninos Santos" way. She organizes the women of her village who create the most beautiful hand sewn clothing.

Fig. 2.1 Julieta Casimiro's Bio from Thirteen Indigenous Grandmothers website

lived in Huautla, Julieta employed a network of children and outsider hangers-on who actively recruited clients as they arrived in town, and in 2000, she was invited to an international conference in Switzerland. In 2003, she became a member of the International Council of Thirteen Indigenous Grandmothers, a group of First Peoples women who periodically meet in different locations.

The bio for Julieta on the Thirteen Grandmothers (2017) website demonstrates the way her image circulates globally (Fig. 2.1). She is totally removed from her local social, cultural, and political context through generic imagery of commodified indigenousness and generic "native wisdom" about protecting the environment; an always already hybridized curing tradition is described as "ancient" and "pre-Hispanic"; cosmopolitan Huautla is misrepresented as a "village"; and Julietta's economic activities are mystified as a benevolent organization of "village women."

In fact, Julieta and her family are powerful figures in a complex local and regional politics, closely tied to the PRI, the formerly dominant political party. In 2004, her son, known as El Diablo, was photographed beating a retired teacher to death because he was involved in a political protest against the gubernatorial candidate (Agencia Reforma, 2013). El Diablo was never arrested and is still politically active, and a frequent presence in Julieta's household, along with her cosmopolitan clients. She has been able to creatively translate each of the themes of outsider discourse—mushroom use as the preserved past, the curer as female, and the lack of interest in actual Mazatec life—into a long and successful career.

Visitors' Mushroom Experiences in Huautla

In most cases, visitors describe their experiences with mushrooms as very positive and often express warm and grateful feelings toward their Mazatec interlocutors. While their accounts overlap with those of my Mazatec informants, their stories stress different themes, and some curers have adapted their practices to accommodate these concerns.

One theme is a certain ambivalence about the trappings of ritual and a re-inscription of difference between the individualist Westerner and ritualist Indians. A Dutch traveler emailed me that he participated in a mushroom ritual in Huautla "but was largely bemused by the experience," concluding "that my white skin and Western mind would forever deny me experiences of the 'archaic' kind." Then, he ate more mushrooms, alone in the city. "There was no ritual," he wrote, "no observation of purity rites, no healer present. I took them for 'fun' and nothing else. To my astonishment, I had what I can only call a profound 'spiritual experience'. . .. I remain unconvinced either way, suspended in disbelief, agnostic if you will."

This story of a profound experience that results, ultimately, from the individualist triumph of the visitor is fairly frequent and emphasizes the contrast between the "self-oriented search for meaning" that characterizes contemporary Western spirituality and the emphasis on collective subjectivity and the social in Mazatec healing (Gomez-Barris, 2012, p. 73). These narratives depict the local intermediary as someone confined in a bounded culture limited by the trappings of ritual and convention. While the curer provides access to native culture as an object of consumption, the spiritual experience comes precisely from the visitor's ability to transcend the particularities of culture.

Some Mazatec curers have embraced a customer service model in response to the preferences of mushroom tourists. Inés Cortés has been participating in veladas with foreigners since she was a young girl, though she had learned some chants and songs from her curandero uncle. But in describing her birth as a curer, it is not her uncle that she emphasizes but the psychologist Salvador Roquet, who she met hanging out at the Posada Rosaura, then the only hotel in Huautla and a setting of intercultural exchange that she remembers with profound nostalgia. Roquet invited her to the veladas he organized with large groups of his urban clients and had her clean the mushrooms and sing. She was enthralled and began hosting ceremonies herself as a young mother in the late 1980s. Her emphasis on the intercultural essence of curing is not "inauthentic" but is itself a version of the Mazatec link between shamanism and intercultural relationships and borders (Feinberg, 2003).

When I met Inés, in 1993, she would require that her clients obey various rules, such as fasting, wearing light colors, removing watches, and staying in the dirt-floored, cave-like altar room of her house where she would sing and chant to them throughout the night. Today, her practice has changed. She has embraced a more individualistic and customer service model. Shamans, she argues, can't really see their clients' issues or cure them; only the client can do that. She also has dropped the rules—"why tell them to do something," she asks me, "that makes them uncomfortable?" She has used her experience to develop a series of national stereotypes about her customers, many of whom are Japanese, as she was highlighted in a Japanese travel blog. "My *japonesitos*," she says, "don't like being in the altar room, and don't like it when I sing. They would rather be in the corridor and left alone." This shows another distinction: while the auditory experience of the shaman's voice is a key element in Mazatec shamanism, foreigners comment more on visual and inner experience, rarely commenting on the language of the curer. In January of 2017, I observed two separate Japanese visitors she hosted and, in fact, both asked to be left alone on the roof of her house, where they took photographs of the town and selfies to share with friends.

Inés's story demonstrates the possibility of intercultural dialogue and connection but also the asymmetrical nature of contemporary tourist encounters. In a context of inequality and competition for a dwindling tourist market, practitioners like Inés are led, whether intentionally or not, to voluntarily relinquish signs of their authority and redefine themselves as hosts of a bed and breakfast-like service experience.

Observations and Implications: From Huautla to Oakland

I met a scientific researcher in Huautla for the first time in 1994. He had conducted experiments with mushrooms with volunteer subjects in Europe in laboratory conditions but had come all the way to Mexico to try them for himself for the first time. I spoke with him over coffee in Inés's kitchen, as he purchased a bag of the child saints, and then the next day, after he had consumed them alone in his hotel room, I asked why he chose to do that: why he had come so far to have his experience by himself instead of seeking a local intermediary. He replied that he wanted to be "in this place" but felt that he had nothing to gain from talking to anyone (he couldn't speak Spanish anyway)—that he wanted to experience everything "in my own brain." His story shows how the scientific discourse about psychedelics is itself a complex and contradictory space. While research has brought undeniable enhancements to scientific knowledge, it also cannot help but continue to traffic in the same powerful patterns of representing indigenous cultures used by spiritual tourists. In this case, the researcher, like other visitors to Huautla before him, sought to claim the sign of indigenousness as a marker of authenticity while insisting on the authority of Western models of individualized experience and transcendence that reject any possibility of mutual exchange.

The current renaissance in the scientific understanding of psychedelic substances is an opportunity to break with the false image of Mazatecos as belonging only to the past and recognize the value of Mazatec knowledge. But we should not underestimate the enduring power of these representations and remain alert to the ways that they permeate dominant representations, including those linked to scientific research. We often still see a contrast between local experiences bound within a static context and Western experiences represented as universal discoveries about medicine.

My ethnographic observations from the Psychedelic Science conference in April 2017 demonstrate these continuities. I approached this field site as a naïve outsider, and I cannot claim any sort of deep knowledge of my host community and its history, and my observations—puzzling over abstracts and wandering through hallways and exhibition halls—must be taken as tentative and speculative, for now.

The multiple and contested meanings at the conference can be looked at through the scholarly presentations, the audience reception, and commercial elements such as those on display in the exhibition hall. The academic portion of the conference was divided into three tracks: Clinical Research, Interdisciplinary Research, and Plant Medicine. The Plant Medicine track operated as a sort of counter-discourse to the more visible frameworks of biomedicine and spiritual tourism, as it included the voices and perspectives of a much more diverse and international array of presenters, including many more women (unlike the male-dominated clinical and interdisciplinary tracks) and some representatives of First Peoples. The diverse presentations in this track offered numerous challenges to the conventional wisdom. In this section, however, I am going to focus only on those elements of the conference that relate most closely to the cultural politics I have described in this chapter.

While some of the abstracts for the Plant Medicine track located psychedelic practices within distinct cultural contexts, others did not, focusing instead on the universal effects of a plant after an initial legitimizing and ahistorical reference to an indigenous group that used the substance "for thousands of years." In fact, the representation of psychedelic practices as "plant medicine" has the potential to erase people from the equation. While Mazatec curers could tell you, if in different ways at different times, that the ceremonial ingestion of the "child saints" is medicinal, they would be invoking a view of curing that goes beyond the fungus and the individual brain and body but involves, at a fundamental level, other people; and the idea of "medicine" often implies, like the "spiritual" narratives of earlier Western visitors to Huautla, a purely individual experience that can be isolated from its social context, bracketing out issues like social inequality and marginalization.

Outside the Plant Medicine track, the absence of an awareness of human diversity was starker: only 1 of the 58 abstracts in the Clinical and Interdisciplinary tracks (a presentation on psilocybin research on religious leaders) located psychedelic experience within the context of a particular cultural setting. Instead, where people were mentioned, they were described in pan-cultural universals—as "individuals," "people," or "patients"—or else as carriers of a particular defined psychological condition (addiction, depression, PTSD, etc.).[1] While there is a great deal of evidence that culture influences how people think about and experience mental illness, through the different ways that "they categorize and prioritize the symptoms, attempt to heal them, and set expectations for their course and outcome," the research presentations assumed the universality of Western labels, and thus the universality of the psychedelic treatments (Watters, 2010, location 50).

---

[1]Williams and Leins (2016) point out that people of color have been significantly underrepresented as subjects for research on the therapeutic effects of psychoactive drugs.

While these research presentations excluded non-Western experiences, conference participants constructed indigenous people in various ways that sought to provide them with legitimacy. After my presentation about the Sierra Mazateca, an audience member asked me if I could confirm a story that a psychedelic researcher had provided María Sabina with synthetic psilocybin and that she had reported that it was "the same" as mushrooms. This story, which was told by Albert Hoffman (1980) about his visit to Huautla in 1962, was new to me, as it would have been of little interest to most Huatecos but apparently functioned as an important authenticating myth for some psychedelic researchers in the tradition of the myths of Pocahontas and La Malinche, in which indigenous women provide legitimacy for future generations of non-Indians to occupy their territory.

Indigenous people also provide legitimacy for some members of the White psychedelic community through their traditional role as undifferentiated objects of charity. After my presentation, an audience member asked me if she could interview me for a presentation she was making. Her only question was "how can we help the 'tribe' you were talking about?" In the exhibition hall, the booth of a business that offered ayahuasca retreats in the Peruvian rainforest ("ancient wisdom for the modern world") included a poster promoting the way it provides outreach and jobs for local Indians. When I asked what this consisted of, the staffer told me that they "educate local people" and employ 23 locals who clean, cook, and carry supplies. Promotional materials for this program described local residents as "gentle" and "caring" and "embodying the wisdom and sincerity of their people." Local culture is presented here as ancient, undifferentiated, and feminized. It embodies characteristics that perfectly suit a service economy; Indians are passive and grateful recipients of help, who contribute to the healing experiences of spiritual tourists without challenging their individualizing interpretations of what constitutes curing.

A final way in which White participants can use indigenous people to generate authenticity is, ironically, through rejecting their "White privilege." I do not have space here to give justice to the politics of cultural appropriation, except to observe that these are complex and may be adapted to different types of representations. After two different Plant Medicine sessions dealing with peyote, the same young White woman came to the microphone to publicly announce that she had made the personal decision never to use peyote, as the value of this substance as the property of indigenous cultures was more important than her bucket list of drug experiences. At both sessions, audiences responded to this confession with a round of applause, a ritual that affirmed their righteousness as culturally sensitive allies of the Lakota and Huichol. While this would appear to be a rejection of racist appropriation, I would argue that it remains within the patterns I have described, bracketing off indigenous people as "other" through an effortless gesture that reinforces the universalized individualistic experience of the Western self, and reduces political and cultural complexity and exploitation to acts of individual consumer choice. Significantly, repudiations of White privilege occurred at presentations dealing with indigenous practices; rather than research presentations that treated psychedelic users through universalized liberal categories of "people" and "individuals."

Ethan Watters (2010, location 3537) writes, "The ideas we export to other cultures often have at their heart a particularly American brand of hyperintrospection and hyperindividualism... [that has] encouraged us to separate the health of the individual from the health of the group." But it is the insights about the essentially social nature of health and disease that I find most alluring in Mazatec mushroom curing, and that can be obscured by sciencifying narratives about the "effects" that psilocybin has on (Western) individuals. The history of Huautla provides lessons for current psychedelic researchers. We can learn from indigenous people, but only if we recognize that treating them as iconic reminders of an ancient past is no more helpful than ignoring them and pretending that the world is composed of individualized patients. Both of these approaches prevent us from embracing a kind of "cultural humility" (Sevelius, 2017) and thoughtful, imperfect engagement that can lead us past our cultural assumptions that what matters most about drugs takes place "in our own brains."

References

Abse, E. (2007). *Toward where the Sun hides: The rise of sorcery and transformations of Mazatec religious life (Doctoral dissertation)*. Charlottesville: University of Virginia.

Agencia Reforma. (2013, March 26). El Diablo quiere la alcaldía de Huautla. *NVI Noticias*. Retrieved from http://old.nvinoticias.com/oaxaca/general/143566-diablo-quiere-alcaldia-huautla

Babb, F. E. (2012). Theorizing gender, race, and cultural tourism in Latin America: A view from Peru and Mexico. *Latin American Perspectives, 39*(6), 36–50.

Biafra, J., & Greenway, J. (1979). *California über alles (recorded by Dead Kennedys)*. San Fransisco: Optional Music.

Bourdieu, P. (1984). *Distinction: A social critique of the judgement of taste*. Cambridge, MA: Harvard University Press.

Broad, K., & Feinberg, B. (1995). Perceptions of ganja and cocaine in urban Jamaica. *Journal of Psychoactive Drugs, 27*(3), 261–276.

Dawson, A. S. (2015). Salvador Roquet, María Sabina, and the trouble with jipis. *Hispanic American Historical Review, 95*(1), 103–132.

Dawson, A. S. (2018). Peyote's race problem. In B. C. Labate & C. Cavnar (Eds.), *Plant medicines, healing and psychedelic science: Cultural perspectives*. Cham: Springer.

D'Emilio, J. (1983). Capitalism and gay identity. In A. Snitow, C. Stansell, & S. Thompson (Eds.), *Powers of desire: The politics of sexuality* (pp. 100–113). New York, NY: Monthly Review Press.

Estrada, A. (1981). *María Sabina: Her life and chants*. Santa Barbara, CA: Ross-Erikson.

Feinberg, B. (1997). Three Mazatec wise ones and their books. *Critique of Anthropology, 17*(4), 411–437.

Feinberg, B. (2003). *The Devil's book of culture: History, mushrooms, and caves in southern Mexico*. Austin: University of Texas Press.

Feinberg, B. (2009). A symbol of wisdom and love? Contesting María Sabina in counter-cultural tourism in Huautla, Oaxaca. In M. Baud & A. Ypeij (Eds.), *Cultural tourism in Latin America: The politics of space and imagery* (pp. 94–114). Amsterdam: Brill.

Gomez-Barris, M. (2012). Andean translations: New Age tourism and cultural exchange in the Sacred Valley, Peru. *Latin American Perspectives, 39*(6), 68–78.

Hoffman, A. (1980). *LSD, my problem child*. New York: McGraw-Hill.

Lancaster, R. (1997). On homosexualities in Latin America (and other places). *American Ethnologist, 24*(1), 193–202.

Löfgren, O. (2004). The global beach. In S. B. Gmelch (Ed.), *Tourists and tourism: A reader* (pp. 35–53). Long Grove, IL: Waveland Press.

Lora, A. (1989). *María Sabina [Recorded by El Tri]. On 21 años después, Alex Lora y El Tri [CD]*. Mexico City, Mexico: WEA.

Lutz, C. A., & Collins, J. L. (1993). *Reading National Geographic*. Chicago, IL: University of Chicago Press.

Mathers, K., & Hubbard, L. (2009). Doing Africa: Travelers, adventurers, and American conquest of Africa. In L. A. Vivanco & R. J. Gordon (Eds.), *Tarzan was an eco-tourist... and other tales from the anthropology of adventure* (pp. 197–214). New York, NY: Berghahn Books.

Morris, H. (Director). (2016). Shepherdess: The story of salvia divinorum [Television series episode]. In H. Morris (Producer), *Hamilton's pharmacopeia*. New York, NY: VBS.tv.

Munn, H. (1973). The mushrooms of language. In M. J. Harner (Ed.), *Hallucinogens and shamanism* (pp. 86–122). London: Oxford University Press.

Pineda Casmiro, J. N. (2007). Doña Julia Julieta Casimiro. *Bomb, 98*. Retrieved from http://bombmagazine.org/article/2880/do-a-julia-julieta-casimiro

Provine, D. M. (2007). *Unequal under law: Race in the war on drugs*. Chicago: University of Chicago Press.

Schwartz, C. (2017, May 6). Molly at the Marriott: Inside America's premier psychedelics conference. *The New York Times*. Retrieved from https://www.nytimes.com/2017/05/06/style/psychedelic-drug-resurgence-daily-life.html?_r=0

Secretaría de Turismo. (2016, May 13). Pueblos mágicos, herencia que impulsan turismo [Magical villages, heritage that drives tourism]. *Secretaría de turismo blog*. Retrieved from http://www.gob.mx/sectur/articulos/pueblos-magicos-herencia-que-impulsan-turismo

Sevelius, J. (2017, July 25). *How psychedelic science privileges some, neglects others, and limits us all*. Chacruna.net. Retrieved from http://chacruna.net/how-psychedelic-science-privileges-some-neglects-others/

Tedlock, D. (1985). *Popul Vuh: The definitive edition of the Mayan book of the dawn of life and the glories of gods and kings*. New York, NY: Simon & Schuster.

Thirteen Indigenous Grandmothers. (2017). *Thirteen Indigenous Grandmothers*. Retrieved from http://www.grandmotherscouncil.org/

Turner, V. (1977). *The ritual process: Structure and anti-structure*. Ithaca, NY: Cornell University Press.

Wasson, R. G. (1957, May 13). Seeking the magic mushroom. *Life*, 100–120.

Wasson, R. G. (1981). Retrospective essay. In A. Estrada (Ed.), *María Sabina: Her life and chants* (pp. 13–22). Santa Barbara, CA: Ross-Erikson.

Watters, E. (2010). *Crazy like us: The globalization of the American psyche*. New York, NY: Simon and Schuster.

Weismantel, M. (2001). *Cholas and pishtacos: Stories of race and sex in the Andes*. Chicago: University of Chicago Press.

Williams, M. T., & Leins, C. (2016). Race-based trauma: The challenge and promise of MDMA-assisted psychotherapy. *MAPS Bulletin, 26(1)*. Retrieved from http://www.maps.org/news/bulletin/articles/407-bulletin-spring-2016/6106-race-based-trauma-the-challenge-and-promise-of-mdma-assisted-psychotherapy

Zolov, E. (1999). *Refried Elvis: The rise of the Mexican counterculture*. Berkeley: University of California Press.

Chapter 4
The Use of *Salvia divinorum* from a Mazatec Perspective

Ana Elda Maqueda

> *Some say it is a sensual and tactile thing. Some say it's about temporality and dimensionality, that it's about time travel. Some say it's about the Root Energy Network or that it's about becoming a plant. This plant is the great secret of our tradition. Consciousness has to do with energy and light. It is really very simple; neither animals nor people have consciousness. It is plants that have consciousness: Animals get consciousness by eating plants*
> [Dale Pendell about *Salvia divinorum*, from his book *Pharmako/Poeia* (1995, p. 158)].

Abstract *Salvia divinorum* is a medicinal and psychoactive plant endemic to the Sierra Madre Oriental of Oaxaca, Mexico. The Mazatec people have been using the leaves for centuries in ceremonies for its psychoactive properties and as a treatment for arthritis and inflammation, gastrointestinal problems, headaches, and addictions, among other uses. The active principle of *Salvia divinorum*, the terpene salvinorin A, is a uniquely potent and highly selective kappa-opioid receptor agonist and, as such, has enormous potential for the development of valuable medications. Among them, the most promising include safe and nonaddictive analgesics, neuroprotectors, short-acting anesthetics that do not depress respiration, antidepressants, anti-inflammatories, medications for the treatment of addiction to stimulants and alcohol, and drugs to treat disorders characterized by alterations in perception. The Mazatec consider *Salvia divinorum* to be a very powerful plant spirit that should be treated with utmost respect, and the preparation for the ceremony requires a strict regimen. They chew the fresh leaves at night while chanting and praying. In the Western use, the dry leaves are potentiated in extracts to be smoked. A lack of information about the appropriate doses and other considerations while smoking the extracts could result in overwhelming

A. E. Maqueda (✉)
Human Neuropsychopharmacology Research Group, Hospital de la Santa Creu y Sant Pau, Avenida Sant Antoni M Claret, Barcelona, Spain
e-mail: ana@maqueda.org

© Springer International Publishing AG, part of Springer Nature 2018   55
B. C. Labate, C. Cavnar (eds.), *Plant Medicines, Healing and Psychedelic Science*,
https://doi.org/10.1007/978-3-319-76720-8_4

experiences due to the high potency and fast onset of the substance. For the Mazatec, smoking the plant is not the preferred mode. How could we create a bridge between the two perspectives? In this chapter, I will try to clarify the best ways to use *Salvia divinorum* for medicinal, psychotherapeutic, and inner exploration purposes.

Natural History of *Salvia divinorum*

Of the more than 1000 species of salvia that exist in the world, none has evoked as much fascination and curiosity as *Salvia divinorum*. It is a perennial and hydrophyte plant belonging to the mint family (Lamiaceae). It has a square and hollow stem, with decumbent secondary stems that allow it to propagate vegetatively, rooting from the nodes and internodes, and can regrow from the ground from senescent stems. This mysterious herb that loves to hide in moist and shadowy places is endemic to the Sierra Madre Oriental of Oaxaca, Mexico. The Mazatec people, who have been using *S. divinorum* for its medicinal and psychoactive properties for hundreds of years, know the plant in their language as "ska pastora" [sic]. As the Mazatec language is a tonal one, the word "ska" (meaning herb or leaf) has been reproduced in the literature as it sounds. Nevertheless, it seems that a more appropriate form of writing herb in Mazatec, closest to the actual sound of the word, would be *xkà* (Carrera, 2011). The Mazatec also refer to this plant with names in Spanish like "hierba de María" (Mary's herb) or "hojas de la pastora" (shepherdess' leaves). The names are related to the Virgin Mary, who they believe is incarnated in the plant. The lack of an indigenous name and the fact that there were no shepherds in Mexico before the arrival of the Spaniards suggest that *S. divinorum* could be a postcolonial introduction or that the original name in Mazatec could have been modified by Christian influence (Ott, 1995).

During the 1930s, various anthropological expeditions toured the Mazatec Sierra, which led to the rediscovery of the use of hallucinogenic mushrooms in the remote hamlet of Huautla de Jiménez. The anthropologist Jean Basset Johnson, who was part of the expeditions, discovered that the Mazatec used the juice of the leaves of a plant called "hierba de María" for divination, in what constitutes the first academic report on the existence of *S. divinorum* (Johnson, 1939). Johnson also knew that the Mazatec employed "semillas de la Virgen" (seeds of the Virgin) in their ceremonies (Johnson, 1939), which were later identified as seeds of the plant ololiuhqui, or morning glory, *Turbina corymbosa*. These seeds contain ergine (LSA), an alkaloid similar in structure to lysergic acid diethylamide (LSD) (Hofmann & Tscherter, 1960). In 1945, the anthropologist Blas Pablo Reko mentioned the use by the Mazatec and the Cuicatec of a "divination leaf," which, in all likelihood, was *S. divinorum* (Reko, 1945). Seven years later, the anthropologist Robert J. Weitlaner reported the therapeutic and divinatory use among the Mazatec of Jalapa de Díaz of a potion made by rubbing in water between 50 and 100 leaves of "hierba de María," the highest dose being used for alcohol addicts. In addition to curing, Weitlaner observed that the leaves were employed to guess where an animal or person had been lost or who had committed a robbery (Weitlaner, 1952). Finally, the Mexican biologist and botanist Arturo Gómez Pompa classified, for the first time, *S. divinorum* as belonging to the *Salvia* genus but could not make a complete identification due to the absence of flowering material (Gómez Pompa, 1957).

The first flowering specimens of *S. divinorum* were collected by Robert Gordon Wasson and Albert Hofmann (Wasson, 1962) and sent to the greatest *Salvia* genus expert at the time, Carl Epling, for identification. In the description (Epling & Játiva, 1962), *S. divinorum* was classified within the section Dusenostachys, whose specimens are mostly endemic to Southern and Central Mexico. However, in a study using a molecular phylogenetic approach by DNA sequencing conducted in 2010 (Jenks, Walker, & Kim, 2010), samples of *S. divinorum* and 52 other *Salvia* species were compared within the subgenus *Calosphace*, to which *S. divinorum* belongs. No evidence was found to include *S. divinorum* in the Dusenostachys section proposed by Epling and Játiva or to consider the plant a hybrid. Also, in the botanical classification performed by Epling and Játiva, the flowers of *S. divinorum* are described with blue chalice and corolla (they are violet), an error that has persisted in the literature, including in the *Hallucinogenic Plants* by Richard Evan Schultes, and in the first edition of *Narcotic Plants* by William Emboden, among others. The official description was corrected by Aaron S. Reisfield in 1993, who described thoroughly the parts of the plant and performed exhaustive fieldwork in the Mazatec Sierra (Reisfield, 1993). Although the exact origin of *S. divinorum* remains a mystery, the results of the 2010 phylogenetic study suggest that *Salvia venulosa*, a rare perennial plant native to a small region of the Colombian Andes, is the closest relative of *S. divinorum*. Thyme (*Thymus vulgaris*), common sage (*Salvia officinalis*), mint (*Mentha piperita*), and basil (*Ocimum basilicum*) are other relatives of *S. divinorum* in the plant kingdom.

The first specimens of living and flowering *S. divinorum* that came out of Mexico and constitute the common strain of the plant that has spread throughout the world were collected at the Mazatec Sierra by psychiatrist and ecologist Sterling Bunnell, who introduced them to the United States in 1962. Bunnell deposited one in the Herbarium of the University of California at Berkeley, grew others in his home, and propagated them among botanists and friends like the chemist Alexander Shulgin. Therefore, the most common variety of *S. divinorum* commercially distributed around the globe is the "Bunnell variety," not the "Wasson and Hofmann variety," which in fact doesn't exist, because the specimens that they collected were dried and pressed, remaining in Mexico (Siebert, 2003).

Until the 1980s, it was believed that the production of seeds was extremely rare and that they were practically unfeasible, so that the reproduction of the plant was exclusively vegetative or by cuttings. This belief was based on the fact that the Mazatec reproduce the plant by seeding cuttings, and in the first expeditions by the Sierra, no populations of *S. divinorum* were found growing wild. Although today it is known that this belief is incorrect, since several researchers in the world have successfully managed to germinate new plants from seeds (Hanna, 1999; Siebert, 1999), their production is certainly scarce, and they seem to have a low rate of germination and survival. However, some Mazatec have stated that the plant does indeed grow wild in the Sierra and that these plants produce seed that can be planted to grow *S. divinorum* (Valdes, Hatfield, Koreeda, & Paul, 1987).

Traditional Use

From the articles published by the researchers who later visited the Mazatec Sierra and participated in ceremonies with *S. divinorum* (see the review of literature from Valdes, Diaz, & Paul, 1983), we know that the Mazatec use the plant, in addition to the aforementioned uses, as a treatment for arthritis and inflammation, headaches, and gastrointestinal problems, for the treatment of eliminatory dysfunctions, and for treating alcohol addiction. Also mentioned is the employment of the leaves for general relief or as a tonic for the sick, the anemic, or the dying. About its shamanic uses, we know from the early reports that *S. divinorum* is the initiation plant or training herb for the future healer (it is considered the plant that is easiest to handle, with the least psychoactive power), followed by the "seeds of the Virgin" (named *naxole natjaoná* in Mazatec) and, finally, by the management of hallucinogenic mushrooms.

During my own fieldwork conducted in the Mazatec Sierra, I have learned that the leaves are applied in poultices to treat insect bites, eczema, and fungi. My feminine informers also remarked that *S. divinorum* is a wonderful plant for women as a remedy for candidiasis and other vaginal diseases, cystitis, and menstrual cramps. I spent some months living with a family in a Mazatec town, in which the older son had become addicted to inhalants and cocaine. The father, a well-known healer, treated his son successfully using *S. divinorum* in ceremonies, as well as with the administration of fresh leaves on alternate days for 1 month.

For the treatment of internal ailments, the bitter juice of 40 leaves or more is drunk right before going to sleep, to avoid the strong psychedelic effects of such a high dose and to obtain the therapeutic benefits on physical problems. The users that I interviewed reported vivid dreams and a significant and lasting remission of symptoms of pain, bronchitis, fever, back contractures, water retention, and inflammation after the night of treatment. The Mazatec say that the plant is a female doctor that works within their bodies to restore their health. I knew also that it is employed for treating symptoms similar to what we call depression or low mood, by eating a small pair of fresh leaves in the morning (the leaves are always consumed in pairs, which represent the human element of man and woman, symbolizing the dual principle of creation and procreation). As we will see later in this chapter, all the medicinal applications of the Mazatec are well supported by recent pharmacological findings.

The way in which the Mazatec consume the leaves depends on their application. In the case of ceremonies, they are well chewed and swallowed, or the mixture of crushed leaves with water is drunk for a softer effect. The number of leaves given to the patient will depend on the physical constitution, previous experience, and the nature of the problem to be treated. The healer and the patient must follow a strict diet by refraining from eating certain foods, drinking alcohol and cold beverages, avoiding certain situations like funerals, and not having sex for a period ranging from several days to several weeks. During the ceremonies, which last for 4 or 5 h and take place in front of an altar at night in complete darkness, chants and prayers are sung. The healer asks questions of the patient, who expresses aloud his or her discoveries about the problem that elicited the consult. The effects appear after 20 or 30 min and consist of feelings of well-being; a sensation of internal peace and calm that lasts for days after the ceremony; out-of-body experiences; physical sensations of floating and of being touched or twisted or massaged; becoming a plant; organic visions of nature elements, animals, and other people; auditory experiences (listening to a soft female voice that responds or advises); and a clear sensation of a loving and gentle feminine presence. Some Mazatec believe this presence to be the Virgin Mary, while others believe her to be the goddess of plants and animals or the soul of Mother Nature itself. Other elements used during the ritual are beeswax candles, cocoa beans (considered a spiritual payment for the healing obtained), a mixture of lime and pulverized tobacco leaf called "San Pedro," and fresh flowers.

Both with sacred entities and with the rest of the beings, alive and dead, the Mazatec establish relations of reciprocity that allow them to unite the divine with the earthly things and to maintain the balance between the different forces and entities with which they share the territory. Well-being is asked of these entities in complex rituals where the *chjota chjine*, "the wise person who heals," or the *chjota chjine xkà*, "the wise person who cures with herbs," serves as a mediator between the worlds. For the Mazatec, disease is produced by an energy imbalance, a rupture in the established order, and a violation of the implicit agreement existing between humans and the settlers of the supernatural world, originated by negative feelings and thoughts or by entities that inhabit nature (Incháustegui, 1994). Women and men of knowledge feed the sick with fungi and plants, causing an altered state of consciousness that allows the individual, with the help of the healer, to become aware of and to detect the origin of their imbalance and to be restored using their will.

Nowadays, the Mazatec know that *S. divinorum* is smoked around the world, but some of them consider this to be wrong and against the spirit of the plant that should never be burnt. They believe that this practice is behind the misunderstandings regarding this herb and that it could be the cause of it being outlawed in some countries. When the Mazatec are asked about the addiction potential of the plant or about toxic or harmful effects, they clearly state that they and their ancestors have consumed *S. divinorum* for centuries, sometimes in amounts up to 100 pairs of leaves, without any problems, intoxications, or addictive behaviors. On the contrary, it is an invaluable source of healing for them. I also asked them about symptoms of paranoia or psychosis after its use, and I received the same answer: this never happened to them. But, for the Mazatec, the shamanic use of *xkà pastora* has to be taken seriously and approached carefully. One must have an honest intention of healing oneself or another or a plan to do good things with its use. A ritual with a beginning and end should be performed, and, even if the purpose is just to navigate internal realms or to get to know the herb better, one must ask for permission of the spirit of the plant before cutting the leaves, be thankful, and show respect to its power.

Salvinorin A

S. divinorum owes its psychoactive properties to its active ingredient, the terpene salvinorin A (SA). SA was isolated and identified for the first time in 1982 in Mexico by Alfredo Ortega and his team, and shortly after by Valdés and his collaborators (Ortega, Blount, & Manchand, 1982; Valdes, Butler, Hatfield, Paul, & Koreeda, 1984). Daniel Siebert was the first researcher to investigate SA in humans (Siebert, 1994).

Pharmacological studies have shown that SA is a highly selective and potent kappa-opioid receptor (KOR) agonist (Roth et al., 2002). In fact, the exact structure of this receptor was described in detail thank to the highly precise binding of SA (Wu et al., 2012). The KOR and its endogenous ligands, the dynorphins, regulate the perception of pain in the human body; change in consciousness, mood, and control of the internal sensations of the body (interoception); and, in interaction with other systems, regulate the reward system of addictions (Chavkin, 2013, Schwarzer, 2009). SA is the only natural non-nitrogen compound currently known capable of acting as an agonist at the level of these opioid receptors. It is also one of the most potent psychoactive substances of natural origin known, being about 20 times more potent than psilocybin (the psychoactive component in numerous species of fungi), and in the range of potency of LSD. On the other hand, SA differs from other compounds capable of modifying perception, the so-called classic hallucinogens, such as mescaline, psilocybin, and LSD. The latter are alkaloids (nitrogenous compounds) and have affinity for the $5-HT_{1A}$ and $5-HT_{2A}$ receptors of serotonin. In my laboratory research administering SA to 32 volunteers, we have demonstrated, for the first time in humans, the involvement of opioidergic neurotransmission, rather than serotonergic, in the effects of SA in perception, cognition, and emotion (Maqueda et al., 2016).

About the subjective effects of the compound, in our laboratory studies, the inhalation of pure vaporized SA led to dose-dependent psychotropic effects of fast onset (less than 1 minute) and short duration (20 min). This is in contrast with the slow instauration and long duration of the effects following the Mazatec method of chewing the fresh leaves.

Perceptual modifications included the visual domain, and, in contrast with $5-HT_{2A}$ agonists, auditory hallucinations were very common. As one volunteer wrote in the trip report, "It was like a group of people shouting, especially female voices, and music was also playing." A special type of visual-bodily synesthesia was also observed. While visual-auditory synesthesia is common with serotonergic and non-serotonergic substances, visual-proprioceptive synesthesia is rarely described (Luke & Terhune, 2013) and seems to be another unique feature of *S. divinorum*.

This effect was explained as seeing external modifications in reality like a wave that affects or folds the volunteer's body, or objects perceived with eyes open or closed were felt as being associated with the body: "A force was pressing the right side of my body . . . so my sensation was being a square. Visually I wasn't seeing any image, but that square was conceptually present in my mind." We observed lateralization of the effects, coming from a specific side of the body or reality: "I had the sensation that the effects of the substance were approaching me from the left." Also, in contrast with the classical serotonergic psychedelics, the loss of contact with external reality is prominent and dose-dependent. At the low (0.25 mg) and medium (0.50 mg) doses, there was an increase in bodily sensations, which means that the subjects experienced their body as safe and reliable, being able to pay more attention to the connection between emotions and physical states. A volunteer reported, "Warmth. I felt my body heavier, relaxed, with a subtle tingle on the neck and the head. My mind was also relaxed. I was connected with my body and with the sensations I was feeling. Very pleasant."

In contrast, high doses (1 mg) increased dissociation and loss of contact with the body and out-of-body experiences, like "I wasn't feeling that in that world I had a physical body. I was an energetic being." Our results suggest that KOR may play a previously underestimated role in the regulation of sensory perception, the interoception, and the sense of body ownership in humans. Other subjective effects reported included, in correlation with that of the Mazatec, physical sensations of being twisted, touched, or pushed and sensations of movement and of presences of beings or entities. Childhood memories were common and sensations of being in two realities at the same time: "I really wanted to be fully in that other reality, it was very familiar, like the reality of my childhood." The visions are not as organic as when the leaves are chewed; instead, volunteers refer to metallic objects, plastic surfaces, and mechanical artifacts. In our experiments, we also observed that SA increases the secretion of prolactin, antidiuretic hormone, and cortisol, and its subjective and physiological effects were blocked by the opioid antagonist naltrexone (Maqueda et al., 2015).

SA experience is clearly unique, with some correspondence with other psychedelics. As reported in an experiment led by Peter H. Addy, using dry leaves of *S. divinorum* potentiated with SA, the subjects compared the experience as similar to dreaming (43%); LSD (13%); psilocybin (10%); marijuana (10%); MDMA (10%); altered states of consciousness such as meditation, trance, or yoga (7%); or NMDA antagonists such as dextromethorphan (DXM) and ketamine (7%) (Addy, 2012).

In regard to safety of inhaled SA, laboratory studies show that doses of up to 12 mg of pure SA are safe in terms of physiological measures (Ranganathan et al., 2012). Of the 112 subjects in total, adding the participants of all the studies carried out in the world up to the present, from six laboratories of six different countries, adverse reactions were not found. On the contrary, volunteers reported liking the good effects and having positive and significant experiences. In general, the somatic side effects induced by SA, if they occur, are transient and do not cause excessive discomfort. These somatic-dysphoric effects are subjective changes in body temperature and sensations of electricity and tingling in the body, which are similar to those of classic hallucinogens.

However, there is a lack of long-term studies. One of the reasons for this could be the low number of users that consume the plant repeatedly. Several surveys have revealed that nontraditional use of *S. divinorum* is sporadic and unremarkable due to unpleasant effects for the typical recreational consumption (Addy, Garcia-Romeu, Metzger, & Wade, 2015). There are two retrospective surveys of recurrent recreational users (Kelly, 2011; Nygård, 2007). Thirteen users (77% males) reported a greater connection with others, increased creativity, and connection with nature, as well as a greater understanding of the nature of reality (Nygård, 2007). However, these reports are limited because of their retrospective nature, relatively small sample size, and possible bias in recall. In one laboratory study with SA (MacLean, Johnson, Reissig, Prisinzano, & Griffiths, 2013), the researchers followed up 1 month after the experiment. Assessments showed no evidence of lasting negative effects, such as depression, anxiety, psychiatric symptoms, or visual impairment. In the open reports, no participant indicated lasting negative effects. Half of the participants reported specific positive changes which they attributed to the experience with SA, including increased self-confidence, a feeling of greater physical comfort and calm, less emotional reactivity, improved interpersonal relationships, and a renewed interest in daily responsibilities. Bücheler and colleagues (Bücheler, Gleiter, Schwoerer & Gaertner, 2005) reported the case of a 19-year-old man in Germany who was a user of *S. divinorum*. The young man smoked or chewed the leaves twice a week for 6 months, without detrimental effects on his health and social or academic life. He described having experienced effects of floating, feelings of having solved personal or philosophical problems, itching, and ringing in the ears. He did not report any negative psychological effects and described a gradual tolerance over the 6-month period.

We have also investigated the neurophysiological correlates of SA effects in humans, measuring spontaneous brain oscillations (EEG) before and after the administration of 1 mg of vaporized SA. The results showed a unique pattern of neurophysiological effects. SA suppressed the alpha rhythm and markedly increased slow delta activity. Less prominent effects included increases in the theta and low gamma bands. While SA shares with serotonergic psychedelics the alpha-suppressing action, its main neurophysiological signature is an atypical enhancement of slow delta activity.

About the neural substrates of SA, in the brain are high levels of KOR in the neocortex, in the thalamus, and in the ventral tegmental area. The agonism of the KOR in the temporal and parietal cortex could be the cause of the visual and auditory modifications (temporal cortex) and of the altered experience of the body (parietal cortex). In addition, the medial posterior parietal cortex is a key structure within the default mode network (DMN), which has been proposed as associated with the inner sense of self (Raichle, 2011; Raichle et al., 2001) or with the embodied self. The claustrum, a layer of neurons near the insula, also shows high levels of KOR. From studies with SA, researchers have proposed that SA could interrupt the processes of brain integration that take place at this level and lead to the effects of disconnection with reality, naming the claustrum as "the gate of consciousness" (Stiefel, Merrifield, & Holcombe, 2014).

In the leaves of *S. divinorum* are other terpenes, such as divinatorins, salvinorins, salvinicins, and salvidivins, whose role in the pharmacological effects is not yet elucidated. They also contain loliolide (a potent ant repellent); hardwickiic acid and (E)-phytol, both with antimicrobial and antibacterial (*Staphylococcus aureus* and *Candida albicans*) properties; and nepetoidin B, with antifungal properties (Casselman, Nock, Wohlmuth, Weatherby, & Heinrich, 2014).

Therapeutic Potential

KOR agonists such as SA have applications for multiple ailments, and SA is extremely affine, potent, and precise when it comes to binding to these brain receptors. Some of the valuable medications that could be developed from *S. divinorum* are:

- Safe analgesics without addictive properties: The efficacy of SA as an analgesic has been demonstrated in animal studies (Guida et al., 2012). In current medical practice, sometimes very powerful analgesics like morphine are used, which are habit forming and produce dependence. This is not the case with SA. In fact, research has shown that SA has anti-addictive properties (Serra et al., 2015).
- Anti-inflammatories: It has been demonstrated in animal studies that SA has ultra-potent effects on macrophages via the KOR and CB1 receptors and exerts an important attenuation of inflammation and antipruritic effects. SA inhibits intestinal motility and reduces abdominal pain in the irritable bowel syndrome. In recent studies with mice, SA has been shown to inhibit the leukotriene-mediated inflammatory response. Leukotrienes are crucial in various autoimmune and inflammatory conditions such as urticaria, bronchial asthma, allergic rhinitis, and cardiovascular problems (Aviello et al., 2011; Rossi et al., 2016).
- Medications to treat different types of cancer: When there are tumors in the brain, one of the difficulties of therapeutics is to get the drugs through the blood-brain barrier and reach the tumor. The terpene SA is able to cross the blood-brain barrier and reach the brain and structures of the CNS in less than a minute. SA analogs have demonstrated antiproliferative properties, inhibiting the growth of 77–86% of tumor cells in breast cancer (Vasiljevik, Groer, Lehner, Navarro, & Prisinzano, 2014).
- Medications for disorders such as schizophrenia, bipolar disorder, and Alzheimer's disease: It is clear that the KOR-dynorphin system plays a key role in modulating perception and human consciousness. This suggests the possibility that new compounds derived from SA could be effective for the treatment of these disorders that are manifested by alterations of perception (Butelman & Kreek, 2015; Tejeda, Shippenberg, & Henriksson, 2012).

- Antidepressants: Animal studies have shown antidepressant properties of SA, and it has been proposed as an ideal candidate for the treatment of major depressive disorder (Taylor & Manzella, 2016). Regarding human subjects, K. R. Hanes (Hanes, 2001, 2003), in Australia, presented a case report of a 26-year-old woman with a long treatment-resistant depression who showed improvement after taking sub-psychoactive oral doses of *S. divinorum* leaves. The patient chewed and held in the mouth 0.5 to 0.75 grams of dry leaf for 15–30 min, two or three times per week. The patient also claimed to benefit from occasional psychoactive doses of *S. divinorum* consisting of 2–4 g of leaves taken following the same method as the previous one. Dr. Hanes reported on the patient's total remission of depressive symptoms in the past 6 months, in addition to a considerable improvement in self-esteem and psychospiritual development. Later, Hanes wrote a follow-up report in which he described six additional patients who reported obtaining complete remission of symptoms in treatment-resistant depression using the leaves of *S. divinorum*. Sadly, Australia was the first country to outlaw *S. divinorum* in 2002.
- Medication to treat psychostimulant abuse: Animal research has revealed that SA reduces dopamine levels in parts of the basal ganglia, disrupting many of the effects of cocaine and the addiction cycle. In the experiments with rats, SA does not seem to suppress their movement, the action of pushing the lever to drink, or their motivation before stimuli. In contrast, SA appears to specifically suppress cocaine-related behaviors and motivations (Dos Santos, Crippa, Machado-de-Sousa, & Hallak, 2015). Western medicine has developed—with questionable success—pharmacological treatments for the abuse of opiates, alcohol, and tobacco, but there is currently no treatment for the abuse of psychostimulants, so research with SA hold the promise to help millions of addicts. However, it is very important to remember that the traditional use of *S. divinorum* by the Mazatec to successfully treat a complex and multifaceted problem like addiction is part of a ritual and a much larger, organic, and inclusive worldview than our compartmentalized interventions and that the properties of this herb cannot be reduced to the pharmacological mechanism of just one isolated component in the form of a pill.
- Assisting psychotherapy: *S. divinorum* has several properties that would make it effective as an adjunct to psychotherapy. As we have seen, in low and medium doses, it helps to increase awareness of the body and of the interconnectedness of emotions and mental states. It also produces a state of deep introspection, facilitates the recall of biographical episodes, and offers access to areas of the psyche that are not easily attainable ordinarily. This possible psychotherapeutic use is not new; even if shamanism and psychotherapy are not the same thing, during the ceremonies with this particular plant, the Mazatec establish a dialogue between patient and healer, posing questions during the ceremony until the problem and the possible solution are elucidated. Also, low doses have been used for enhancing meditation work, finding unusual clarity of mind, and enhancing the ability to concentrate (Soutar & Strassman, 2000). From the trip reports

from volunteers in one of our studies, "The state of peace obtained allowed me to think in a very lucid way" (Maqueda et al., 2015).

Other promising medications are neuroprotectors for a number of acute brain pathologies accompanied by a vasoconstrictive event (Su, Riley, Kiessling, Armstead, & Liu, 2011) and short-term anesthetics that do not depress breathing, safer than the anesthetics that are used today (McCurdy, Sufka, Smith, Warnick, & Nieto, 2006).

How to Use *Salvia divinorum*

Learning from the Mazatec, in the best possible scenario, somebody interested in using *S. divinorum* for medicinal, psychotherapeutic, or inner exploration purposes should grow their own cuttings at home. This would create a direct relationship with them, as we both are living beings in mutualistic existence, like humans and plants have always coexisted. Cuttings can be bought online, and they are relatively easy to grow. Nursing and touching them, witnessing them growing (and maybe flowering), and honoring this teacher plant that is giving us so much would be the fundamental relationship that we could create at home to approximate the loving appreciation of the Mazatec toward *S. divinorum*. To perform a ritual before harvesting and consuming the leaves, with simple constitutive elements and personal thoughts, would simulate the Mazatec "set and setting" by an act that opens and closes the ingestion of a mind-altering herb that gives access to the unknown.

To chew its crunchy and velvety fresh leaves is an ideal method of consumption to begin with; it provides a very rich and totally unique experience and is easily manageable. Sounds and lights can interrupt the trip, and the effects start very subtly. Therefore, it is very important to remain in a meditative state and in complete darkness and to wait for the effects. The sounds heard in the Sierra are of a forest at night, running water, and usually rain. There is some inverse tolerance, so if the effects are not attained in the first tries, they could be achieved in consecutive attempts. The Mazatec microdose with small leaves when feeling low energy levels or to enhance mood, and the microdosing approach could be a good way to prepare the body for a ceremony with more leaves. The quantity of SA per leaf can vary depending on the size of the leaves and on the potency of the strain, and since individual sensitivity is highly variable too, due to genetic and gender differences with the KOR (Schmidt et al., 2005), it is better to start with small amounts until the personal sensitivity to the substance is known. Peltate glandular trichomes, which contain SA, are present only on the abaxial surface of the leaves (Siebert, 2004).

As bigger amounts of leaves are required to attain stronger effects or to follow a weekly treatment, dry leaves can also be bought online. In my own practice with the Mazatec, I have had noticeable psychedelic effects with 6–8 leaves of medium size. My chewing method could be applied for dry leaves too: to break the leaves in little pieces with the incisors and moisten them well with saliva while moving them with the tongue all around the inside of the mouth. The leaves could be eaten in pairs of two like a sandwich bent in the middle, accumulating the well-chewed wet plant material in the upper gums and eating the next two leaves and so on. The excess of saliva that will be produced could be used to moisten again the plant material accumulated in the gums instead of being swallowed. More leaves can be eaten as desired for bigger effects or to prolong the effect, but keep in mind that the effects will appear in about 20–30 min or more. Before chewing the leaves, it could be useful to brush the mouth to remove dead cells and to use a mouthwash with alcohol, to increase the permeability of the mucous membranes. External applications of poultices can be previously moistened in water or applied with alcohol as the Mazatec do.

Strong and high-quality tinctures can be bought online or can be made at home following extraction methods of variable difficulty. They are a good way of experiencing the effects like the traditional Mazatecs, with effects starting slowly and remaining longer. To attain psychedelic effects, the leaves or tinctures must be in contact with the oral mucosa, because enzymes in the intestinal tract rapidly degrade SA. Interestingly, pure SA alone is not sublingually active, but it is when the leaves are chewed. Could some of the other terpenes present in the leaf work as a catalyst? More research is needed to unveil *S. divinorum*'s mysteries and to investigate further the greater bioavailability of SA in other solvents. Future work might test other dosage forms, like patches targeting the oral mucosa for rapid delivery of high doses when it's therapeutically needed, which may allow maintenance of therapeutic drug levels in the brain (Orton & Liu, 2014).

In regard to the most potent and fastest method of attaining psychedelic effects, that is, smoking SA-enhanced leaves, or potentiated extracts, we should know by now that *S. divinorum* and SA can be dangerous if used irresponsibly, like any other substance that alters consciousness. It is one of the most potent psychedelics, and smoking high doses can make one forget that one has a body while navigating internal landscapes. From our neurophysiological results, we know that 1 mg of pure SA puts the brain for a few minutes in a deep sleep state, but the body is still able to move. So it is imperative to be accompanied by a sober and attentive sitter. While smoking plain dry leaf, it can be difficult to achieve strong effects because of the large quantities of smoke that must be inhaled. This is easier to achieve with the SA-enhanced leaves. For managing the potentiated extracts, it is very important to have a precision scale to measure milligrams and to start with the lowest strength. Starting with low doses and slowly dosing up is a really good way to become familiar with the effects. Patience, information, and the precision scale are all what is needed to have an enjoyable and unique experience smoking this extraordinary herb while visiting what is called by psychonauts around the globe "the *Salvia* space." This plant is high technology for the mind, an invaluable tool to put to test the fabric of reality and to explore the wonders of human consciousness. As D. M. Turner put it in his book, *Salvinorin: The Psychedelic Essence of Salvia divinorum* (1996, para. 1), "If there is a physical counterpart to consciousness, memory or identity in humans, and if it could be extracted from our brains, I think we would find something similar to salvinorin."

I strongly recommend visiting the *Salvia divinorum* Research and Information Center, managed by the expert Daniel Siebert, to learn how to calculate dosing and other important details to take into account when smoking.[1] Some extraordinary reports written by a highly experienced psychonaut smoking very high doses of potentiated extracts that may be of interest can be found in the blog, A World Out of Mind.[2] Trip reports of experiences with fresh leaves and other methods and ideas of consumption can be found in the special journal of *The Entheogen Review* dedicated to *S. divinorum* and SA (Aardvark, 2002). I have created the nonprofit "Xkà Pastora," dedicated to the ethnobotanical conservation of *S. divinorum*, where my fieldwork can be followed.[3] The Mazatec Sierra, the natural sanctuary of *Salvia*, still has secrets to unveil. How many different varieties could have wildly emerged from seeds during the centuries, and with what properties? Current research is studying only one of them! What are the long-term effects of *Salvia* among the Mazatec? Is there a Mazatec elder that still remembers the native name of the herb? Are there any particular chants sung during ceremonies with the plant? Ideas that are worth consideration for future explorers.

References

Aardvark, D. (Ed.) (2002). *Salvia divinorum* and salvinorin A. In *The best of Entheogen Review 1992–2000* (2nd ed.). Sacramento, CA: Entheogen Review.

Addy, P. H. (2012). Acute and post-acute behavioral and psychological effects of salvinorin A in humans. *Psychopharmacology, 220*(1), 195–204.

Addy, P. H., Garcia-Romeu, A., Metzger, M., & Wade, J. (2015). The subjective experience of acute, experimentally-induced *Salvia divinorum* inebriation. *Journal of Psychopharmacology (Oxford), 29*(4), 426–435.

Aviello, G., Borrelli, F., Guida, F., Romano, B., Lewellyn, K., De Chiaro, M., . . . Capasso, R. (2011). Ultrapotent effects of salvinorin A, a hallucinogenic compound from *Salvia divinorum*, on LPS-stimulated murine macrophages and its anti-inflammatory action in vivo. *Journal of Molecular Medicine (Berlin), 89*(9), 891–902.

Bücheler, R., Gleiter, C. H., Schwoerer, P., & Gaertner, I. (2005). Use of nonprohibited hallucinogenic plants: Increasing relevance for public health? A case report and literature review on the consumption of *Salvia divinorum* (Diviner's Sage). *Pharmacopsychiatry, 38*(1), 1–5.

Butelman, E. R., & Kreek, M. J. (2015). Salvinorin A, a kappa-opioid receptor agonist hallucinogen: pharmacology and potential template for novel pharmacotherapeutic agents in neuropsychiatric disorders. *Frontiers in Pharmacology, 6*, 190.

Carrera Guzmán, C. (2011). *Acercamiento gramatical a la lengua mazateca de Mazatlán [Grammatical approach to the Mazateca language of Mazatlan]*. Villa de Flores, Oaxaca, Mexico: INALI.

Casselman, I., Nock, C. J., Wohlmuth, H., Weatherby, R. P., & Heinrich, M. (2014). From local to global: Fifty years of research on *Salvia divinorum*. *Journal of Ethnopharmacology, 151*(2), 768–783.

---

[1]The *Salvia divinorum* Research and Information Center, sagewisdom.org

[2]A World Out of Mind, salviaspace.blogspot.com

[3]Center for Research and Ethnobotanical Conservation of *Salvia divinorum*, xkapastora.org

Chavkin, C. (2013). Dynorphin – still an extraordinarily potent opioid peptide. *Molecular Pharmacology, 83*(4), 729–736.

Dos Santos, R. G., Crippa, J. A., Machado-de-Sousa, J. P., & Hallak, J. E. (2015). Salvinorin A and related compounds as therapeutic drugs for psychostimulant-related disorders. *Current Drug Abuse Reviews, 7*(2), 128–132.

Epling, C., & Játiva-M., C. D. (1962). A new species of *Salvia* from Mexico. *Botanical Museum Leaflets, Harvard University, 20*(3), 75–76.

Gómez Pompa, A. (1957). *Salvia divinorum herbarium sheets. A. Gómez Pompa 87556 and 93216.* Mexico, D.F: National Herbarium (UNAM).

Guida, F., Luongo, L., Aviello, G., Palazzo, E., De Chiaro, M., Gatta, L., … Maione, S. (2012). Salvinorin A reduces mechanical allodynia and spinal neuronal hyperexcitability induced by peripheral formalin injection. *Molecular Pain, 8,* 60.

Hanes, K. R. (2001). Antidepressant effects of the herb *Salvia divinorum. Journal of Clinical Psychopharmacology, 21*(6), 634–635.

Hanes, K. R. (2003). *Salvia divinorum:* Clinical and research potential. *MAPS Bulletin, 13*(1), 18–20.

Hanna, J. (1999). Growing *Salvia divinorum* from seed. *The Entheogen Review, 8*(3), 110–124.

Hofmann, A., & Tscherter, H. (1960). Isolation of lysergic acid alkaloids from the Mexican drug ololiuqui (Rivea corymbosa (L.) Hall.f.) *Experientia, 16,* 414.

Incháustegui, C. (1994). *La mesa de plata: cosmogonía y curanderismo entre los mazatecos de Oaxaca [The silver table: Cosmogony and quackery among the Mazatecos of Oaxaca].* Oaxaca, Mexico: Instituto Oaxaqueño de las Culturas.

Jenks, A. A., Walker, J. B., & Kim, S. C. (2010). Evolution and origins of the Mazatec hallucinogenic sage, *Salvia divinorum* (Lamiaceae): A molecular phylogenetic approach. *Journal of Plant Research, 124*(5), 593–600.

Johnson, J. B. (1939). The elements of Mazatec witchcraft. *Göteborgs Etnografiska Museum. Etnologiska Studier, 9,* 119–149.

Kelly, B. C. (2011). Legally tripping: A qualitative profile of *Salvia divinorum* use among young adults. *Journal of Psychoactive Drugs, 43,* 46–54.

Luke, D. P., & Terhune, D. B. (2013). The induction of synaesthesia with chemical agents: A systematic review. *Frontiers in Psychology, 4,* 753. https://doi.org/10.3389/fpsyg.2013.00753

MacLean, K. A., Johnson, M. W., Reissig, C. J., Prisinzano, T. E., & Griffiths, R. R. (2013). Dose-related effects of salvinorin A in humans: Dissociative, hallucinogenic, and memory effects. *Psychopharmacology, 226*(2), 381–392.

Maqueda, A. E., Valle, M., Addy, P. H., Antonijoan, R. M., Puntes, M., Coimbra, J., … Riba, J. (2015). Salvinorin-A induces intense dissociative effects, blocking external sensory perception and modulating interoception and sense of body ownership in humans. *International Journal of Neuropsychopharmacology, 18*(12), pyv065. https://doi.org/10.1093/ijnp/pyv065

Maqueda, A. E., Valle, M., Addy, P. H., Antonijoan, R. M., Puntes, M., Coimbra, J., … Riba, J. (2016). Naltrexone but not Ketanserin antagonizes the subjective, cardiovascular, and neuroendocrine effects of Salvinorin-A in humans. *International Journal of Neuropsychopharmacology, 19*(7), pyw016. https://doi.org/10.1093/ijnp/pyw016

McCurdy, C. R., Sufka, K. J., Smith, G. H., Warnick, J. E., & Nieto, M. J. (2006). Antinociceptive profile of salvinorin A, a structurally unique kappa opioid receptor agonist. *Pharmacology, Biochemistry, and Behavior, 83*(1), 109–113.

Nygård, E. A. (2007). *Listening to the sage: The experience of learning from the Salvia divinorum altered state* (Unpublished doctoral dissertation). Institute of Transpersonal Psychology, Palo Alto, CA.

Ortega, A., Blount, J. F., & Manchand, P. S. (1982). Salvinorin, a new trans-neoclerodane diterpene from *Salvia divinorum* (Labiatae). *Journal of the Chemical Society, Perkin Transactions, 1*(0), 2505–2508.

Orton, E., & Liu, R. (2014). Salvinorin A: A mini review of physical and chemical properties affecting its translation from research to clinical applications in humans. *Translational Perioperative and Pain Medicine Journal, 1*(1), 9–11.

Ott, J. (1995). Ethnopharmacognosy and human pharmacology of *Salvia divinorum* and salvinorin A. *Curare, 18*(1), 103–129.

Raichle, M. E. (2011). The restless brain. *Brain Connectivity, 1*(1), 3–12.

Raichle, M. E., MacLeod, A. M., Snyder, A. Z., Powers, W. J., Gusnard, D. A., & Shulman, G. L. (2001). A default mode of brain function. *Proceedings of the National Academy of Sciences of the United States of America, 98*(2), 676–682.

Ranganathan, M., Schnakenberg, A., Skosnik, P. D., Cohen, B. M., Pittman, B., Sewell, R. A., & D'Souza, D. C. (2012). Dose-related behavioral, subjective, endocrine, and psychophysiological effects of the κ opioid agonist Salvinorin A in humans. *Biological Psychiatry, 72*(10), 871–879.

Reisfield, A. S. (1993). The botany of *Salvia divinorum* (Labiatae). *SIDA, 15*(3), 349–366.

Reko, B. P. (1945). *Mitobotanica Zapoteca.* Tacubaya, Mexico: Private printing.

Rossi, A., Pace, S., Tedesco, F., Pagano, E., Guerra, G., Troisi, F., … Capasso, R. (2016). The hallucinogenic diterpene salvinorin A inhibits leukotriene synthesis in experimental models of inflammation. *Pharmacological Research Journal, 106,* 64–71.

Roth, B. L., Baner, K., Westkaemper, R., Siebert, D., Rice, K. C., Steinberg, S., … Rothman, R. B. (2002). Salvinorin A: A potent naturally occurring nonnitrogenous kappa opioid selective agonist. *Proceedings of the National Academy of Sciences of the United States of America, 99*(18), 11934–11939.

Schmidt, M. D., Schmidt, M. S., Butelman, E. R., Harding, W. W., Tidgewell, K., Murry, D. J., … Prisinzano, T. E. (2005). Pharmacokinetics of the plant-derived kappa-opioid hallucinogen salvinorin A in nonhuman primates. *Synapse, 58*(3), 208–210.

Schwarzer, C. (2009). 30 years of dynorphins – new insights on their functions in neuropsychiatric diseases. *Pharmacology & Therapeutics, 123*(3), 353–370.

Serra, V., Fattore, L., Scherma, M., Collu, R., Spano, M. S., Fratta, W., & Fadda, P. (2015). Behavioral and neurochemical assessment of Salvinorin A abuse potential in the rat. *Psychopharmacology, 232*(1), 91–100.

Siebert, D. J. (1994). *Salvia divinorum* and salvinorin A: New pharmacologic findings. *Journal of Ethnopharmacology, 43*(1), 53–56.

Siebert, D. J. (1999). Clones of *Salvia divinorum.* Retrieved from http://www.lycaeum.org/salvia/clones.html

Siebert, D. J. (2003). The history of the first *Salvia divinorum* plants cultivated outside of Mexico. *The Entheogen Review, 12*(4), 117–118. Retrieved from http://www.sagewisdom.org/salviahistory.html

Siebert, D. J. (2004). Localization of salvinorin A and related compounds in glandular trichomes of the psychoactive sage, *Salvia divinorum. Annals of Botany, 93*(6), 763–777.

Soutar, I., & Strassman, R. (2000). *Meditation with Salvia divinorum/Salvinorin A.* Retrieved from http://www.maps.org/researcharchive/salvia/sdmeditation.html

Stiefel, K. M., Merrifield, A., & Holcombe, A. O. (2014). The claustrum's proposed role in consciousness is supported by the effect and target localization of *Salvia divinorum. Frontiers in Integrative Neuroscience, 8,* 20.

Su, D., Riley, J., Kiessling, W. J., Armstead, W. M., & Liu, R. (2011). Salvinorin A produces cerebrovasodilation through activation of nitric oxide synthase, κ receptor, and adenosine triphosphate-sensitive potassium channel. *Anesthesiology, 114*(2), 374–379.

Taylor, G. T., & Manzella, F. (2016). Kappa opioids, Salvinorin A and major depressive disorder. *Current Neuropharmacology Journal, 14*(2), 165–176.

Tejeda, H. A., Shippenberg, T. S., & Henriksson, R. (2012). The dynorphin/kappa-opioid receptor system and its role in psychiatric disorders. *Cellular and Molecular Life Sciences, 69*(6), 857–896.

Valdes, J. L., III, Butler, W. M., Hatfield, G. M., Paul, A. G., & Koreeda, M. (1984). Divinorin A, a psychotropic terpenoid, and divinorin B from the hallucinogenic Mexican mint *Salvia divinorum*. *Journal of Organic Chemistry, 49*, 4716–4720.

Valdes, J. L., III, Diaz, J. L., & Paul, A. G. (1983). Ethnopharmacology of ska Maria Pastora (*Salvia divinorum* Epling and Jativa-M). *Journal of Ethnopharmacology, 7*(3), 287–312.

Valdes, J. L., III, Hatfield, G. M., Koreeda, M., & Paul, A. G. (1987). Studies of *Salvia divinorum* (Lamiaceae), an hallucinogenic mint from the Sierra Mazateca in Oaxaca, Central Mexico. *Economic Botany, 41*(2), 283–291.

Vasiljevik, T., Groer, C. E., Lehner, K., Navarro, H., & Prisinzano, T. E. (2014). Studies toward the development of antiproliferative neoclerodanes from Salvinorin A. *Journal of Natural Products, 77*(8), 1817–1824.

Wasson, R. G. (1962). A new Mexican psychotropic drug from the mint family. *Botanical Museum Leaflets Harvard University, 20*(3), 77–84.

Weitlaner, R. J. (1952). Curaciones mazatecas [Mazatec cures]. *Anales del Instituto Nacional de Antropologia e Historia, 4*, 279–285.

Wu, H., Wacker, D., Katritch, V., Mileni, M., Han, G. W., Vardy, E., ... Stevens, R. C. (2012). Structure of the human kappa opioid receptor in complex with JDTic. *Nature, 485*(7398), 327–332.

Chapter 5
Examining the Therapeutic Potential of Kratom Within the American Drug Regulatory System

O. Hayden Griffin, III

Abstract Kratom is a plant native to Southeast Asia. It has been used for hundreds, if not thousands, of years in traditional medicine within that region. Kratom is a rare substance, due to it having both stimulant and narcotic properties. Kratom use has spread to regions outside of its native geographic range, and these countries are simultaneously considering both the benefits kratom could hold for patients and the misuse that could occur among drug users. Within the United States, after reports of increasing kratom use, the Drug Enforcement Administration (DEA) announced its intention to regulate the plant on an emergency basis. After considerable public and legislative backlash, the DEA backed off of this decision. To date, no federal regulation exists within the United States, and only a few states have regulations. This chapter discusses kratom use within Southeast Asia and the growing body of research documenting the potential medical benefits as well as the abuse liability of kratom. It concludes by discussing the drug regulation system within the United States and the potential hurdles kratom might face before becoming a recognized part of American pharmacopeia.

Introduction

The world is getting smaller; at least that is what some people will say. While there is little evidence to support the notion that the Earth is actually shrinking, in an age of globalization, people are exposed to much more than they were only a few years ago. Such a process began with better transportation and then proceeded with improved forms of communication; perhaps the most important of which is the Internet. As globalization has increased, so has access to different types of drugs. In some instances, this will simply mean that traditional drug traffickers (peddling the traditionally trafficked, such as heroin, cocaine, and cannabis) are able to import greater quantities of drugs to existing markets or branch out to new ones. In other

O. Hayden Griffin, III (✉)
Department of Criminal Justice, University of Alabama at Birmingham, Birmingham, AL, USA
e-mail: hgriffin@uab.edu

© Springer International Publishing AG, part of Springer Nature 2018 71
B. C. Labate, C. Cavnar (eds.), *Plant Medicines, Healing and Psychedelic Science*,
https://doi.org/10.1007/978-3-319-76720-8_5

instances, the so-called novel psychoactive substances (NPS) are introduced. Some of these substances are actually newly discovered synthetic or perhaps rediscovered synthetic substances. Respective examples of this are spice (some refer to it as synthetic marijuana) and MDMA. However, in many instances, these NPS are not newly discovered substances but instead substances that have been traditionally used since time immemorial. The only thing novel about these substances is that they are simply introduced to a new region. There are two reasons that this latter process occurs. The first is simply that someone or some people decided to sell a traditional drug to a new market. The second is that many traditional drugs are not regulated in emerging markets. Thus, sellers might have some window of time to sell these traditional drugs until drug regulators are aware and control these newly introduced (but traditional elsewhere) substances. The growth of the Internet and the ability of sellers to peddle these substances without engaging in a normal drug distribution process, such as selling drugs in "head shops" or on street corners, have greatly aided drug users' knowledge and availability of new substances. In some instances, NPS are introduced simply so that recreational users will have another substance to use. In other cases, the introduction of a NPS might be due to people who find the therapeutic utility of available substances lacking and are seeking new treatments for maladies from which they suffer. A recent example of this, within the United States, is a plant indigenous to Southeast Asia: kratom.

Kratom

In Southeast Asia, the Korth tree (*Mitragyna speciosa*) grows. Many people refer to the plant (or substances that come from the plant) as "kratom" or "ketum." The stem of the tree is not very thick, which to some observers may lead them to refer to the plant as a shrub rather than a tree. Typically, the plant grows in marshy areas. Usually, kratom only grows to 6 to 9 feet tall, but specimens have been found to grow more than 40 feet in height. Branches on the plant point upward and contain green oval-shaped leaves that range from about 8 to 12 centimeters. The leaves are broad and have narrow pointed tips. Yellow flowers grow on the plant in globular clusters, and the seeds are winged (Schultes, Hofmann, & Ratsch, 1998). Throughout the dry season, leaves from the tree will be shed and fall to the ground, and new leaves sprout and grow during the rainy season (Macko, Weisbach, & Douglas, 1972). If a casual observer were looking at the plant, they would probably not find the Korth tree remarkable. Indeed, to someone other than a botanist, there are most likely a great number of plants similar looking to the Korth tree. Yet, looks can be deceiving.

Kratom leaves contain more than 20 alkaloids; many of those alkaloids have psychoactive properties. While this may seem like novel news to people living in the Western hemisphere, to people living in Southeast Asia, especially Thailand and Malaysia, this is indeed old news. The first scientific reference to kratom was made in 1836. For how long people within this region have known of the psychoactive properties of kratom is difficult to ascertain (Jansen & Prast, 1988). Plants have been used by humans for medicinal purposes for millennia, and there are roughly 1000 known plants that are used for their psychoactive properties (Schultes et al., 1998). Yet, even among this many plants, kratom seems slightly special. The two most important psychoactive alkaloids within kratom are mitragynine and 7-hydroxymitragynine (7-OH). Mitragynine is the primary alkaloid found within the kratom plant. It is a partial opioid agonist that has one-fourth the potency of morphine. Mitragynine produces stimulant effects. 7-OH, which is a minor alkaloid within kratom and found in lower quantities than mitragynine, is roughly ten times more powerful than morphine and produces narcotic effects when consumed (Babu, McCurdy, & Boyer, 2008; Kitajima et al., 2006). Thus, while a plant that produces stimulant or narcotic properties would not make it especially rare, the fact that a plant contains both those properties puts kratom in a rare group of plants. Studies have typically found that lower doses of kratom are typically used for the stimulant properties of kratom, while higher doses are typically used for narcotic properties. This is most likely due to the aforementioned higher concentrations of mitragynine and the lower concentrations of 7-OH. To produce narcotic properties, a person will usually have to take a higher dose to receive greater amounts of 7-OH (Babu et al., 2008; Cinosi et al., 2015; Hassan et al., 2013; Jansen & Prast, 1988).

Like many other drugs, kratom has several different routes of administration. The most basic way that kratom can be ingested is by simply chewing the leaves. As Chittrakarn, Penjamras, and Keawpradub (2012) noted, "Thai peasants, laborers, and farmers" have chewed kratom leaves "for decades and perhaps forever" (p. 81). These groups of people chew kratom leaves for their stimulant properties so that they can work for longer hours in a more vigorous fashion. Additionally, kratom produces a pleasant feeling. Furthermore, in addition to producing stimulant effects, users have reported that chewing kratom helps cope with the effects of heat and sunlight common to the region. Chewers of kratom leaves typically prefer to chew fresh leaves. While dried leaves can be chewed, it is more likely kratom users will crush dried leaves so they can be swallowed. People who are regular kratom chewers will chew leaves between three and ten times a day. For those who have developed a tolerance to kratom, a chewer might chew 30 leaves or more a day. The stimulant effects of kratom chewing occur between 5 and 10 min after chewing begins (Jansen & Prast, 1988).

In addition to chewing kratom leaves, kratom users can brew powdered leaves into a tea. Lemon juice can be added to help extract the psychoactive alkaloids from the powder. Sugar and honey are common additives to kratom tea, since some tea drinkers find the taste of the tea bitter. Similarly, dried leaves can be boiled in water until the mixture becomes a syrup. This syrup can be combined with finely chopped palm leaves into a pill form. This pill can be either swallowed or smoked. Some users in Malaysia will smoke this type of kratom pill (which they call a *madatin*) in long bamboo pipes (Hassan et al., 2013).

The composition of kratom plants will often vary depending upon geography, leading to significant differences in the quantities of psychoactive compounds found in these different samples of plants (Kowalczuk, Łozak, & Zjawiony, 2013). Yet, so far, there has not been documented evidence that differences in the type of kratom have different potencies (Griffin, Daniels, & Gardner, 2016). One way to differentiate between different types of kratom is a technique employed by biologists to determine the region from which it originates. Among the regions that kratom germinates within are Bali, Borneo, Indonesia, Indonesian Island, Java, Malaysia, New Guinea, Riau, and Sumatra (Eisenman, 2014). While there has been no documented difference in the pharmacological properties of kratom, users have noted preferences for different types of the plant (Chittrakarn et al., 2012; Suwanlert, 1975).

As far back as 1836, it was documented that people in Malaysia were using kratom as a substitute for opium. By the early 1900s, it was documented that kratom could alleviate the symptoms of opiate withdrawal. Additionally, kratom has been used in the treatment of malaria, cough, hypertension, diarrhea, and depression and reduction of fever, and it can be used as a painkiller (Jansen & Prast, 1988). While some people might view kratom as just another medicine or a drug that can be misused, it is often important to look to the history of regions from which these types of substances originate. As Tanguay (2011) wrote, kratom use has a long tradition in Thailand and Southeast Asia. To many people in this region, the use of kratom is not considered drug use, and there seems to be little stigmatization of or discrimination against users. As Tanguay documents, kratom use is simply a part of life in Southern Thailand and is "closely embedded in the traditions and customs, such as local ceremonies, traditional cultural performances, and teashops" (p. 2). As previously mentioned, kratom is commonly used by laborers, especially those who work on rubber plantations and those who work at sea. An additional consideration is that several provinces in Southeast Asia have significant Islamic populations. Those who abide by religious tenets of the Islamic faith are forbidden from drinking alcohol. The use of kratom can often serve as a substitute for that which is not allowed by their faith. According to Tanguay, to many people in Southeast Asia, using kratom is no different from drinking coffee.

Abuse Liability of Kratom

One of the most frequent, and perhaps controversial, topics concerning kratom is its abuse potential. As Tanguay (2011) has documented, kratom has been used in traditional medicine in Southeast Asia for generations. Many of these traditional users do so to work longer or as an alternative to opiates. According to Jansen and Prast (1988), reports in the 1930s referred to chronic kratom users as "thin, and to have dry skin and a darker complexion" (p. 455). Reports of dependence were first documented in the medical literature in the 1950s, with a case report of a "chronic user who had a marked withdrawal on cessation, but who nevertheless remained in good health despite heavy use, being mentally and physically 'normal'" (p. 455). While there have been many studies of kratom users, most researchers acknowledge that the abuse liability of kratom is still poorly understood.

In more recent years, many researchers have attempted to obtain better documentation of the number of people using kratom and profiles of those users. One study conducted by Vicknasingam, Narayanan, Beng, and Mansor (2010) surveyed a total of 136 active users of kratom who resided in northern Malaysia. The researchers found that the average age of users was 38.7 years. Thus, users were typically older than one would expect from users of similar substances. Among the long-term users of kratom (those with more than 2 years or more of use), these users were more likely to be married and have a healthy appetite. According to the results of the study, many of the short-term users were likely to be using kratom as a substitute for opiates. Most users reported their use for instrumental purposes (e.g., opiate substitute, to work harder, be more active, and improved sexual performance), and only a few users (5.6–12.5%) reported that they used kratom for the recreational purpose of merely getting high. A few years later, Vicknasingam was part of a similar study that focused on incidents of kratom dependence and withdrawal. Singh, Müller, and Vicknasingam (2014) conducted a cross-sectional survey of 293 regular kratom users who resided in three different northern states in the peninsula of Malaysia. They found that more than half of these users showed signs of severe kratom dependence, and 45% showed moderate dependence. Regular users who consumed three or more glasses of kratom a day were more likely to become dependent. Among the reported withdrawal symptoms were muscle spasms and pain, trouble sleeping, watery eyes or nose, hot flashes, fever, a decrease in appetite, diarrhea, restlessness, tension, anger, sadness, and nervousness.

In a different study, Ahmad and Aziz (2012) conducted 562 face-to-face interviews of kratom users (using snowball sampling methods for recruitment) in a border town between two states in northern Malaysia. Most of the respondents (88%) used kratom daily, and 90% of users consumed kratom as a tea. Users from the study were also older than typical substance users with the mean reported age of initiation of kratom at 28.3 years. While users reported very similar motives for use as Vicknasingam and colleagues, Ahmad and Aziz found that 87% of the people they interviewed reported they were dependent upon kratom and could not stop using. Interestingly, users with lower education levels were more likely to be able to stop using kratom than users with more education.

As has already been alluded to and will be discussed in more depth later in the chapter, kratom has made its way to the United States. Grundmann (2017) sent an anonymous survey in October 2016 to 10,000 active kratom users through social media and online resources available from the American Kratom Association; 8049 of those 10,000 people completed the survey. Similar to the aforementioned results, Grundmann found that kratom users were typically older than typical substance users. In this case, kratom users were primarily 31–50 years of age. Additionally, most users made more than $35,000 or more a year. Just like previous studies, users primarily reported instrumental use: 68% reported kratom use for self-treatment of pain, and 66% reported that they used kratom to treat emotional or mental conditions. Many users used kratom to treat withdrawal symptoms associated with opioids. Two other findings were that many kratom users had no problem admitting to kratom use, with 40% discussing their use to healthcare providers and a very low

0.65% reporting that at some time they suffered from kratom-related toxicity that required medical treatment.

One common way that the abuse liability of drugs is tested is through trials with animals. Indeed, to get approval from the Food and Drug Administration (FDA), the results of animal studies need to be reviewed and approved by the agency before human trials can begin (Hawthorne, 2005). Yet, these results always need to be put into context. Care needs to be taken that animal testing is conducted with species that present good comparisons with humans and that animals do not receive dosage equivalents that would not be witnessed in humans (Ator & Griffiths, 2003). Animal testing is often relied upon because testing regulations require that humans take drugs as directed in safe dosages; thus, in clinical settings, it is difficult to ascertain how humans might misuse drugs or react to high or dangerous doses (Griffiths, Bigelow, & Ator, 2003). In one very recent study, Yusoff et al. (2016) studied the effects of kratom on rats and mice. After testing, they concluded, "we describe an addictive profile and cognitive impairments of acute and chronic mitragynine administration, which closely resembles that of morphine" (p. 98). Among the findings was that withdrawal signs occurred after 12 h of cessation and increased levels of anxiety after 24 h. This led Yusoff and colleagues to conclude that kratom could be classified "as a harmful drug" (p. 98).

While a picture is emerging of the dependence potential of kratom, how toxic it may be and whether kratom has the ability to kill users are still a subject of debate. More evidence still needs to be gathered, but there is some evidence that kratom use can lead to seizures, coma, and even the death of users (Boyer, Babu, Adkins, McCurdy, & Halpern, 2008; Nelsen, Lapoint, Hodgman, & Aldous, 2010; Rosenbaum, Carreiro, & Babu, 2012). In one case study, Karinen, Fosen, Rogde, and Vindenes (2014) recounted the death of a Norwegian man. In postmortem testing, traces of mitragynine, 7-OH, zopiclone, citalopram, and lamotrigine were found in his system. The latter three substances were found at therapeutic levels. The deceased, who was found dead at his home, had a history of drug abuse and mental illness. Karinen and colleagues concluded from the circumstances that this consti- tuted an "accidental poisoning" of kratom (p. e29). Three drugs were found at therapeutic levels, and there reported to be "high concentrations" of mitragynine and 7-OH (p. e29). In another incident, a 17-year-old White man was found unresponsive in bed. When emergency medical technicians arrived, they pro- nounced the young man dead at the scene; aside from evidence that he had vomited, there were no other signs of trauma. An "investigation team" later arrived at the scene, and the young man's girlfriend provided investigators with an empty bottle of kratom which the girlfriend said her deceased boyfriend had taken the night before. Within the investigation, it was found that the young man had both a history of heroin use and suffered from chronic back pain. His use of kratom was reported to be self-medication for the two conditions. After an autopsy was performed, traces were found of mitragynine, over-the-counter cold medications, and benzodiazepines. These circumstances led the medical examiner to conclude that "possible kratom toxicity" occurred, and the young man's death was ruled an accident (Neerman, Frost, & Deking, 2013). Thus, in these case studies, both which involve patients with histories of drug abuse and who had used multiple substances, both men appeared to have accidentally died after ingesting kratom. Whether either man would have died from merely ingesting kratom is unclear.

Polydrug abuse is one of the biggest dangers from drugs and still seems to represent the biggest danger of kratom toxicity within the literature. Nelsen et al. (2010) documented the case of a 64-year-old male who suffered seizure and coma after ingesting a tea made with kratom and *Datura stramonium* (commonly known as jimsonweed or Devil's snare and a member of the nightshade family). From the case study, it is not made clear if the case involved a presold combination product; however, it has become increasingly clear that some kratom combination products have been sold with deadly results. One such product is krypton, a combination of powdered kratom leaves and O-desmethyltramadol. The latter substance is the active metabolite of tramadol, which is a commonly prescribed painkiller. Kronstrand, Roman, Thelander, and Eriksson (2011), while conducting autopsies in Sweden, found evidence that as many as nine deaths were caused in 1 year by the ingestion of krypton.

While krypton is only a mix of two substances, another kratom product shows the lengths to which some people will go to risk getting high. As Tungtananuwat and Lawanprasert (2010) have documented, within Thailand, some young people have begun to consume a drink referred to as "4 × 100." The researchers were not aware of the origin of the name but speculated that it might be due to the four ingredients within the concoction. The three major ingredients of the cocktail are boiled kratom leaves, a cola-based soft drink, and cough syrup that contains either codeine or diphenhydramine. Tungtananuwat and Lawanprasert assert that the fourth ingredient is essentially up to whoever is making the drug. According to them, among the substances that have been used are mosquito coils, anxiolytic drugs, antidepressants, painkillers, methadone, cannabis, methamphetamine, herbicide, or "the powder peeled from the inside of fluorescent light bulbs" (p. 43). In their report, they document the death of a 21-year-old Islamic man. The man's family did not consent to a full autopsy, but from blood and urine samples, it was determined that the young man had ingested kratom, caffeine, diphenhydramine, alprazolam, nortriptyline, methadone, tramadol, and methamphetamine. Tungtananuwat and Lawanprasert noted "interpretation of the cause of death in this cause was limited" (p. 46) but concluded, "based on the toxicological findings, the cause of death in this case study seemed likely to be due to multiple drugs intoxication" (p. 47). Tanguay (2011) speculated that 4 × 100 use began in Thailand sometime around 2006. In one district, Tanguay found that 21 out of 39 villages reported use of 4 × 100. Unlike kratom, there seemed to be some stigma associated with 4 × 100, so users seemed to use the substance in clandestine settings. While there was some stigma attached to use, Tanguay stated that the stigma attached to 4 × 100 was "far milder than for yaba or heroin users" (p. 3).

In sum, while research on kratom is certainly ongoing, studies generally show a lack of fatalities involving the substance, and, while there is clear evidence that kratom can be habit-forming and produce dependence, it seems mild compared to other substances. The main problem associated with kratom, which is indicative of a great many drugs, is that, when kratom is combined with other substances (many of which are either legal or available via a physician's prescription), harm can result. What is clear is that kratom by itself *is not* a substance that should be simply removed from legal pharmacopeia before it can be properly studied by medical research.

Legal Status of Kratom

While kratom has been used for generations in Southeast Asia, controls of the substance are more recent. Thailand first placed controls on various forms of kratom in 1943. In 1976, kratom was placed into Schedule 5 of the Thai Narcotics Act. According to Hassan et al. (2013), Schedule 5 is the most lenient category of the Act; however, the legislation still prohibits the purchase, sale, import, or possession of kratom. Furthermore, it is prohibited to plant or cultivate kratom, and existing kratom plants are supposed to be removed. As an example of kratom enforcement in Thailand, in 2009, 20,877 kg of kratom were seized in 5485 cases, which led to the arrests of 7388 people (Tanguay, 2011). Additionally, as Hassan et al. (2013) noted, in Malaysia, the other country in which kratom has a long history, kratom was inserted into the country's Poison Act during 2003. According to the law, distribution of kratom products is punishable with "a penalty and/or jail sentence" (p. 141). Many other countries have controlled or regulated kratom including Australia, Bhutan, Denmark, Finland, Lithuania, Myanmar, Poland, and Sweden.

Within the United States, kratom has had a short but interesting history. Exactly when kratom appeared in the United States is unclear. Boyer, Babu, Macalino, and Compton (2007) documented a case study of a man who was reported to use kratom as a tool in desisting from hydromorphone use. In a Google news search, the first article in the United States appeared in *PC World* magazine with the title "Lab Tests of Drugs Purchased Online Reveal Risks" (Spring, 2009). According to Swogger et al. (2015), a search of PubMed conducted in early 2015 found only ten published medical case reports involving kratom. By 2013, the Drug Enforcement Administration (DEA) had listed kratom as a drug of concern, a move Hassan et al. (2013) speculated "suggests that the agency may eventually try to ban it in the US once more reliable data on its addictive properties and/or health hazards become available" (p. 141). The DEA would eventually move to prohibit kratom, but not for the reasons Hassan and colleagues suggested.

By 2016, Griffin et al. (2016) noted that the states of Alabama, Indiana, Tennessee, Vermont, and Wisconsin had placed controls on kratom. Legislation was pending to control kratom in Michigan and New Jersey, while efforts to control kratom in Arizona, Florida, Illinois, Louisiana, and Oklahoma had failed. Since that time, according to the American Kratom Association, Arkansas has prohibited kratom as well. While the DEA at least had its eye on kratom since 2013, the agency began to take action in 2016. In that year, the Center for Disease Control and Prevention (CDC) released a report on July 29. The report noted that, from 2010 to 2015, poison control centers in the United States had received a total of 660 calls within that time period. In the first year, 2010, only 26 calls were received, while in 2015, 263 calls were received. According to Anwar and Schier (2016), the authors of the report, since the number of calls to poison control had increased, this should be a cause for concern, and the American public, as well as American healthcare providers, should be aware of the potential dangers of kratom. As Griffin and Webb (in press) noted, the report from the CDC received some attention in the media, but not much. A Google search in August of 2016 found a total of 10 media articles and 51 blogs discussing kratom during that month. A search of LexisNexis only produced 10 media articles. Indeed, it is probably not hard to see why the report received so little attention. As Mowry, Spyker, Brooks, McMillan, and Schauben (2015) documented, in 2014 alone, there were 2,890,909 calls to poison control centers. More than 300,000 of those calls were for drugs of various forms. Thus, by comparison, 263 calls across the United States concerning kratom probably did not appear too newsworthy. Yet, the DEA seemed to have paid attention.

On August 30, 2016, the DEA announced their intention to classify mitragynine and 7-OH as Schedule I drugs using their emergency scheduling powers. By statute, Schedule I substances within the Controlled Substances Act are supposed to be drugs that have both no accepted medical use and a high potential for abuse. In justifying the decision, the DEA noted the aforementioned CDC report and also noted that law enforcement agencies had seized 55,000 kilograms of kratom products from February 2014 to July 2016, and an additional 57,000 kilograms were confiscated during the importation process into the United States. What, if any, overlap existed between those two seizure amounts was not indicated, and the DEA offered no evidence indicating that kratom abuse was either prevalent or a problem within the United States (Griffin & Webb, in press).

The action of emergency scheduling a drug into Schedule I is a serious matter. Placing a drug into Schedule I of the CSA prevents any physician from prescribing the drug and places severe restrictions on research (Griffin, Miller, & Khey, 2008). As Jaffe (1985) noted, placing a drug into Schedule I can essentially end the medical utility of a drug in the United States. That the DEA would use its emergency scheduling power on flimsy evidence is not novel. Multiple researchers have recounted how despite clear evidence of medical utility, the DEA insisted that MDMA had no medical utility, despite clear evidence to the contrary. Instead, the DEA primarily focused on the dangers that became associated with MDMA: young adults using the drug at raves and several groups of distributors engaging in the mass wholesale of the drug before prohibition took place (Beck & Rosenbaum, 1994; Eisner, 1989; Griffin, 2012; Rosenbaum & Doblin, 1991). Another example is cannabis in the United States. Despite clear evidence that the plant is not toxic and over half of American states having provisions for medical cannabis (including eight states where the recreational use and sale are legal), the DEA still stubbornly holds the view that cannabis belongs in Schedule I and has no accepted medical value (Griffin, 2017). Thus, when the DEA announced that kratom would be placed into Schedule I, it appeared, based upon past history, that kratom might be one in a string of many drugs that essentially ended up in the pharmacological scrap heap of

American drug regulation. Yet, so far, kratom has not merely gone quietly into the night.

One of the first organizations to protest the decision was the Drug Policy Alliance (DPA). The group, which until very recently was led by Ethan Nadelmann, is a policy think tank that engages in activism and lobbying based upon harm reduction policies and a call to end drug war policies. The DPA was a natural fit to protest the DEA's decision regarding kratom and produced several articles and blog entries critical of the DEA's decision. Additionally, the lobbying group provided an electronic form so that people could easily submit complaints to members of Congress regarding the decision. The DPA, which was formed in 2000 from the merger of the Lindesmith Center (founded by Nadelmann in 1994) and the Drug Policy Foundation (founded in 1987 by Arnold Trebach and Kevin Zeese), has a long history of conducting research and lobbying for drug policy reform. That the DPA would be on the forefront criticizing and lobbying against the actions of the DEA was natural. Indeed, the advocacy groups have a long history of doing so; however, a very new grassroots organization would add its voice to the fight.

In 2014, Susan Ash began the work to form the American Kratom Association (AKA). The group officially launched in 2015. Ash began her career as a park ranger and naturalist at Bryce Canyon National Park. Since that time, she has been an environmental advocate and engaged in many different charitable and advocacy endeavors. In 2011, Ash had to leave a job in Norfolk, Virginia, due to complications with Lyme disease. In a search to mitigate the harm she suffered from her illness, Ash found that kratom was able to manage the symptoms that afflicted her. Ash founded the AKA as a means to try to preserve her access (and that of others) to kratom. As a group, the AKA disseminates information about kratom and employs a law firm, a lobbying firm, and a public relations firm to provide information and lobby different government officials. While it is difficult to measure the true effect of a lobbying group, the AKA at least managed to get under one state legislator's skin. As Gancarski (2017) documented, State Representative Kristin Jacobs, a Democrat representing Coconut Creek in Florida, had introduced legislation on several occasions to schedule mitragynine and 7-OH within the State of Florida Controlled Substances Act. When asked about the AKA, Jacobs had very pointed words to describe the organization. Among the highlights was "They have a story... Just like Hitler believed if you tell a lie over and over again, it becomes the truth" and "lie machine...a powerful lobby with a lot of money" (para. 3).

Along with the lobbying efforts of the DPA and AKA, media attention surrounding kratom increased substantially. According to Griffin and Webb (in press), the number of articles accessed from Google News and LexisNexis increased from 10 to 113 and 10 to 28, respectively, from the months of August to September. Additionally, more than 140,000 people signed a petition to the White House protesting the kratom scheduling decision, and a bipartisan group of 51 members of the House of Representatives submitted a letter to the administrator of the DEA arguing that the emergency scheduling decision was premature and should be delayed until there is sufficient evidence that such an action was indeed warranted. The scheduling of kratom was supposed to take effect on September 30, but the DEA delayed their decision and ultimately withdrew their intent to emergency schedule kratom on October 12, 2016.

Many people thought the decision by the DEA to withdraw the intent to schedule kratom was the right call; however, based upon past history, it is probable that most people believed that the DEA would still not make it. Regarding the decision, it seemed as if, among the most surprised people, were the people of the DEA. While speaking to members of the press, DEA spokesperson Russ Baer described the action as "unprecedented" and stated that the agency had never before withdrawn an emergency scheduling order. In describing the actions of the DEA, Baer stated that the agency did not want to be perceived as "a group of government bureaucrats" who lacked any concern for the health and safety of the American people. After the DEA withdrew the order, the agency stated that they would solicit comments from the American public regarding the decision. That process was supposed to last 6 weeks (Chen, 2016). Since that time, the DEA has not made any substantive comments nor made their future intent known regarding kratom.

Imagining the Medical Utility of Kratom in the United States

As documented, kratom has been used in traditional Southeastern Asian medicine for a long time, and there is a growing literature suggesting that while kratom has signs of causing dependence, the abuse liability of the plant is lower than many existing medications, especially, many of the opiates/opioids. While the United States allows the dispensation of both methadone and buprenorphine on a maintenance basis to opiate/opioid users who have difficulty quitting through traditional abstinence methods, there have been many critics of such policies. Some people simply believe that methadone and buprenorphine are just other opioids to be misused, and others who have embraced this type of treatment note that it can have limitations (Miller, Griffin, & Gardner, 2016). Furthermore, one of the great quests of research, and many policymakers, is replacing opiates/opioids with other painkillers that have a lower abuse liability profile (Acker, 2002). Such a goal becomes increasingly relevant as the number of deaths from opiates/opioids continues to climb in the United States.

While Hassan et al. (2013) have questioned whether the hopes associated with kratom as an alternative to opiates/opioids have been primarily driven by sellers of kratom looking for expanded sales, there is literature available, before Internet sales of anything existed, suggesting that kratom could be used as an alternative or substitute for opiates/opioids. Furthermore, groups such as the AKA and DPA have pushed against kratom prohibition in the United States, and it seems a sizeable group of citizens and legislators are willing to give kratom a chance as well. However, before one can imagine a future with pain patients drinking a glass of kratom tea rather than swallowing an opioid pill, there is one major hurdle: the United States drug regulatory system.

Today, the drug regulatory system is known to some people as being too lenient, while others find the system too strict (Hawthorne, 2005). It did not begin this way. As Sutherland (1940) argued, the federal government was not able to thwart the lobbying attempts of the pharmaceutical companies until 1906, when the Pure Food and Drug Act was passed. It had only taken 30 years of effort and 140 failed bills before Congress until one of those bills finally broke through, was signed, and became law. It would take one tragedy and one close call (at least in the United States) before the regulatory structure took hold. In 1937, a drug called Elixir Sulfanilamide was available for just 4 weeks. In that amount of time, 105 patients who had taken the drug died (34 of whom were children). A year later, the Food, Drug, and Cosmetic Act required that, before any drug could be sold in the United States, it needed to receive FDA approval and, before that could be given, a pharmaceutical company needed to prove that the drug was safe for consumption. In 1962, the Act was amended again. The amendments required that not only must a pharmaceutical company prove their drugs were safe but any approved drug must be proven effective as well. The legislative action was taken due to the high number of pregnant women in Europe miscarrying children and birth defects in those children who survived after their mothers had taken thalidomide (to reduce morning sickness). Richardson-Merrill, the manufacturer of thalidomide, had applied for FDA approval in the United States, but a particularly diligent investigator, Dr. Frances Kelsey, had repeatedly demanded more information from the company. Right after the company realized FDA approval would not be given, they pulled their application. Shortly thereafter, reports of the damage that thalidomide had caused became widely known (Hawthorne, 2005).

The American drug regulatory system, which keeps many people safe, may be the very thing that could keep kratom from the pharmaceutical market. This is not because kratom could not potentially be proven to be safe for human consumption or effective for the treatment of certain ailments. Instead, the problem is the cost of bringing the product to market. Getting a drug through the FDA approval can cost millions. The reason that pharmaceutical companies go through this process is so that they can make money. One important part of this process is having some proprietary interest or patent rights, so that a company can make the money back that they spent during the approval process. The problem is that kratom is a plant that has been around for many centuries. Thus, the grand payoff—and the fear that other producers might come into the market after potential FDA approval has been granted—could prevent anyone from ever filing a New Drug Application with the FDA for kratom. Practically all FDA applications involve new drugs, not plants that have been around for eons.

Realizing the difficulties in the FDA approval process, or perhaps just wanting to maintain the status quo, the AKA seems to be plotting another path. In 1994, Congress passed the Dietary Supplement Health and Education Act (DSHEA). The Act established procedures for marketing and advertising dietary supplements in the United States, which do not have to go through FDA approval (Knapik et al., 2016). The AKA has gone to great lengths to portray kratom as a natural substance. This and other languages the organization has used might indicate that it is their hope to have kratom regulated by the lesser standard of dietary supplements. While kratom certainly is a natural substance, there are countless other substances (cannabis immediately comes to mind) that are heavily regulated. It seems a positive step that kratom was not emergency scheduled, but while the DEA has backed off from emergency scheduling, it seems that kratom will eventually be placed into some schedule and FDA approval will have to come at some point in time for the use of kratom in the United States to continue. Until then, it is difficult to see or guess what medical potential kratom could have in the United States and what benefits it could have; certainly, though, the potential is there; how much, if any, is the only question. At the very least, it seems like kratom may be given a chance of legitimacy in American pharmacopeia that other psychedelics never properly received. Although Timothy Leary and his contemporaries demonstrated that LSD and psilocybin had medical utility, their subsequent actions thoroughly stigmatized LSD and psilocybin in the United States (Lee & Shlain, 1985). DMT had a similar fate in the United States, and, so far, only the First Amendment protection of religious freedom has allowed religious groups who consume ayahuasca during religious rituals to do so (Griffin, 2014). Anything beyond the spiritual use of ayahuasca in the United States may prove difficult, despite promising evidence suggesting that ayahuasca might fit within the rigid definitions of medical utility within the CSA. MDMA had once seemed a promising drug, but its association with rave culture caused great harm to its therapeutic potential in the United States (Griffin, 2012). Perhaps the greatest hope for kratom is that it never receives a similar association.

References

Acker, C. J. (2002). *Creating the American junkie: Addiction research in the classic era of narcotic control*. Baltimore, MD: Johns Hopkins University Press.

Ahmad, K., & Aziz, Z. (2012). Mitragyna speciosa use in the northern states of Malaysia: A cross-sectional study. *Journal of Ethnopharmacology, 141*(1), 446–450.

Anwar, M., & Schier, J. (2016). Notes from the field: Kratom (Mitragyna speciosa) exposures reported to poison centers—United States, 2010–2015. *Morbidity and Mortality Weekly Report, 65*, 748–749.

Ator, N. A., & Griffiths, R. R. (2003). Principles of drug abuse liability assessment in laboratory animals. *Drug and Alcohol Dependence, 70*(3), S55–S72.

Babu, K. M., McCurdy, C. R., & Boyer, E. W. (2008). Opioid receptors and legal highs: *Salvia divinorum* and kratom. *Clinical Toxicology, 46*(2), 146–152.

Beck, J., & Rosenbaum, M. (1994). *Pursuit of ecstasy: The MDMA experience*. Albany, NY: SUNY Press.

Boyer, E. W., Babu, K. M., Adkins, J. E., McCurdy, C. R., & Halpern, J. H. (2008). Self-treatment of opioid withdrawal using kratom (Mitragyna speciosa Korth). *Addiction, 103*(6), 1048–1050.

Boyer, E. W., Babu, K. M., Macalino, G. E., & Compton, W. (2007). Self-treatment of opioid withdrawal with a dietary supplement, kratom. *American Journal on Addictions, 16*(5), 352–356.

Chen, A. (2016, October 17). What's next for kratom after the DEA blinks on its emergency ban? *Scientific American*. Retrieved from https://www.scientificamerican.com/article/what-s-next-for-kratom-after-the-dea-blinks-on-its-emergency-ban/

Chittrakarn, S., Penjamras, P., & Keawpradub, N. (2012). Quantitative analysis of mitragynine, codeine, caffeine, chlorpheniramine and phenylephrine in a kratom (Mitragyna speciosa Korth.) cocktail using high-performance liquid chromatography. *Forensic Science International, 217*(1), 81–86.

Cinosi, E., Martinotti, G., Simonato, P., Singh, D., Demetrovics, Z., Roman-Urrestarazu, A., … Li, J. -H. (2015). Following "the roots" of kratom (Mitragyna speciosa): The evolution of an enhancer from a traditional use to increase work and productivity in Southeast Asia to a recreational psychoactive drug in Western countries. *BioMed Research International, 2015, 968786*.

Eisenman, S. W. (2014). The botany of Mitragyna speciosa (Korth.) Havil. and related species. In R. B. Raffa (Ed.), *Kratom and other Mitragynines: The chemistry and pharmacology of opioids from a non-opium source* (pp. 57–76). New York, NY: CRC/Taylor & Francis.

Eisner, B. (1989). *Ecstasy: The MDMA story*. Berkeley, CA: Ronin Publishing.

Gancarski, A. G. (2017, January 9). Kristin Jacobs: Kratom lobby "just like Hitler." *Florida Politics*. Retrieved from http://floridapolitics.com/archives/230018-kristin-jacobs-kratom-lobby-just-like-hitler

Griffin, O. H. (2012). Is the government keeping the peace or acting like our parents? Rationales for the legal prohibitions of GHB and MDMA. *Journal of Drug Issues, 42*(3), 247–262.

Griffin, O. H. (2014). The role of the United States Supreme Court in shaping federal drug policy. *American Journal of Criminal Justice, 39*(3), 660–679.

Griffin, O. H. (2017). A democracy deficit within American drug policy. *Southern California Review of Law and Social Justice, 26*, 103–130.

Griffin, O. H., Daniels, J. A., & Gardner, E. A. (2016). Do you get what you paid for? An examination of products advertised as kratom. *Journal of Psychoactive Drugs, 48*(5), 330–335.

Griffin, O. H., Miller, B. L., & Khey, D. N. (2008). Legally high? Legal considerations of *Salvia divinorum. Journal of Psychoactive Drugs, 40*(2), 183–191.

Griffin, O. H., & Webb, M. E. (in press). The scheduling of kratom and selective use of data. *Journal of Psychoactive Drugs*. https://doi.org/10.1080/02791072.2017.1371363

Griffiths, R. R., Bigelow, G. E., & Ator, N. A. (2003). Principles of initial experimental drug abuse liability assessment in humans. *Drug and Alcohol Dependence, 70*(3), S41–S54.

Grundmann, O. (2017). Patterns of kratom use and health impact in the US: Results from an online survey. *Drug and Alcohol Dependence, 176*, 63–70.

Hassan, Z., Muzaimi, M., Navaratnam, V., Yusoff, N. H., Suhaimi, F. W., Vadivelu, R., … Muller, C. P. (2013). From kratom to mitragynine and its derivatives: Physiological and behavioural effects related to use, abuse, and addiction. *Neuroscience & Biobehavioral Reviews, 37*(2), 138–151.

Hawthorne, F. (2005). *Inside the FDA: The business and politics behind the drugs we take and the food we eat*. Hoboken, NJ: John Wiley & Sons.

Jaffe, J. H. (1985). Impact of scheduling on the practice of medicine and biomedical research. *Drug and Alcohol Dependence, 14*(3), 403–418.

Jansen, K. L., & Prast, C. J. (1988). Psychoactive properties of mitragynine (kratom). *Journal of Psychoactive Drugs, 20*(4), 455–457.

Karinen, R., Fosen, J. T., Rogde, S., & Vindenes, V. (2014). An accidental poisoning with mitragynine. *Forensic science international, 245*, e29–e32.

Kitajima, M., Misawa, K., Kogure, N., Said, I. M., Horie, S., Hatori, Y., … Takayama, H. (2006). A new indole alkaloid, 7-hydroxyspeciociliatine, from the fruits of Malaysian Mitragyna speciosa and its opioid agonist activity. *Journal of Natural Medicines, 60*(1), 28–35.

Knapik, J. J., Steelman, R. A., Hoedebecke, S. S., Austin, K. G., Farina, E. K., & Lieberman, H. R. (2016). Prevalence of dietary supplement use by athletes: Systematic review and meta-analysis. *Sports Medicine, 46*(1), 103–123.

Kowalczuk, A. P., Łozak, A., & Zjawiony, J. K. (2013). Comprehensive methodology for identification of kratom in police laboratories. *Forensic Science International, 233*(1), 238–243.

Kronstrand, R., Roman, M., Thelander, G., & Eriksson, A. (2011). Unintentional fatal intoxications with mitragynine and O-desmethyltramadol from the herbal blend Krypton. *Journal of Analytical Toxicology, 35*(4), 242–247.

Lee, M. A., & Shlain, B. (1985). *Acid dreams: The complete social history of LSD: The CIA, the sixties, and beyond.* New York City, NY: Grove Press.

Macko, E., Weisbach, J., & Douglas, B. (1972). Some observations on the pharmacology of mitragynine. *Archives Internationales de Pharmacodynamie et de Therapie, 198*(1), 145.

Miller, J. M., Griffin, O. H., & Gardner, C. M. (2016). Opiate treatment in the criminal justice system: A review of crimesolutions.gov evidence rated programs. *American Journal of Criminal Justice, 41*(1), 70–82.

Mowry, J. B., Spyker, D. A., Brooks, D. E., McMillan, N., & Schauben, J. L. (2015). 2014 Annual report of the American Association of Poison Control Centers' National Poison Data System (NPDS): 32nd annual report. *Clinical Toxicology, 53*(10), 962–1147.

Neerman, M. F., Frost, R. E., & Deking, J. (2013). A drug fatality involving kratom. *Journal of Forensic Sciences, 58*(s1), S278–S279.

Nelsen, J. L., Lapoint, J., Hodgman, M. J., & Aldous, K. M. (2010). Seizure and coma following kratom (Mitragyna speciosa Korth) exposure. *Journal of Medical Toxicology, 6*(4), 424–426.

Rosenbaum, C. D., Carreiro, S. P., & Babu, K. M. (2012). Here today, gone tomorrow. . . and back again? A review of herbal marijuana alternatives (K2, Spice), synthetic cathinones (bath salts), kratom, *Salvia divinorum*, methoxetamine, and piperazines. *Journal of Medical Toxicology, 8*(1), 15–32.

Rosenbaum, M., & Doblin, R. (1991). Why MDMA should not have been made illegal. In J. A. Inciardi (Ed.), *The drug legalization debate* (pp. 135–146). Newbury Park, CA: Sage.

Schultes, R. E., Hofmann, A., & Ratsch, C. (1998). *Plants of the Gods: Their sacred, healing, and hallucinogenic powers.* Rochester, VT: Healing Arts Press.

Singh, D., Müller, C. P., & Vicknasingam, B. K. (2014). Kratom (Mitragyna speciosa) dependence, withdrawal symptoms and craving in regular users. *Drug and Alcohol Dependence, 139*, 132–137.

Spring, T. (2009, February 1). Lab tests of drugs purchased online reveal risks. *PC World.*

Sutherland, E. H. (1940). White-collar criminality. *American Sociological Review, 5*(1), 1–12.

Suwanlert, S. (1975). A study of kratom eaters in Thailand. *Bulletin on Narcotics, 27*(3), 21–27.

Swogger, M. T., Hart, E., Erowid, F., Erowid, E., Trabold, N., Yee, K., . . . Walsh, Z. (2015). Experiences of kratom users: A qualitative analysis. *Journal of psychoactive Drugs, 47*(5), 360–367.

Tanguay, P. (2011). *Kratom in Thailand.* Retrieved from http://speciosa.org/wp-content/uploads/2016/03/Transitional-Institutes-Analysis-Legislative-Reform-of-Drug-Policies-Addresses-Kratom-Law-Reform-in-Thailand.pdf

Tungtananuwat, W., & Lawanprasert, S. (2010). Fatal 4×100: Homemade kratom juice cocktail. *Journal of Health Research, 24*(1), 43–47.

Vicknasingam, B., Narayanan, S., Beng, G. T., & Mansor, S. M. (2010). The informal use of ketum (Mitragyna speciosa) for opioid withdrawal in the northern states of peninsular Malaysia and implications for drug substitution therapy. *International Journal of Drug Policy, 21*(4), 283–288.

Yusoff, N. H., Suhaimi, F. W., Vadivelu, R. K., Hassan, Z., Rümler, A., Rotter, A., . . . Navaratnam, V. (2016). Abuse potential and adverse cognitive effects of mitragynine (kratom). *Addiction Biology, 21*(1), 98–110.

Chapter 6
Bubbling with Controversy: Legal Challenges for Ceremonial Ayahuasca Circles in the United States

Kevin Feeney, Beatriz Caiuby Labate, and J. Hamilton Hudson

Abstract The use of ayahuasca has been spreading rapidly worldwide; however, no current statistics are available to provide a comprehensive understanding of the scope or pace of this expansion. In the United States, the expansion has included the appearance of the Brazilian ayahuasca religions Santo Daime and União do Vegetal (UDV), underground ceremonial circles, workshops with itinerant Amazonian shamans, and spiritual retreat centers. This trend has included the recent emergence of groups and organizations that publicly advertise "legal" ayahuasca ceremonies and retreats. This chapter maps the existence of a series of organizations and actors who have controversially claimed legal protection through incorporation as "branches" of the Native American Church (NAC). The legality, religious character, and sincerity of these churches are reviewed in light of governing law, such as the First Amendment of the US Constitution, the Religious Freedom Restoration Act (RFRA), the Controlled Substances Act (CSA), and pertinent court cases involving the UDV and the Santo Daime, as well as ethnographic accounts of the historical Native American Church. Finally, it examines a petition for a religious exemption from the CSA from Ayahuasca Healings and speculates on the possibilities of the future of ayahuasca legality in the United States.

K. Feeney (✉)
Central Washington University, Ellensburg, WA, USA
e-mail: feeneyk@cwu.edu

B. C. Labate
East-West Psychology Program, California Institute of Integral Studies (CIIS), San Francisco, CA, USA

Center for Research and Post Graduate Studies in Social Anthropology (CIESAS), Guadalajara, Mexico
e-mail: blabate@bialabate.net

J. H. Hudson
Tulane University, New Orleans, USA

Interdisciplinary Group for Psychoactive Studies (NEIP), Brazil/USA, Boulder, CO, USA
e-mail: jhudson2@tulane.edu

© Springer International Publishing AG, part of Springer Nature 2018   87
B. C. Labate, C. Cavnar (eds.), *Plant Medicines, Healing and Psychedelic Science*,
https://doi.org/10.1007/978-3-319-76720-8_6

Introduction

Public advertisements for "legal" ayahuasca ceremonies have recently begun surfacing in the United States, a development that has caused consternation among researchers, activists, and others working strategically to develop a legal framework to protect ceremonial ayahuasca use. Some of these emergent groups offer the spiritual benefits of an ayahuasca ceremony in a local environment, with "guaranteed" legal protections for their customers. However, while two of the main Brazilian ayahuasca religions have secured legal protections to use ayahuasca as a sacrament in the United States, ayahuasca contains a highly regulated Schedule I substance, the use and possession of which is prohibited outside the confines of these specific religious organizations. Advertisements for "legal" ayahuasca pose legal and financial risks for unknowing members of the public and threaten to undermine legitimate efforts to protect the religious and spiritual use of this sacramental brew.

While indigenous peoples of the Upper Amazon have used ayahuasca from time immemorial, ayahuasca has recently gained a worldwide following with different modalities of use, including religious, therapeutic (e.g., the treatment of depression, anxiety, and substance use problems, among others), and in the context of neo-shamanic circles for personal healing and spiritual development (Labate & Cavnar, 2014a, 2014b; Labate, Cavnar, & Gearin, 2017; Labate & Jungaberle, 2011). Typically prepared by boiling the spiraling liana, *Banisteriopsis caapi*, together with the leaves of either the shrub *Psychotria viridis* or the liana *Diplopterys cabrerana*, ayahuasca contains the substance N,N-dimethyltryptamine (DMT), which is partially responsible for the psychoactive effects of this brew. DMT is a Schedule I drug under the US Controlled Substances Act (CSA) and regulated internationally under the 1971 United Nations Convention on Psychotropic Substances (Labate & Feeney, 2012; Sánchez & Bouso, 2015; Tupper & Labate, 2012).

We begin with a brief discussion of ayahuasca use in the United States, followed by a description of the Brazilian ayahuasca religions, União do Vegetal (UDV) and Santo Daime, and their successful legal battles to protect their sacramental ayahuasca use. The resulting scope and structure of these individualized rights is then examined. Next, based on fieldwork and media research, we address other groups that identify as "churches" that have followed the lead of the UDV and Santo Daime in claiming their own rights to use ayahuasca as a sacrament. These include the Oklevueha Native American Churches (Ayahuasca Healings, AYA Quest, Peaceful Mountain Way, and Soul Quest) and other unaffiliated churches, like the Arizona Yagé Assembly (AYA). Next, we consider the role of the First Amendment's free-exercise clause, the Controlled Substances Act (CSA), and the Religious Freedom Restoration Act (RFRA) in determining the rights of religious groups in relation to ayahuasca. Finally, we examine a petition for a CSA religious exemption submitted to the Drug Enforcement Agency (DEA) by Ayahuasca Healings in 2016. Throughout this chapter, we attempt to provide the reader with two things: a brief overview of new ayahuasca circles in the United States and an understanding of the legal obstacles faced by groups seeking religious exemptions for their ayahuasca practices.

Ayahuasca Use in the United States

Over the last 30 years, interest in ayahuasca in the United States has grown from an obscure curiosity, mostly known from the writings of William Burroughs and Allen Ginsburg (Burroughs & Ginsburg, 1963) or the works of ethnobotanist Richard Evans Schultes, into mainstream awareness, with references popping up on network television, in Hollywood films, and reports printed in widely read publications. Indeed, the knowledge and use of ayahuasca seem to have spread all over the United States, with weekend ceremonies being held in large- and medium-sized cities around the country. According to our fieldwork, the current underground ceremonial circles are usually small and are frequently led by itinerant indigenous shamans, nonindigenous practitioners trained (to various degrees) in Amazonian shamanism or former Santo Daime and UDV members.[1] Most of these groups have a fluctuating number of followers and frequently charge some fee for participation. Some groups have incorporated as NGOs or as religious organizations (usually not mentioning the use of ayahuasca), and others present themselves as branches of the Native American Church, a Native American peyote religion that has received an exemption from Congress to pray with their sacrament and spiritual "medicine," peyote (*Lophophora williamsii*).

Recreational use of ayahuasca appears to be minimal, with most groups operating in ceremonial settings and adhering to certain ritual protocols. Frequently, these groups follow similar ritual patterns and share certain practices and beliefs, suggesting that, although autonomous and independent of one another, they are characteristic of larger social and cultural trends. Similarities between these groups and their ceremonies include the belief that ayahuasca is some kind of "plant teacher," "sacrament," or "medicine"; facilitation by a trained leader; screening and orientation for participants; limiting ayahuasca consumption to ceremonial contexts; employment of symbols in the ceremonial setting; ritual parameters for the frequency and amount of ayahuasca served; and provision of some sort of counseling or integration for participants following a ceremony. One notable trend seems to be the regular fragmentation and creation of new groups, as well as a fluid membership.

Ayahuasca-drinking groups in the United States exist on a legal spectrum ranging from the permitted to the prohibited. At one end of the spectrum is the UDV, which is the only ayahuasca religion permitted to use ayahuasca throughout the country. Next is Santo Daime, branches of which have permission to use ayahuasca in its ceremonies in Oregon, California, and Washington State. All other ayahuasca groups in the United States, as we will see, lack legal protections for the sacramental or ceremonial use of ayahuasca. While the proliferation of these groups suggests a strong degree of interest in the perceived healing and spiritual properties of this

---

[1] Author Beatriz C. Labate conducted fieldwork with various underground ceremonial circles in the United States between 2007 and 2017 and has also conducted fieldwork with US branches of the Santo Daime and UDV.

brew—a considerable phenomenon that should be taken seriously by policy makers—we limit ourselves here to examining these groups within the current legal framework.

The Brazilian Ayahuasca Religions: União do Vegetal and Santo Daime

Both of the major Brazilian ayahuasca religions, the União do Vegetal (UDV) and the Santo Daime, trace their origins to the twentieth-century boom and bust of the rubber-tapping industry in Brazil. The boom brought hordes of working class Brazilians into the jungles of the Amazon, where they encountered local indigenous and mestizo communities who used ayahuasca. Through the combination of Amerindian shamanism with Catholicism, African religiosity, and European esotericism, these new religious movements arose. With the collapse of rubber prices in the 1940s, many of these Brazilians returned to their home communities, some of whom brought awareness of ayahuasca and a newfound faith back with them.

The UDV was founded in 1961 by Brazilian rubber tapper José Gabriel da Costa in the state of Rondônia, Brazil, and the Santo Daime was founded by a Brazilian rubber tapper named Raimundo Irineu Serra and was formally established in 1945 in the State of Acre. Both the Santo Daime and the UDV have Christian doctrines, religious hierarchies, and special ritual clothing and calendars. Both rely on oral traditions, and neither have a central religious text. The UDV's services are characterized by preaching and the sharing of stories containing spiritual teachings, whereas Santo Daime worship is characterized by the singing of religious hymns that are spiritually received and sung collectively. Of the two, the UDV is more structured and hierarchical, with a strong conservative ethos. In both contexts, ayahuasca is syncretized with the figure of the religion's founder (Mestre Irineu for Santo Daime and Mestre Gabriel for UDV) and Christian symbols and is considered a central sacrament, the *sine qua non* condition of communion with the divine.

União do Vegetal in the United States

The UDV arrived in the United States in 1988, when its first sessions were held in Norwood, Colorado. In 1999, US custom agents seized a batch of *hoasca* (ayahuasca) arriving from Brazil and threatened members of the UDV with prosecution under the CSA (Bronfman 2007, 2011). In response, the UDV sought an injunction preventing the federal government from enforcing the CSA against them.

In 2006, the Supreme Court granted the UDV an injunction temporarily preventing the DEA from enforcing the CSA against their sacramental ayahuasca use. The court's ruling, while momentous, did not end the dispute. The DEA was left with the option to continue to gather evidence and build a case against the UDV, and risk a more serious precedent-setting loss, or to exert its power in shaping a limited exception specific to the UDV. Ultimately, the DEA and UDV entered into an agreement allowing the UDV to import and distribute hoasca for UDV religious ceremonies under the watchful eye of the DEA (Labate, 2012; UDV v. Holder, 2010). Under the terms of the agreement, every UDV congregation that directly imports hoasca must apply for DEA registration and must give 2 weeks advanced notice of shipments entering the United States (UDV v. Holder, 2010). Records must be maintained and submitted for DEA inspection, and any congregation wishing to cultivate plants for the production of hoasca must register with the DEA as a manufacturer of controlled substances. While the UDV won a significant victory, the freedoms enjoyed by the UDV were achieved through collaboration with law enforcement and are subject to a number of regulations and controls.

Santo Daime in the United States

Santo Daime's first US branch was founded in Boston, Massachusetts, in 1988. Like the UDV, Santo Daime's legal troubles also began in 1999, following the apprehension of a shipment of *daime* (ayahuasca) from Brazil. Santo Daime's court controversies came later than the UDV's, and they were able to benefit from the precedent set by the UDV. Santo Daime's legal controversies, however, have been lower profile and more localized than the UDV's.

In 2008, two Oregon Santo Daime branches, Church of the Holy Light of the Queen and Church of the Divine Rose, filed jointly in the Federal District Court of Oregon for injunctive relief from enforcement of the CSA against their religious use of daime. The following year the Court granted relief under RFRA, ordering a permanent injunction prohibiting the DEA from threatening the church with prosecution (Church of the Holy Light of the Queen v. Mukasey, 2009). The DEA appealed, and 2 years later the Ninth Circuit affirmed the injunction (Church of the Holy Light of the Queen v. Holder, 2011).

In 2014, driving the point home, the Ninth Circuit ordered the government to pay Santo Daime's attorney fees (Church of the Holy Light of the Queen v. Holder, 2014). The scope of these legal successes, however, is limited to the involved congregations and their activities in the state of Oregon and does not apply to congregations in other states. Consequently, new congregations must apply separately for permits. This type of localized effort was part of the Santo Daime's original legal strategy, and other chapters have since followed suit with successful petitions for exemptions in both California and Washington.

Roy Haber (2011), one of Santo Daime's attorneys for the case, later shared that the federal government had encouraged Santo Daime to submit a petition for an exemption from the CSA rather than file a lawsuit (just as the DEA would later encourage Ayahuasca Healings, Soul Quest, and others to submit their own petitions, as we detail in this chapter). According to Haber, filing such a petition would have been unfavorable to Santo Daime, since the reviewing agency, the DEA, has as its primary purpose the enforcement of federal drug laws, a reality that should raise questions about the impartiality and fairness of the petition process. Haber encouraged Santo Daime to file a lawsuit, not a petition, because a lawsuit would be heard in a neutral court of law by an impartial judge, rather than by the agency designated with enforcement of the nation's drug laws. While the Oregon chapters of Santo Daime found victory in court, chapters in California and Washington have subsequently found success through the petition process.

The New Ayahuasca "Native American Churches" in the United States

Currently, a variety of ayahuasca circles are proliferating in the United States. We will focus here on one aspect of this phenomenon: the emergence of ayahuasca circles that identify themselves as branches of the Native American Church. Like the Santo Daime and the UDV, these organizations are also driven by a group of people united around the ceremonial use of ayahuasca; however, these groups typically have significantly looser organizational structures and membership and tend to lack a concrete religious doctrine. Significantly, these groups appear to lack cultural, historical, and political ties to the Native American Church, an indigenous institution that developed among tribal peoples of the continental United States during the late nineteenth century. The practice of incorporating as a "Native American Church" has been promoted among non-Natives by James "Flaming Eagle" Mooney, founder of the Oklevueha NAC (ONAC), as a means for these groups to acquire "legal" protection for their ayahuasca use. However, this promotion has relied upon a misrepresentation of the law, the history, and the nature of the NAC, as well as ONAC's legitimacy as part of this unique pan-Indian institution.

A little background on the NAC and its religious exemption for ceremonial peyote use is required to understand the source of ONAC's legal claims and why they are unfounded. The Native American Church, first formally incorporated in 1918, has its roots in the nineteenth century removal of Native peoples from their traditional territories and onto reservations in the United States. This forced relocation was the coup de grâce for Native American peoples and their cultures, ultimately leading to a collapse in the social, economic, and political structures that held these communities together. The peyote religion emerged during the Reservation Era as a mechanism for rebuilding Native communities, creating new social structures and solidarity between disparate tribes and providing a sense of hope and meaning, as well as a mechanism for building and maintaining a distinctive Native identity (Feeney, 2007; Slotkin, 1956). The peyote religion has continued to be an important Native institution, offering healing, spiritual guidance, social support, and other benefits for its adherents. The importance of this religious institution was recognized by the federal government when, in 1965, an exemption for the religious use of peyote was provided to "members of the Native American Church" and, again in 1994, when federal protections for Native peyote religions were adopted by Congress (Code of Federal Regulations [CFR], 1971; Feeney, 2007).

The NAC is not hierarchical like some religious institutions but rather is a confederation of loosely associated churches with localized leadership. While there is some variation in the ritual, protocol, and cosmology between different chapters, the core structure of the rituals and belief systems are consistent, including the manner in which one becomes a Roadman or ceremonial leader of the Church. The other commonality is that, while some chapters are multiracial, NAC chapters arise out of Native communities and are predominantly peopled by members of these communities (Feeney, 2014).

Within this context, ayahuasca churches in the United States identifying as branches of the "Native American Church" can be seen as both appropriating the NAC name as well as attempting to exploit the special protections provided to members of the NAC. The basis for claiming the NAC title appears to be grounded upon two key, but misguided, beliefs: (1) that the specific exemption for NAC ceremonial peyote use extends to other sacraments designated as controlled substances in the United States and (2) that anyone can start, lead, or be a member of a NAC branch. Another apparent justification for the creation of simulated Native American Church branches is the questionable belief that individuals are justified in appropriating the NAC title due to the perceived unfairness of Native Americans being granted certain rights that are denied to non-Natives. And a variation on this belief, equally disputable, is that many people feel justified in using any and all mechanisms to legitimize their practices due to a perception that US drug laws themselves are either unfair or unjust.

The proliferation of non-Native NACs (non-NACs) and ayahuasca-NACs has been promoted by James "Flaming Eagle" Mooney, an individual with disputed claims to Native American ancestry, who started his own branch of the NAC, Oklevueha Native American Church (ONAC), in the late 1990s, and has since turned its expansion into a business model. Part of Mooney's success has to do with a victory in the Utah Supreme Court that found ONAC's use of peyote to be protected (State of Utah v. Mooney, 2004). The court determined that state law deferred to a federal regulation exempting "members of the Native American Church" from criminal prosecution (see CFR, 1971) and found that the plain language of the regulation protected members of any organization carrying the name "Native American Church," regardless of the structure, history, or nature of the organization. However, the laws of Utah were revised in 2006 to apply specifically to "members of federally recognized tribes" and to exclude organizations like Mooney's ONAC (Utah Controlled Substances Act, 2017). Despite this fundamental legal change, Mooney turned his defunct court victory into an advertising campaign for the commercialization of ONAC, as well as the right to use and possess controlled substances that, he claims, ONAC membership confers (Feeney, 2014).

Though ONAC has been publicly denounced as illegitimate by most Native American Churches (National Council of Native American Churches, 2016), Mooney runs a website where one can purchase an ONAC membership card for a "contribution" of $200, pronouncing, "Being a member of ONAC qualifies this card-holder to carry and/or possess bird of prey feathers and Native American Church sacraments (Peyote, Ayahuasca, Cannabis, etc.)" (ONAC, 2017). Despite the fact that ayahuasca and cannabis are not NAC sacraments and that several ONAC members have been arrested and prosecuted for possession, cultivation, and distribution of cannabis (Carpenter, 2014), the use of ONAC cards for "legal protection" appears to be relatively widespread.

In addition to selling membership cards, ONAC had a long-standing practice of selling church chapters, which included Articles of Incorporation, among other things. For the price of $2495, individuals could start their own chapter of ONAC and, according to the ONAC website, establish legal "protection to worship with any and all earth-based Sacraments" (ONAC, 2000–2012). For many, $2495 appeared a small price to pay for an exemption from the CSA, and an opportunity to set up their own ayahuasca-based churches. While ONAC appears to have discontinued publicly advertising the sale of church branches, the proliferation of ONAC churches continues to gain momentum.

Over 200 branches of ONAC-affiliated churches have been incorporated since the Mooneys' first established their church in 1997, with no fewer than 35 chapters established since 2013 (Callicott, 2017).[2] The exact number of ONAC branches is hard to estimate, as many of these groups fluctuate in size and duration and frequently multiple chapters are associated with a single individual or group of individuals. More research is needed in this area to determine the actual scope and influence of ONAC and its affiliates. Similarly, it is unclear how many of these churches are ayahuasca-based, rather than cannabis or peyote oriented, but our preliminary research findings demonstrate that at least four ONAC-affiliated churches use ayahuasca as their primary "sacrament."

While some ONAC branches and affiliates are overtly commercial, advertising their services online for a fee, others fly under the radar. These churches generally claim a mixed Native American and Christian spiritual heritage, with ayahuasca-oriented branches additionally claiming links to one of the Brazilian ayahuasca religions or to indigenous shamans from Peru, Colombia, Brazil, or Ecuador. Some use multiple substances, and some incorporate North American indigenous rituals, such as the sweat lodge or vision quest, as well. Notably, four of the five organizations discussed below have specifically identified as an ONAC chapter at some point in its timeline.

---

[2]While we have been able to identify over 200 ONAC-affiliated churches, Mooney himself estimates the total number to be nearer to 300 (Brown 2016).

Ayahuasca Healings

A British man named Marc "Kumbooja Banyan Tree" Shackman formed Ayahuasca Healings in 2015 with a former Internet marketer from Toronto, Canada, named Christopher "Trinity" de Guzman. Their goal was to "bring this sacred medicine of Ayahuasca to the American public" by establishing "more than 200" ayahuasca churches throughout the United States (McGivern, 2016, p. 2). Initially a branch of a now-defunct ONAC chapter, the New Haven Native American Church (NHNAC), Ayahuasca Healings developed its church premises in Elbe, Washington, and professed, on its website and in various advertisements and press releases, to be "the first public legal ayahuasca church in the United States" (Callicott, 2017). A 2015 promotion for Ayahuasca Healings garnered tens of thousands of "likes" and "shares" on the social media website Facebook.

Ayahuasca Healings' radical claims about their legal status caused both excitement and suspicion among those with an interest in ayahuasca. Online investigations into the backgrounds of de Guzman and Shackman, as well as the history of Mooney and ONAC, began to emerge (Callicott, 2017; Highpine, 2015a, 2015b; Hudson, 2015), and the high-profile rollout of Ayahuasca Healings began to unravel. An anonymous Facebook group called "Ayahuasca Healings is NOT legal" was started to warn interested parties about the dubious claims of Ayahuasca Healings. As the controversy reached a boiling point, ONAC founder James "Flaming Eagle" Mooney contacted Ayahuasca Healings and convinced them that ONAC's legal protections were stronger than NHNAC. Ayahuasca Healings dumped NHNAC and adopted a direct affiliation to ONAC, changing its name to ONAC-Ayahuasca Healings. Despite this change, Ayahuasca Healings legitimacy issues remained unresolved and its troubles continued (for a history of this controversy, see Callicott, 2017).

On February 29, 2016, 5 weeks after Ayahuasca Healings officially began operations, it held its final retreat. On March 8, a public letter was released announcing that Ayahuasca Healings was temporarily suspending its operations (Callicott, 2017). What the statement did not disclose was that Ayahuasca Healings had received a forceful letter from the DEA, warning that possession and distribution of ayahuasca are criminal offenses in the United States and informing it that if it wished to continue operations, it should first submit—and have approved—a petition for a religious exemption from prosecution under the CSA.[3]

After ceasing operations, Ayahuasca Healings began consultation with a local attorney to develop a legal strategy for acquiring an exemption to serve ayahuasca at their ceremonial retreats. On April 4, 2016, Ayahuasca Healings filed a petition for a religious exemption from the CSA (McGivern, 2016). At the time of this writing, no response from the DEA had been received; nevertheless, an analysis of the legal

---

[3]This document was briefly posted on the Internet. Unfortunately, it was removed before the authors were able to catalogue it, and it is no longer publicly available.

merits of this petition may prove instructive to others. We will examine this petition at greater length below.

Soul Quest

Chris Young and his wife Verena Young founded Soul Quest Church of Mother Earth ("Soul Quest"), based in Orlando, Florida, in 2014 (Soul Quest, 2016). It was initially a branch of ONAC but cuts ties with ONAC in 2016. Chris Young is an active public leader for the young organization, attending psychedelic conferences, engaging in debates on social media, giving media interviews, and participating in a documentary film ("From Shock to Awe") detailing the experiences of American war veterans in Soul Quest ayahuasca retreats. Similar to Ayahuasca Healings, Soul Quest advertises widely and charges a fee for participation in its ayahuasca ceremonies. Perhaps unsurprisingly then, Soul Quest received a letter from the DEA in August 2016, advising it to cease and desist the use of ayahuasca (Milione, 2016a). In its letter, the DEA advised Soul Quest to cease its use of several other sacraments as well, including *sananga*, which the DEA stated contains the Schedule I substance ibogaine, and *San Pedro*, which contains the Schedule I substance mescaline. Soul Quest responded, claiming to be a "hybrid of Native American spirituality and Christianity" and "very much akin" to the UDV, and therefore justified in its "religious" practices (Brett, 2016, p. 1). Unlike the UDV, however, Soul Quest advertised fee-based ceremonies online; ceremonies involving multiple plant and animal-derived substances, including *kambô* (venom from the bicolor tree frog [*Phyllomedusa bicolor*]), *rapé* (a tobacco-based snuff with varying admixtures), and *sananga* (probably *Tabernaemontana undulata*).[4] Despite Soul Quest's claims to have "Native American" and Brazilian roots, there is little to no known documentation of their religious practices or beliefs. On a webpage titled "Church Doctrine," Soul Quest refers interested parties to a document titled "Ayahuasca Manifesto," an anonymous document circulated online since 2011 that outlines "the moral standard and spiritual guidance" for ayahuasca use (Anonymous, 2011, p. 46).

Soul Quest initially responded to the DEA by challenging the exemption process itself. Its criticism of the exemption process was two-fold: first, the process gives the DEA too much discretion with too little oversight; and second, the process has no clear timetable for completion (Brett, 2016). The DEA replied on December 21, 2016, stating that its exemption process fully complies with the law (Milione, 2016b).

---

[4]The DEA claims *Tabernaemontana undulata*, like *Tabernanthe iboga*, contains the Schedule I drug, ibogaine, but this is disputed.

Despite Soul Quest's initial rejection of the exemption process, the submission of a formal DEA petition was announced to their membership in August 2017.[5]

Other New Ayahuasca Native American Churches

Besides Ayahuasca Healing and Soul Quest, we have identified two other, relatively conspicuous, ayahuasca-oriented ONAC affiliates. One of these organizations, Aya Quest Native American Church in Kentucky, advertises itself as "a place to take the journey to source and to meet who you really are for the very first time" (Aya Quest, 2015). Steven Hupp, founder of Aya Quest, claims to have been trained by a "South American shaman" on how to brew ayahuasca and acts as the group's "chief medicine man." Aya Quest offers ayahuasca retreats from between $395 and $995 and also offers kambô workshops for $260 (Aya Quest, 2015). The second church, known as ONAC of the Peaceful Mountain Way, was established in 2015 and is also based in Kentucky. The Peaceful Mountain Way offers both group and private ceremonies, ranging in price from $375 to $1050 (Peaceful Mountain Way, 2015–2017). Peaceful Mountain Way, as well as Mooney's parent ONAC Church, is currently the subject of a wrongful death lawsuit following the death of a young woman tied to an ayahuasca ceremony held by the church in the fall of 2016 (Kocher, 2017).

Another organization, Arizona Yagé Assembly (AYA), while not under the ONAC umbrella, appears to be inspired by their model. AYA, based in Tucson, espouses a mission "to bring people in communion with divine love through the sacrament of ayahuasca" (AYA, 2017). AYA advertises extensively and currently holds ceremonies around the United States, from St. Louis, Missouri, to Tucson, Arizona, and San Francisco, California, with participation fees ranging from $150 to $250 (Aya Guide, 2015). According to our fieldwork, this group has also expressed intentions to petition for an exemption from the DEA.

Ayahuasca Law in the United States

One of the two ingredients of ayahuasca, *P. viridis*, known by its Quechua name *chacruna*, contains the substance N,N-dimethyltryptamine (DMT). DMT is classi-fied as a Schedule I substance under the CSA, meaning that DMT has no currently

---

[5]We have not had a chance to access this document; however, we have continued to observe the unfolding of the controversy, which included Soul Quest announcing that instead of using ayahua-sca, it was using "vine only" (only *Banisteriopsis caapi*) in their ceremonies (see https:// ayahuascachurches.org/schedule/). This would probably be seen by the DEA as evidence that "feasible alternatives" are available, and DMT-containing ayahuasca is not sufficiently "important" to Soul Quest's practices to warrant an exemption (see Table 6.1).

accepted medical use and has a high potential for abuse (CSA, 1970). Because the ayahuasca preparation contains DMT, a Schedule I substance, ayahuasca is also considered a Schedule I substance under US law (DEA, 2016; Gonzáles v. UDV, 2016).

The UDV's legal right to use ayahuasca in religious ceremonies is based on, and supported by, the Religious Freedom Restoration Act (RFRA). Congress passed RFRA in 1993 in response to the notorious 1990 Supreme Court decision in *Employment Division v. Smith* that overturned decades of First Amendment jurisprudence and left the free-exercise clause a shell of its former self. The opinion, written by the late Justice Antonin Scalia, claimed that the First Amendment only protects religious freedoms if a religious practice is intentionally targeted for discriminatory treatment. Laws that "incidentally" burden religious practices, according to this ruling, are valid Constitutional restrictions on religious practices. Under this interpretation, so-called "neutral" laws, laws that burden religious practices without necessarily intending to do so, constitute valid restrictions on religious practices.

In the *Smith* controversy, two NAC members were fired and denied unemployment compensation based on their religious use of the peyote cactus. They challenged the denial of unemployment benefits as a violation of their free-exercise rights under the First Amendment. The Supreme Court, finding no evidence that Congress intended to burden Native American religious practices when scheduling peyote, determined that the Controlled Substances Act was "neutral" toward all religions and therefore did not violate the free-exercise clause.

Religious groups around the country recognized the implications of the *Smith* decision, and a diverse political coalition was quickly assembled, with members as disparate as Pat Robertson's American Center for Law and Justice and the American Civil Liberties Union, in order to pressure Congress for reform (Epps, 2001). In response, Congress passed RFRA, which restored the Compelling Interest test, a balancing test used for decades by courts, prior to *Smith*, in order to weigh the religious interests of practitioners against the regulatory interests of government. Under this test, a religious practitioner wishing to challenge a government regulation must demonstrate that the regulation in question substantially burdens a religious practice that is based on sincere belief. In response, the government carries the burden to prove two things: first, that there is a compelling governmental interest behind the challenged regulation, and second, that the regulation in question is the least restrictive means of furthering that compelling governmental interest (RFRA, 1993).

In *Gonzales v. O Centro Beneficente União do Vegetal* (2006), the Supreme Court found that the sacramental use of hoasca by the UDV was substantially burdened by the CSA, a finding that required the government to demonstrate a compelling interest in prohibiting ayahuasca use and showing that the CSA is *narrowly tailored* to achieve that goal. The federal government put forward three goals it argued constituted compelling government interests: (1) protecting the health and safety of UDV members, (2) preventing diversion of hoasca to the black market, and (3) remaining compliant with US obligations under the Convention on Psychotropic Substances (CPS). The government failed on all three counts. First, the court found scientific evidence of harm to be inconclusive, particularly in light of evidence offered by the UDV demonstrating the safety of hoasca when used in a controlled ritual setting. Second, the government failed to provide sufficient evidence of either a black-market demand or instances of diversion. Finally, the court determined that being a signatory of CPS, by itself, was not sufficient to constitute a compelling government interest. It was the outcome of this decision that ultimately led to the arrangements between the UDV and DEA to permit the sacramental use of hoasca with DEA regulatory oversight.

Since the UDV's RFRA victory in 2006, a number of groups proclaiming religious use of various substances have attempted to establish their own legal rights. The first of these to receive a DEA response was the Church of Reality, a cannabis-based church in California. The Church of Reality's RFRA petition merits discussion, particularly since the DEA laid out a lengthy 33-page roadmap for RFRA petitions in its denial of the Church's petition.

The Church of Reality's Petition

In 2007, shortly after the victory of the UDV at the Supreme Court, the Church of Reality contacted the DEA to proclaim its sacramental use of marijuana and acquire an exemption from the CSA. A lengthy back and forth ensued, while the DEA tried to establish what information they needed to determine whether a group had a meritorious legal claim under RFRA. In 2008, the DEA issued its denial (Rannazzisi, 2008) and outlined the elements required for a successful RFRA petition (Table 6.1).

First, in order to invoke RFRA, a religious organization must demonstrate that the challenged law or regulation substantially burdens a religious practice based in sincere belief. This means that the organization must demonstrate that the practice in question is (1) religious in nature, (2) based in sincere belief, and (3) substantially burdened by a specific government regulation. An organization that satisfies these three criteria is considered to have established what is known as a *prima facie* case, which means the group has presented a meritorious claim that is likely to be successful. Once this is done, the government carries the burden of refuting the organization's claim.

In its rejection of the Church of Reality's petition, the DEA found that the Church of Reality did not qualify as a *true* religion, that it's beliefs were *insincere*, and that its purported religious practices were not substantially burdened by the CSA. Problematically, RFRA provides no definition for "religion"; thus, courts have been left to develop their own criteria. The DEA outlined five guidelines for determining whether a particular group's practices and beliefs qualify as religious, three of which it applied to the Church of Reality's petition. The first guideline addressed whether a group's beliefs involve "fundamental and ultimate ideas that address reality beyond the physical world" (Rannazzisi, 2008, p. 7); the second, whether a group's beliefs represent a comprehensive moral and ethical system; and

Table 6.1 Elements of a prima facie case under RFRA, specifically for challenges to the Controlled Substances Act (*Gonzales v. UDV, 2006; Rannazzisi, 2008; United States v. Meyers, 1995; United States v. Quaintance, 2006*)

1. **Exercise of religion** (criteria for evaluating religion):
(a) Fundamental & ultimate ideas
(b) Metaphysical beliefs
(c) Moral or ethical system
(d) Comprehensive belief system
(e) Accoutrements (structural characteristics) of religion
2. **Religious beliefs sincerely held** (criteria for evaluating sincerity):
(a) Ad hoc beliefs
(b) Quantity of controlled substance
(c) Evidence of commerce
(d) Lack of ceremony or rituals
(e) Use of other controlled substances
3. **Religious exercise substantially burdened by government regulation** (Inquiries for evaluating the degree of burden):
(a) Is burdened practice "important"?
(b) Are "feasible alternatives" to the practice available?
When the above elements are met, the burden shifts to the government to prove a "Compelling Interest" in the challenged regulation, and to show that the regulation is "Narrowly Tailored" to meet that goal.

the third, whether a group has structural characteristics "that may be analogized to accepted religions" (2008, p. 10, citing *Africa v. Commonwealth* 1981, p. 1035). This analysis comes before the question of "sincerity" and whether government regulations pose a substantial burden on a religion's practices.

Expounding on the "fundamental and ultimate ideas" criterion, the DEA quoted from the decision in *Meyers* involving another cannabis church, explaining that religious beliefs generally "address a reality which transcends the physical and immediately apparent world" (Rannazzisi, 2008, p. 7, citing *Meyers*, p. 1502). Deeper, such beliefs "address a fear of the unknown, the pain of loss, a sense of alienation, feelings of purposelessness, the inexplicability of the world, and the prospects of eternity" (2008, p. 7, citing *Meyers*, p. 1505). The DEA found the Church of Reality's proclamation that its beliefs are "based on the acceptance of the axiom that our existence is important and that expanding our understanding of reality has value," and that its explanation that "the Church of Reality is a new breed of religion that is based on reality rather than mythology," "does not appear to differentiate the Church's pursuits from that of science or philosophy" (2008, pp. 7–8). Lacking any metaphysical belief system, or any beliefs addressing life's great questions, the Church of Reality's belief system did not address fundamental or ultimate ideas about life and reality.

Next, the DEA assessed whether the Church of Reality's beliefs included a comprehensive moral and ethical system. The DEA focused on whether the Church of Reality prescribed a certain way of life, categorizing certain behavior as good or evil, right or wrong, and just or unjust, and provided answers to many of the human problems and concerns. Citing the District Court in *United States v. Quaintance* (2006), the DEA explained that a comprehensive moral or ethical system "should create duties imposed by some higher power, force or spirit, and should have religious consequences if the principles are not followed" (Rannazzisi, 2008, p. 9). Finding no evidence of spiritual or religious inspiration for the Church of Reality's "Sacred Principles," and based on the Church's own admission that the "Sacred Principles were generated in order to obtain 501(c)(3) tax exempt status," the DEA determined that the Church's "Sacred Principles" could not be characterized as "religious" (2008, p. 9).

Weighing the third criterion, structural and external characteristics of religions, the DEA considered whether the Church of Reality exhibited structural and external signs characteristic of accepted religions. These signs may include:

> formal ceremonies or rituals, gathering places, clergy and/or prophets, structure and organization, important writings, observance of holidays, efforts at propagation, diet or fasting, prescribed clothing and appearance, and other similar manifestations associated with traditional religions. (Rannazzisi, 2008, p. 10)

The DEA found that this "internet-based" religion lacked structure and organization, did not have clergy or prophets in any traditional sense, and specifically disavowed rituals on its website. Based on these deficits, the DEA determined that the Church of Reality did not have sufficient "accoutrements" of religion.

While the Church of Reality failed to demonstrate its religiousness, the DEA proceeded to evaluate the remaining elements of a prima facie RFRA case: (1) sincerity of belief and (2) a substantial government burden on "religious" practices. Addressing the issue of sincerity, the DEA outlined five separate bases for evaluating the sincerity of religious beliefs involving use of controlled substances: ad hoc beliefs, lack of ceremony or ritual, use of other illegal substances, evidence of commerce, and quantity of the substance involved (*United States v. Quaintance,* 2006). The DEA addressed the first three bases of sincerity in its response to the Church of Reality's petition.

The first of these bases, ad hoc beliefs, refer to beliefs that appear to be "manufactured on an *ad hoc* basis to justify [a] lifestyle" (Rannazzisi, 2008, p. 11). Several issues worked against the Church on this criterion, but perhaps the most significant was a long-standing practice of secular marijuana use, predating the founding of the Church, and an admission in its petition of using RFRA to "trump" federal law on issues with which the Church disagrees. The DEA determined that the Church failed the ad hoc test of sincerity, stating that the Church of Reality's "newfound religious beliefs appear to be rationalizations designed to justify [its] long-held political and medical views about the alleged benefits of marijuana use" (2008, p 12).

The second basis for insincerity, lack of ceremony or ritual, also worked against the Church of Reality, which offered no mention of ritual—a religious practice that the Church publicly disavows on its website. Thirdly, the DEA addressed the Church's use of other controlled substances in evaluating the sincerity of the

Church's religious beliefs. The DEA noted that in its petition, the Church described how members used other drugs, including "LSD, Mushrooms, Peyote and Hoasca," and also proclaimed that "Although our request at this time is for the use of marijuana, we are not limiting ourselves to just that one drug" (Rannazzisi, 2008, p. 13). Based on these statements, the DEA determined that the Church's "request is driven by a desire to use illegal substances, rather than a sincere religious belief" (2008, p. 13).

Finally, the DEA asked whether its prohibition on the Church of Reality's use of cannabis was a substantial burden on its religion. The DEA's question boiled down to whether the use of cannabis was "important" to the church's religious practice and whether feasible alternatives were available in the practice of the Church's professed religion. When the Church of Reality admitted that there were alternative ways for achieving its stated religious goal of "fostering creative thinking," and explained that Church of Reality members were permitted to use those alternatives, it failed to prove that marijuana prohibition posed a substantial burden on its "religious" practice (Rannazzisi, 2008, p. 13).

The DEA letter denying the Church of Reality's RFRA petition stands as an important document, as it clearly and substantively outlines the position and thinking of the DEA when it comes to sacramental drug use. In 2009, the DEA developed and published specific guidelines for individuals and organizations seeking a CSA exemption for religious use of a controlled substance. The document seeks to streamline the exemption process and presumably to prevent litigation of spurious claims. The process allows self-identified religious groups to make their case under RFRA by submitting a petition to the DEA demonstrating that its controlled substance use is based on a (1) sincere (2) religious practice that is (3) substantially burdened by the CSA (DEA, 2009). To aid in the evaluation of a group's request, the DEA requires petitions to include detailed information about:

(1) the nature of the religion (*e.g.* its history, belief system, structure, practice, membership policies, rituals, holidays, organization, leadership, *etc.*);
(2) each specific religious practice that involves the manufacture, distribution, dispensing, importation, exportation, use or possession of a controlled substance;
(3) the specific controlled substance that the party wishes to use; and
(4) the amounts, conditions, and locations of its anticipated manufacture, distribution, dispensing, importation, exportation, use or possession.(2009, p. 1)

The combination of the Church of Reality denial letter and the DEA-issued guidelines should provide religious ayahuasca groups a foundation for determining whether their beliefs and practices might qualify for a CSA exemption. Below, we consider how these required elements of the petition might benefit or disqualify different ayahuasca-using groups in the United States.

Ayahuasca Healings' Petition

Ayahuasca Healings filed a petition for an exemption from prosecution under the CSA pursuant to RFRA on April 4, 2016 (McGivern, 2016). Beginning its proof in earnest, Ayahuasca Healings looked to establish a prima facie case under RFRA (Table 6.1), by demonstrating the authenticity of its religion, the sincerity of its beliefs, and that its religious practices are substantially burdened by the CSA. To substantiate its religious authenticity, Ayahuasca Healings sought to demonstrate the presence of (1) fundamental and ultimate questions that address a reality beyond the physical world, (2) a comprehensive moral and ethical system, and (3) structural characteristics of religions in general, three criteria, as we have seen, that were used by the DEA in its evaluation of the Church of Reality.

For the first criterion, fundamental and ultimate questions, Ayahuasca Healings described its beliefs in a reality that transcends the physical world—the metaphysical spirit world into which Mother Ayahuasca enables entry; its belief in a transcendent Great Spirit, similar to a theistic Supreme Being, like God, Hashem, or Allah; and its understanding of the purpose of human life as serving something greater—the Great Spirit, Mother Earth, and Collective Humanity, its belief in reincarnation, and its philosophy of "filial piety through environmental stewardship" (McGivern, 2016, p. 6).

Ayahuasca Healings quoted extensively from its website, where de Guzman wrote "I have walked this path for countless years, or really, countless lifetimes, and this is all about one thing. . . Our Global Awakening" (McGivern, 2016, p. 6). At the heart of that awakening, for Ayahuasca Healings, appears to be the understanding that "we are all serving something so much greater than [ourselves]" (2016, p. 6).

For the second criterion, a comprehensive moral and ethical system, Ayahuasca Healings cited its philosophy of environmental stewardship, "a moral duty to act in accordance with the spiritual and ecological needs of the environment" as well as "a moral duty to act in accordance with the spiritual and physical needs of other persons" (McGivern, 2016, p. 7). Ayahuasca Healings described its understanding of the consequences of breaching those moral duties as akin to the Hindu principle of karma: any action one takes against another is simultaneously an action against oneself. Translating karma into Christian terms, Ayahuasca Healings cited Matthew 7:12, "Do unto others as you would have them do unto you" (2016, p. 7). But, in case karma and Matthew 7:12 were not sufficient to constitute a comprehensive moral and ethical system, Ayahuasca Healings added that it had adopted the ONAC Code of Ethics and Code of Conduct, which includes proscriptions for behavior toward women, children, family, and community, and required pledges such as "I commit to making effort to spend time each day in meditation and prayer, drawing closer to the Great Spirit. . ." and "I will never share sacraments or sell medicines to those who are not members of ONAC" (2016, p. 8).

Addressing the third criterion of religion, structural characteristics, Ayahuasca Healings submitted evidence of formal ceremonies and rituals, gathering places, clergy and prophets, organizational structure, efforts at propagation, diet and fasting, and belief in supernatural entities. Its gathering place is a "sacred tipi" erected on its land in Elbe, Washington. Its organizational structure consisted of an executive body with three members: de Guzman, Shackman, and another administrator. De Guzman was the "Visionary Director of the church" serving as spiritual teacher through "sermon-like videos published online" (McGivern, 2016, p. 9). Shackman was the "chief medicine man and church director," coordinating and overseeing on the ground church activities (2016, p. 9). Formal ceremonies and rituals include a "Sweat Lodge," purging or cleansing through the use of emetic and purgative plants, and the ritualized consumption of ayahuasca—which Ayahuasca Healings likened to Catholic Communion. Notably, these rituals have parallels among some indigenous groups of North and South America. Recognized clergy were described as "Medicine Men/Women... who have undergone long and extensive training with *curanderos* in the Amazonian jungles" (2016, p. 9). Dietary proscriptions, described in detail, included the "traditional Peruvian ayahuasca diet" (2016, p. 9). Ayahuasca Healings claimed to believe in supernatural entities like "Mother Ayahuasca, Father San Pedro, Great Spirit," as well as thousands of angels, the "Ascended Masters Buddha and Jesus," and countless animistic plant, animal, and mountain spirits (2016, p. 12).

Having addressed these three criteria of religious authenticity, Ayahuasca Healings set out to demonstrate that its beliefs are "sincerely held." To do so, Ayahuasca Healings addressed each of the five indicators of sincerity: ad hoc beliefs, lack of ceremony or ritual, quantity of controlled substance used, use of other controlled substances, and evidence of commerce. For the first and second indicators, Ayahuasca Healings stated simply that its beliefs were not ad hoc but derived "directly from shamanic, animist religions of the Amazon Rainforest and elements of other belief systems, most prominently that of Christianity" (McGivern, 2016, p. 3) and that Ayahuasca Healings holds frequent ceremonies. More challenging for Ayahuasca Healings was addressing the fourth and fifth indicators of sincerity/insincerity: the use of other controlled substances and evidence of commerce.

Ayahuasca Healings admittedly used another illegal substance, San Pedro, a *Trichocereus* cactus variety that contains the Schedule I controlled substance mescaline (McGivern, 2016, p. 13). To assuage the DEA's potential concerns, Ayahuasca Healings stated that it was not currently seeking an exemption for San Pedro—though it planned on doing so at a later date—and that San Pedro, while important, was not absolutely essential to the practice of their religion, as is ayahuasca. Addressing concerns about commerce arising from their use of advertisements and apparent "pay to pray" business model, Ayahuasca Healings explained, "the contributions the Church has received have gone almost entirely into overhead costs" (2016, p. 13). Addressing its notorious efforts at propagation, Ayahuasca Healings admitted it "went overboard" with marketing. As a concession, it offered the DEA "the right of pre-publication review and authorization for any written or audio/visual materials prepared for publication on AHNAC's [Ayahuasca Healings Native American Church] website" (2016, p. 10). Moreover, Ayahuasca Healings dropped its goal of opening 200 churches, stating that it would focus on developing its Church in Elbe, Washington.

Having submitted its petition, it is now up to the DEA to determine whether Ayahuasca Healings is a legitimate religion, rather than a spiritual retreat center or something else, whether it is sincere in its beliefs and practices, and whether its religious practices are substantially burdened by the CSA. While fulfilling many of the DEA's requirements, the Ayahuasca Healings petition has several significant flaws. Some of these are minor, but others may be insurmountable. A brief analysis follows.

Has Ayahuasca Healings Established a Prima Facie Case?

The first issue concerns whether Ayahuasca Healings can be considered a religion. While there are issues with untangling beliefs that are philosophical versus religious, and questions about the outlined moral system of Ayahuasca Healings, Ayahuasca Healings' structural characteristics present a bigger challenge to its potential identification as a religion. The DEA has provided a number of characteristics that satisfy this criterion, including "formal ceremonies or rituals, gathering places, clergy and/or prophets, structure and organization, important writings," etc., but has indicated that "the absence of one or more" structural characteristics common to known religions "is not determinative" of an organization's religious legitimacy (Rannazzisi, 2008, p. 10). Ayahuasca Healings provides a number of characteristics in its petition to satisfy this criterion, but DEA questions about structure and organization could prove problematic.

Ayahuasca Healings is a small group with no formal membership process. Healing retreats are offered for a fee to those "who come in a good way" and to ONAC members. There is no indication that individuals must accept the tenets of the Church, particularly since "Ayahuasca Healings Native American Church is committed to Honoring all of the spiritual traditions of our ancestors" (Ayahuasca Healings, 2016). And, notably, attendees do not have any clear responsibilities, obligations, or long-term commitments to the Church. All of this suggests that the fee-based retreats are simply transactional, without conferring membership or commitment to the moral and ethical code of the Church, which appears to be optional. The lack of formal membership may not in and of itself be fatal to Ayahuasca Healings but will likely be problematic in combination with other shortcomings in its petition.

Next is the issue of sincerity: Ayahuasca Healings addresses three of the five criteria laid out by the court in *Quaintance*, including (1) ad hoc beliefs, (2) evidence of commerce, and (3) use of other illegal substances. Regarding ad hoc beliefs, a critical point will likely be the incorporation of Ayahuasca Healings as part of NHNAC and later ONAC. The relationship between these organizations seems to have been established for the sole purpose of acquiring "legal protection" to possess and distribute ayahuasca. Ayahuasca Healings' claim to the NAC mantle stands in contrast with the fact that the CSA exemption provided to the Native American Church is based on a special relationship between federally recognized tribes and the federal government and was provided for the benefit of a specific Native American religious tradition. While Ayahuasca Healings claims to use a tipi for its ceremonies, and to perform sweat lodges, there appears to be no significant parallels between Ayahuasca Healings' historical roots and religious doctrine and the traditions of the Native American Church. The appropriation of the NAC moniker appears to be nothing more than a legal strategy to protect otherwise illegal behaviors. Similarly, the adoption of the ONAC Code of Ethics appears to have been for the sole purpose of satisfying DEA criteria for a CSA exemption, "as opposed to being derived from a cohesive moral or ethical imperative"; another reason the DEA dinged the Church of Reality's petition (Rannazzisi, 2008, pp. 9–10).

Evidence of commerce, however, will likely be Ayahuasca Healings' Achilles heel. Whereas the UDV and Santo Daime have a community of members that attend regularly scheduled religious services, Ayahuasca Healings appears to have no such community, other than a small group of organizers, and instead offers one-off retreats to those who "come in a good way" and come with money. Its initial goal of opening 200 churches across the United States, without any formal membership, sounds more like a business plan than spreading church gospel. Ayahuasca Healings insistence in its petition that it has dropped this goal does little to change the apparent commercial structure of its existing organization. While all religious groups have financial considerations, Ayahuasca Healings appears to be organized around a fee-for-service model that aims to build revenue quickly, rather than being invested in building a community of parishioners that will grow organically to financially support the Church.

Finally, the use of another illegal substance, the mescaline-containing San Pedro cactus, is suggestive of a simple interest in averting US drug laws. While Ayahuasca Healings does not ask for an exemption for San Pedro in its petition, stating that it is secondary in importance to ayahuasca, and while the use of San Pedro is traditional in other areas of Peru beyond the Amazon (where ayahuasca comes from), the presence of this second substance in its "religion" likely does not help its case. Rather, it may cause the DEA to draw parallels to the Church of Reality's insistence that, "Although our request at this time is for the use of marijuana, we are not limiting ourselves to just that one drug" (Rannazzisi, 2008, p. 13).

While Ayahuasca Healings has submitted a petition that is substantively stronger than the one submitted by the Church of Reality, the outline of its cosmology and moral code is undermined by the absence of a stable and formal membership, and the ability of anyone to attend ceremonies simply by paying a fee, regardless of any personal investment in Ayahuasca Healings' beliefs, mission, or moral code. The deciding factor for emerging ayahuasca-using groups in the United States may boil down to the following questions: does the religion have a regular congregation? And, if not, is it simply seeking to provide anyone who has money a legal psychedelic experience that "is almost always an indescribably profound religious experience" (2016, p. 4)?

Conclusions

The rapid proliferation of underground ayahuasca circles and churches in the United States over the last two decades demonstrates an immense level of social interest in this Amazonian brew. While there are a multitude of reasons people are drawn to ayahuasca, whether it be for healing, spiritual exploration, or for an exotic experience, the proliferation of these circles and churches reflects much broader cultural and social trends that are beyond our present scope.

Our aim in this chapter has not been to malign or discount the current phenomenon of ayahuasca in the United States but to objectively explore some of the approaches used by different groups to acquire legal protection for their practices, to provide a framework for understanding the legal steps and considerations involved in petitioning the DEA for a CSA exemption, and to explore some of the ethical considerations posed by the emerging trend of appropriating the "Native American Church" title among some nonindigenous new ayahuasca-using groups. Currently, in the United States, the ability to use ayahuasca legally depends on the ability of a group to demonstrate a sincere religious practice that is burdened by US drug laws. While there are other legitimate uses and applications of ayahuasca beyond a religious context, there is no legal pathway at present for these uses to become protected.

The US Constitution (and subsequent statutes like RFRA) was designed to protect a diversity of religions and religious practices, but not spirituality and individual spiritual practices, which potentially includes traditional shamanic and neo-shamanic practices. Currently, RFRA provides the one legal avenue for an organized religion to acquire an exemption from the CSA; however, as we have seen, the statute never defines the term "religion." Instead, courts must look to case law for guidance in evaluating whether a particular group qualifies as religious for purposes of RFRA. The DEA's own guidelines rely on the 10th Circuit Court's decision in *United States v. Meyers* (1996) for determining the religious nature of groups petitioning for a CSA exemption. The criteria are comprehensive and flexible but retain a Western bias and require groups to be structured around very clear principles and belief systems. Groups that come together to share a spiritual experience, but who don't share a common set of a beliefs or moral codes, are likely to have trouble satisfying the *Meyers* Test. Underground circles and groups whose rituals are adapted from indigenous shamanic traditions will likely need to structure and formalize their practices, membership, ethical codes, and belief systems if they wish to satisfy the *Meyers* Test and acquire a legal exemption.

The second obstacle for underground ayahuasca groups is to demonstrate the sincerity of their beliefs and practices. Here, the DEA has adopted the standards set out by the District Court of New Mexico in *United States v. Quaintance* (2006). The primary challenges posed to ayahuasca groups by *Quaintance* are ad hoc beliefs and evidence of commerce. Many groups representing themselves as branches of the NAC appear to be adopting the NAC title for perceived legal benefits and generally lack a comprehensive system of beliefs or a moral code. Here, the act of cultural appropriation and lack of sensitivity towards the protection of Native American rights bodes poorly for "sincerity." It also appears likely that groups that charge for ceremonies and retreats will fail the *Quaintance* test for engaging in economic activity. Calling a fee a "donation" is unlikely to alter this outcome. Groups who can demonstrate ongoing and consistent membership that also request financial support from their members may fair differently, but this would likely be limited to smaller private groups that do not advertise aggressively. While proselytizing is a component of many religions, it is unclear where the line between proselytizing and advertising will be drawn. However, outreach efforts that emphasize fees and services rather than a religious message will likely fail under *Quaintance*.

With the above considerations in mind, Ayahuasca Healings' petition will most likely be denied. The DEA will be narrow and very strict in applying the guidelines they have set out and are unlikely to set a precedent that could potentially open the floodgates for a proliferation of ayahuasca retreat centers around the country.

We have seen in this chapter how new religious movements and spiritual practices seeking legal accommodations in the United States are typically evaluated against commonly "accepted" or "recognized" religions. This means practices that are less structured, less doctrinal, and less group oriented are less likely to be recognized as religions. This is a significant obstacle for many using ayahuasca, who see it as part of their personal spiritual path and who also reject organized religion. It also potentially leads to some absurdities, with Christian-based Brazilian ayahuasca churches, with roots in the twentieth century, achieving legally exempt status, while age-old indigenous shamanic practices are likely to remain prohibited.

While the criteria for religious exemptions in the United States are strict, they are not insurmountable. Both the UDV and Santo Daime have CSA exemptions, and other groups who pray with this sacrament in a sincere way may also be able to acquire their own exemption. As demonstrated by the Brazilian ayahuasca religions, the road to legitimacy in the United States is long but can end in security and legitimacy. For those individuals and circles that prefer a looser structure and independence on their spiritual path and are less concerned with legitimacy in the eyes of the government, we will likely see underground ayahuasca circles continue to flourish.

References

Africa v. Commonwealth of Pennsylvania, 662 F.2d 1025, 1032 (3d Cir. 1981).
Alvarado v. City of San Jose, 94 F.3d 1223, 1229 (9th Cir. 1996).
Anonymous (2011). *Ayahuasca manifesto: The spirit of ayahuasca and its planetary mission*. Retrieved from https://soulquest-6xltrrbaxi24mjo1rc8a.netdna-ssl.com/wp-content/uploads/2016/09/ayahuasca-manifesto_anonymous-4.pdf
Arizona Yagé Assembly [AYA]. (2017). *Arizona Yagé Assembly: About*. Facebook.com. Retrieved from https://www.facebook.com/pg/ayachurchaz/about/
Aya Guide. (2015). *Bringing you into the ayahuasca ceremony*. Retrieved from https://www.aya.guide/

Aya Quest. (2015). Aya quest native American church (A.N.A.C.): Ayahuasca in America. Retrieved from www.ayaquest.com

Ayahuasca Healings. (2016). *ONAC of Ayahuasca Healings: Vision, mission & philosophy.* Retrieved from https://ayahuascahealings.com/ayahuasca-usa-church-vision/

Brett, D. B. (2016, December 6). *Letter from Derek B. Brett, Counsel for Soul Quest, to Joseph T. Rannazzisi, Deputy Assistant Administrator for the Office of Diversion Control, DEA.* Retrieved from http://www.bialabate.net/wp-content/uploads/2008/08/Soul_Quest%E2%80%99s_response_DEA_2017.pdf

Bronfman, J. (2007). The extraordinary case of the United States versus the União do Vegetal church. In J. P. Jarpignies (Ed.), *Visionary plant consciousness: The shamanic teaching of the plant world* (pp. 170–187). Rochester, VT: Park Street Press.

Bronfman, J. (2011). The legal case of the União do Vegetal vs. the Government of the United States. In B. C. Labate & H. Jungaberle (Eds.), *The internationalization of ayahuasca* (pp. 287–300). Zürich: Lit Verlag.

Brown, Karina (2016, April 15). Ruling doesn't settle future of Native American Church. *Courthouse News Service.* Retrieved from http://www.courthousenews.com/2016/04/15/ruling-doesnt-settle-future-of-native-american-church.htm

Burroughs, W. S., & Ginsburg, A. (1963). *The yage letters.* San Francisco, CA: City Lights Books.

Callicott, C. (2017, April 17). *Pandora's brew: The new ayahuasca (Part 1–7).* Savage minds: Notes and queries in anthropology. Retrieved from http://www.bialabate.net/wp-content/uploads/2017/03/Callicot_Pandoras_New_Ayahuasca_Savage_Minds_2017.pdf

Carpenter, K. (2014, July 25). Motion for leave to file brief and brief of amici curiae the National Council of native American churches, the native American Church of North America, the Azee' bee Nahagha of Diné nation, the native American church, state of Oklahoma, and the native American church, state of Sourth Dakota, in support of appellees. Oklevueha native American Church of Hawaii, Inc. v. Holder, et al., ninth circuit court of appeals. No. 14-15143. Retrieved from http://www.bialabate.net/wpcontent/uploads/2008/08/NACNA_Brief_Opposing_Oklevueha.pdf

Church of the Holy Light of the Queen v. Mukasey, 615 F.Supp.2d 1210 (D. Or. 2009), *aff'd* (9th Cir. 2011) *aff'd* (9th Cir. 2014) (awarding Santo Daime attorney's fees). Retrieved from http://www.bialabate.net/wp-content/uploads/2009/04/Decision-9th-Court-Appeal-Santo-Daime-USA-2014.pdf

Church of the Holy Light of the Queen v. Mukasey, 615 F.Supp.2d 1210 (D. Or. 2009), *aff'd* (9th Cir. 2011). Retrieved from http://www.bialabate.net/wp-content/uploads/2009/04/164-32709-amended-judgment.pdf

Code of Federal Regulations [CFR]. (1971). Special exempt persons: Native American Church. Title 21, §1307.31.

Controlled Substances Act [CSA]. (1970). 21 United States Code § 801.

Drug Enforcement Administration [DEA]. (2009). Guidance regarding petitions for religious exemptions from the Controlled Substances Act pursuant to the Religious Freedom Restoration Act. Retrieved from http://www.bialabate.net/wp-content/uploads/2008/08/DEA_Guidelines_for_Petition_for_Religious_Exemptions_to_CSA.pdf

Employment Division v. Smith, 494 U.S. 872 (1990).

Epps, G. (2001). *To an unknown god.* New York, NY: St. Martin's Press.

Feeney, K. (2007). The legal bases for religious peyote use. In M. J. Winkelman & T. B. Roberts (Eds.), *Psychedelic medicine: New evidence for hallucinogenic substances as treatments* (pp. 233–250). Westport, CT: Praeger.

Feeney, K. (2014). Peyote, race, and equal protection in the United States. In B. C. Labate & C. Cavnar (Eds.), *Prohibition, religious freedom, and human rights: Regulating traditional drug use* (pp. 65–88). New York, NY: Springer.

Gonzales v. O Centro Espírita Beneficente União do Vegetal, 546 U.S. 418. (2006).

Haber, R. (2011). The Santo Daime road to seeking religious freedom in the USA. In B. C. Labate & H. Jungaberle (Eds.), *The internationalization of ayahuasca* (pp. 301–317). Zürich: Lit Verlag.

Highpine, G. (2015a, December 22). *Is ayahuasca actually illegal in the United States?* Retrieved from http://www.bialabate.net/news/is-ayahuasca-actually-illegal-in-the-united-states

Highpine, G. (2015b, December 12). *The "legality" of ayahuasca churches under the Oklevueha Native American Church.* Retrieved from http://www.bialabate.net/news/the-legality-of-ayahuasca-churches-under-the-oklevueha-native-american-church

Hudson, J. H. (2015, December 7). *Don't believe the hype about the "legal ayahuasca USA church" going around Facebook—it's not legal, it's dangerous, and here's why.* Retrieved from http://www.bialabate.net/news/dont-believe-the-hype-about-the-legal-ayahuasca-usa-church-going-around-facebook-its-not-legal-its-dangerous-and-heres-why

Kocher, G. (2017, June 14). Suit: Woman's collapse, death due to negligence at Berea church. *Lexington Herald Leader.* Retrieved from http://www.kentucky.com/news/local/counties/madison-county/article156151889.html

Labate, B. C. (2012). Paradoxes of ayahuasca expansion: The UDV-DEA agreement and the limits of freedom of religion. *Drugs: Education, Prevention & Policy, 19*(1), 19–26.

Labate, B. C., & Cavnar, C. (Eds.). (2014a). *Ayahuasca shamanism in the Amazon and beyond.* New York, NY: Oxford University Press.

Labate, B. C., & Cavnar, C. (Eds.). (2014b). *The therapeutic use of ayahuasca.* Berlin: Springer.

Labate, B. C., Cavnar, C., & Gearin, A. K. (Eds.). (2017). *The world ayahuasca diaspora: Reinventions and controversies.* Abingdon, UK: Routledge.

Labate, B. C., & Feeney, K. (2012). Ayahuasca and the process of regulation in Brazil and internationally: Implications and challenges. *International Journal of Drug Policy, 23*(2), 154–161.

Labate, B. C., & Jungaberle, H. (Eds.). (2011). *The Internationalization of ayahuasca.* Zurich: Lit Verlag.

McGivern, B. B. (2016, April 4). Ayahuasca Healings Native American Church's petition for a Controlled Substances Act exemption under the Religious Freedom Restoration Act. Letter from Blaine B. McGivern, Counsel for Petitioners, to Joseph T. Rannazzisi, Deputy Assistant Administrator for the Office of Diversion Control, DEA. Retrieved from http://www.bialabate.net/wp-content/uploads/2008/08/Ayahuasca_Healing_DEA_Exemption_Request_Documents..pdf

Milione, L. J. (2016a, August 22). Letter from Louis J. Milione, Assistant Administrator for the Office of Diversion Control, DEA, to Christopher Young. Retrieved from http://www.bialabate.net/wpcontent/uploads/2017/03/Letter_DEA_Soul_Quest_Aug_2016.pdf

Milione, L. J. (2016b, December 21). Letter from Louis J. Milione, Assistant Administrator for the Office of Diversion Control, DEA, to Derek B.Brett, Counsel for Soul Quest. Retrieved from http://www.bialabate.net/wp-content/uploads/2008/08/DEA_Respose_Soul_Quest_2016.pdf

National Council of Native American Churches. (2016, February 18). *National Council does not condone faux Native American Churches or marijuana use.* Retrieved from https://indiancountrymedianetwork.com/history/events/national-council-does-not-condone-faux-native-american-churches-or-marijuana-use/

O Centro Espirita Beneficente União do Vegetal [UDV] v. Holder. (2010, July 19). Settlement Agreement signed by Nancy Hollander, attorney for Plaintiffs, Jeffrey Bronfman, President of UDV-USA, and Eric J. Beane, Trial Attorney for the U.S. Department of Justice. No. 00-1647 JP/RLP (D. NM 2010). Retrieved from http://www.bialabate.net/wp-content/uploads/2010/07/UDV_Settlement_Agreement_DEA_20101.pdf

Oklevueha Native American Church [ONAC]. (2000–2012). *Acquiring an "Oklevueha NAC membership card."* Retrieved from http://nativeamericanchurches.org/join

Oklevueha Native American Church [ONAC]. (2017). *Oklevueha Native American Church card offering.* Retrieved from https://nativeamericanchurches.org/membership/

Perkel v. U.S. Department of Justice. On petition for review of an order of the Drug Enforcement Administration, No. 08-74457 (9th Cir. 2010). Retrieved from http://www.bialabate.net/wp-content/uploads/2008/08/Appellate_Court_DEA_Religious_Church_of_Reality.pdf

Rannazzisi, J. T. (2008, October 1). Letter from Joseph T. Rannazzisi, Deputy Assistant Administrator for the Office of Diversion Control, DEA, to Marc Perkel, denying The Church of Reality's petition for a CSA exemption pursuant to RFRA. Retrieved from http://www.bialabate.net/wp-content/uploads/2008/08/DEA_Rejection_Church_of_Reality.pdf

Religious Freedom Restoration Act, 42 U.S.C. § 2000bb (1993).

Sánchez, A. C., & Bouso, J. C. (2015). *Ayahuasca: From the Amazon to the global village*, *Drug Policy Briefing, No. 43*. Barcelona: Transnational Institute/ICEERS Foundation.

Slotkin, J. S. (1956). *The peyote religion: A study in Indian-White relations*. Glencoe, IL: The Free Press.

Soul Quest. (2016). *Soul Quest Ayahuasca Church of Mother Earth*. Retrieved from https://ayahuascachurches.org/

State of Utah v. Mooney, 2004 UT 49 (UT 2004).

Tupper, K., & Labate, B. C. (2012). Plants, psychoactive substances and the INCB: The control of nature and the nature of control. *Human Rights and Drugs, 2*(1), 17–28.

United States v. Meyers, 95 F.3d 1475, 1482-84 (10th Cir. 1996).

United States v. Quaintance, 471 F. Supp. 2d 1153 (D.N.M. 2006)

Utah Controlled Substances Act (2017). Prohibited Acts: Penalties. 58-37-8(12)a,b. Amendments adopted in 2006.

Chapter 7
Integrating Psychedelic Medicines and Psychiatry: Theory and Methods of a Model Clinic

Jordan Sloshower

Abstract The past two decades has seen a significant increase in both popular and scientific interest in psychedelic substances and plants as therapeutics for mental illness, addictions, and psychospiritual suffering. Current psychiatric practice privileges a biological paradigm in which the brain is considered the locus of mental illness and symptom-focused treatments are delivered to patients as passive recipients. In contrast, a psychedelic healing paradigm, constructed through examination of different ontologic understandings of plant medicines, is based on a complex multidimensional perspective of human beings and their suffering. This paradigm actively engages the sufferer in addressing root causes of illness through healing on multiple levels of existence, including spiritual and energetic domains. Numerous theoretical, methodological, and ethical challenges complicate the integration of the psychedelic healing paradigm into psychiatric practice. These include developing coherent therapeutic narratives that account for the complex processes by which psychedelic healing occurs and overcoming reductionist tendencies in the medical sciences. Tasked with overcoming such challenges, a model clinic is proposed that seeks to implement and study the psychedelic healing paradigm in a critical, interdisciplinary, and reflexive manner. Such "critical paradigm integration" would employ multimodal patient formulation and treatments, as well as a range of knowledge generation and sharing practices. Outcomes-oriented research would seek to establish an evidence base for the model, while critical dialogues would advance understandings of psychedelic substances and plants and related practices more generally. The clinic would serve as proof of concept for a new model of studying, conceptualizing, and treating mental illness.

J. Sloshower (✉)
Department of Psychiatry, Yale University, New Haven, CT, USA
e-mail: jordan.sloshower@yale.edu

© Springer International Publishing AG, part of Springer Nature 2018
B. C. Labate, C. Cavnar (eds.), *Plant Medicines, Healing and Psychedelic Science*,
https://doi.org/10.1007/978-3-319-76720-8_7

Introduction

How can the use of psychedelic substances and plants[1] help alleviate human suffering? What are the barriers to these medicines becoming part of mainstream mental health treatment? What models could be used to both treat mental disorders with psychedelics and conduct research on their therapeutic uses in a meaningful and ethical way? This chapter attempts to provide some preliminary answers to the above questions. First, it will discuss key differences between current psychiatric treatment and a proposed paradigm of psychedelic healing. Next, it will examine relevant theoretical, methodological, and ethical challenges in integrating the two paradigms. Lastly, it will outline how an integrative psychedelic healing approach could be implemented in a model clinic utilizing "critical paradigm integration."

Psychedelic Medicines in the Era of Biological Psychiatry

My training in psychiatry at Yale University has emphasized a "biopsychosocial" approach to diagnosis and treatment (Engel, 1980), in which biological, psychological, and social factors are thought to contribute to a person's mental illness or suffering. Accordingly, treatment interventions are meant to address problems in each of those domains. The model is fairly comprehensive and often quite effective when a person is able to access and make use of the various possible treatments, such as medications, evidence-based individual and group psychotherapies, and social interventions. Unfortunately, this is too often not the case due to resource limitations and, I would argue, to an overprivileging of biological perspectives and technological interventions in the field of psychiatry in recent decades (Bracken et al., 2012). This shift has occurred for several reasons, including (a) helping psychiatry take its place among other specialties of medicine grounded in the biological sciences; (b) destigmatizing mental illness and addictions by reframing them as chronic treatable illnesses, like diabetes or heart disease, rather than as moral failings or resulting from weak character; and (c) promoting pharmaceuticals as the primary means of addressing mental illness and alleviating everyday suffering (Carlat, 2010; Moynihan & Cassels, 2006).

In the current era of biological psychiatry, mental illnesses like depression and schizophrenia, as well as addictions, are primarily conceptualized as brain diseases resulting from aberrant neural circuitry and chemical imbalances. To address brain-

---

[1]A note about terminology: There are currently debates about how psychedelic substances or molecules are similar to or different from plants or plant-based preparations containing psychoactive (as well as other) compounds. The latter are commonly referred to as "plant medicines" by enthusiasts and some academics. The nuances of this debate are beyond the scope of this chapter, which will give preference to the more neutral and inclusive term "psychedelic substances and plants," as most points being made about psychedelic healing apply to both.

based pathology, psychiatrists commonly prescribe medications and deliver other interventions, such as electroconvulsive therapy (ECT) or transcranial magnetic stimulation (TMS), that primarily target brain circuits and neurotransmitters.[2] The sufferer is largely a passive recipient or consumer of such treatments and, without additional psychotherapy or lifestyle modification, is positioned as a relatively helpless victim of a diseased brain. Evidence-based forms of psychotherapy, which conversely require the active engagement of the sufferer in his or her own healing, are too often unavailable, unaffordable, or not sought out by people suffering with mental disorders. This is largely due to the current structures of insurance coverage and financial incentives for mental health practitioners in the United States and has resulted in a rise in the proportion of patients receiving pharmacotherapy only (Olfson & Marcus, 2010).

Moreover, most pharmacological treatments currently available in psychiatry target symptoms, rather than root causes of psychiatric illness. This is due, on the one hand, to a lack of understanding of the precise biological etiologies of mental illnesses and, on the other, to the inability of conventional pharmaceuticals to address psychological, social, and spiritual or energetic[3] causes of suffering. Symptoms also constitute the focus of most psychiatric or "medication management" patient encounters. This reflects the way in which mental health service provision and reimbursement are currently based on categorical or descriptive diagnoses, which cluster symptoms into disorders. In such a system, mental health providers must elicit symptoms from patients in order to make a diagnosis (as is generally required for reimbursement) and focus treatments on diminishing those symptoms. The result of this approach is often chronic drug administration, associated side effects, partial treatment effectiveness, and patient dissatisfaction (Goff et al., 2017; Samara et al., 2016; Warden, Rush, Trivedi, Fava, & Wisniewski, 2007). This in turn has led to the rise of new paradigms, such as the recovery movement and strengths-based or resilience-based approaches, and to a rapid expansion of complementary and alternative medicine (CAM) in the West (Tindle, Davis, & Phillips, 2005).

Different Ontological Understandings of Psychedelic Medicines

Psychoactive plants have been in relationship with humans for thousands of years (El-Seedi, Smet, Beck, Possnert, & Bruhn, 2005; Torres, 1995), playing various roles in society, culture, religion, and medicine over time. Reflecting this complex

---

[2]Effective clinicians may also imbue these treatments with additional meaning and target patient expectancy in order to boost the placebo effect of the intervention.

[3]By energetic, I refer to Eastern conceptions of physiology and pathophysiology involving energetic channels, meridians, and centers (or chakras), such as in traditional Chinese medicine or Ayurveda, as well as shamanic notions of energy.

historical relationship, there are numerous different ways that psychedelic substances and plants are understood and characterized by different groups of people and academic disciplines. Before outlining tenets of a psychedelic healing paradigm, I will first consider these different "ontologic understandings" (Tupper & Labate, 2014) in order to shed light on different possible ways that psychedelics may exert their therapeutic effects.

Ayahuasca will make a useful example here, given its long history of use among indigenous peoples and more recent expansion into a variety of cultural, spiritual, and scientific contexts. An anthropological or indigenous perspective of ayahuasca may view the brew as a "plant spirit" or "teacher" with which a person or shaman interacts to bring about a desired effect (Luna, 1984). Meanwhile, ayahuasca could be described in strict biomedical terms as a collection of alkaloids and other chemical compounds, primarily a serotonin 2A receptor agonist and monoamine oxidase inhibitor (MAO-I), which alter brain network connectivity and neuroplasticity (Domínguez-Clavé et al., 2016). Perhaps between these views are psychological perspectives of the brew as a "psychedelic" or "cognitive tool" (Tupper & Labate, 2014) capable of eliciting non-ordinary states of consciousness, manifesting aspects of the subconscious, and bringing about insights and change.

There are multiple other ways of conceptualizing ayahuasca that continue to evolve as its use becomes more widespread. Spiritual or religious perspectives may classify it as an "entheogen" or "sacrament," capable of catalyzing profound spiritual or mystical experiences (Richards, 2015). More recent discourses consider ayahuasca to be an "evolutionary tool" that can help our species evolve or live more harmoniously with nature. Finally, ayahuasca and other psychedelic plants are often endearingly called "plant medicines" by contemporary users wishing to highlight their healing effects.

From Ontologies to a Psychedelic Model of Healing

Although different ontologic understandings of psychedelic plants may be based on different modes of knowledge (i.e., empiric scientific investigation versus experiential or intuitive understanding), I do not see them as separate or incompatible. Rather, I would argue they reflect different "mechanisms of action" by which psychedelic medicines exert their effects on the human organism. Unlike with traditional psychopharmaceuticals, psychedelics and psychedelic-assisted therapies are described by the various ontologies as impacting multiple layers of existence (i.e., biological, psychological, social, spiritual, and energetic) both during the acute experience and afterward. Thus, accounting for the various ontologic understandings of psychedelics points toward a particular way of conceptualizing the human condition, namely, that we exist as complex multilayered beings, with brain-minds, bodies, hearts, and spirits, all of which are connected to each other and to our natural and social environments.

The next task is to translate this psychedelically informed perspective of human existence into a healing paradigm. With an eye toward integration of psychedelic healing into mainstream medicine, I believe this could be achieved through revision and expansion of the well-known biopsychosocial model of diagnosis and treatment discussed earlier. First, a psychedelic healing model would level the playing field between the biological and the psychosocial; it would reaffirm psychological and social interventions as valued and worthwhile means of healing. More uniquely, it would expand the model to more explicitly include emotional, spiritual, transpersonal, energetic, and ecological diagnostic perspectives and therapeutic interventions.[4]

In this psychedelic model of healing, mental suffering does not just result from pathology of the brain; suffering and "disease" may arise in any of these layers of existence and can be propagated through them in complex ways. For instance, emotional trauma or chronic social stressors may become internalized throughout the body's psychoneuroendocrine immunologic (PNEI) network, resulting in a range of psychological and physical symptoms (Tafur, 2017). As a result, proper treatments must be capable of intervening on multiple layers of existence. While this ability may be inherent to psychedelic medicines, having a therapeutic effect may not be, especially in those experiencing profound suffering. This is in line with the well-established principle that the effects of psychedelic medicines are idiosyncratically dependent on "set" (psychological state) and "setting" (environment) (Leary, Metzner, & Alpert, 1995). Thus, for people experiencing profound depression or other mental illnesses, healing effects may need to be guided through one or more of layers of existence and outward into interpersonal and social domains. Without discounting the ability of a person's "inner healer" to accomplish this through careful preparation and intention, the process may be made safer and more effective by the guidance and support of a well-trained therapist, perhaps working in collaboration with a shaman, before, during, and after the medicine experience.

The continuation and propagation of healing begun during a psychedelic experience is how I define the increasingly popular term "psychedelic integration." On the one hand, biological changes induced by psychedelic substances, such as heightened neuroplasticity or altered patterns of brain connectivity (Carhart-Harris et al., 2016), may be taken advantage of following an acute experience through ongoing practices that change cognition and neurocircuitry, such as psychotherapy or meditation. On the other hand, a deep insight gained during an acute experience may initiate a process of changing one's daily habits, interpersonal relations, living environment, and relation to society and nature.

In sum, psychedelic healing is not a "magic bullet" intervention, requiring only the passive compliance of a sufferer in ingesting a medication. Rather, it actively engages the sufferer in a multilayered healing process that has the ability to interrupt deep-seated pathological patterns and processes. This targeting of root causes of illness helps explain both the popular excitement behind psychedelic healing and the

---

[4]Details of this approach will be discussed further in the second half of the chapter.

profound and long-lasting therapeutic benefits seen thus far in clinical trials (Bogenschutz et al., 2015; Griffiths et al., 2016, 2011; Johnson, Garcia-Romeu, & Griffiths, 2016; Ross et al., 2016).

Theoretical, Methodological, and Ethical Challenges to Paradigm Integration

Thus far, I have described different ways of understanding how psychedelics impact the human organism and proposed a paradigm of psychedelic healing premised on the profound interconnectedness of biology, psychology, and spirituality. In order to harness the full therapeutic potential of psychedelic substances and plants for the greatest number of people and problems, the field of psychedelic science needs to develop deep understandings of how they operate at each ontological or existential level and, critically, how these levels and processes interact. For instance, we need to understand how the use of music, psychotherapy, and other shamanic practices may alter the effects of a given medicine, both phenomenologically and biologically, in terms of altering neurobiology, physiology, or epigenetics. Thus, as a clinician and academic researcher, I view the primary mission of the emerging field of psychedelic science as integrating previously disconnected and conflicting modes of knowledge and approaches to healing.

This project of knowledge integration is likely to be contested at multiple sites of knowledge production, by various actors, and at various points along its path. I will now highlight pertinent theoretical, methodological, and ethical challenges to integration, especially those I have encountered in the academic setting.

Theoretical Issues Given the multiple ontologies and related terminologies of psychedelics, one primary challenge for practitioners in this field is articulating a coherent narrative or model for psychedelic healing. In my experience, "code switching" (Auer, 2013), or flexibly utilizing different idioms and paradigms to convey concepts of psychedelic healing to different audiences, is a common tactic to negotiate this problem. For instance, the explanatory model offered to scientific colleagues and funders of how ayahuasca may help promote recovery from addictions may differ in tone and terminology from that given to lay audiences or research subjects.

A more significant challenge for clinicians and researchers working in academia arises when attempting to translate the psychedelic healing paradigm into clinical trial protocols. This involves striking a delicate balance in presenting a narrative that is sufficiently scientific to satisfy colleagues and grant-awarding bodies that operate primarily in a biological framework without completely obscuring other ontologic understandings. Succeeding in this is complicated, as healing principles and interventions derived from shamanism or spiritual perspectives are largely foreign to traditional drug development research and involve introducing variables that are difficult to control (see the following section on methodological issues).

An example of this would be in rationalizing the decision to use liquid ayahuasca instead of freeze-dried capsules in a clinical trial protocol or conference presentation. Medical doctors and psychiatrists, who are not trained to see drug-induced altered states of consciousness as therapeutic and are unfamiliar with the traditional use of purgative plants, would be primarily concerned about isolating the "active ingredient," tightly controlling dose, and minimizing side effects. Thus, an explanation that the water in ayahuasca is itself considered an important ingredient for healing and that preserving its natural odor, consistency, and taste are essential for inducing beneficial purgative effects would likely be unsatisfactory. Rather than convey these unconventional ideas in a scientific protocol, one may offer a rationale around "effectiveness"—studying what occurs in the real world—as a scientific justification. Similar problems arise in explaining and operationalizing the concept of "medication-assisted psychotherapy," or in incorporating esoteric healing practices that are foreign to most clinical trials, such as the use of music during experimental sessions.

While operating within a single ontologic understanding of psychedelic medicines or focusing on a particular site of suffering may be appropriate or necessary at certain times and situations, my concern is that an unintegrated language around the use of psychedelics limits our breadth of understanding and narrows their therapeutic potential. This is especially true because differential alignment with particular ontological understandings or theoretical perspectives bias toward particular therapeutic approaches at the exclusion of others. In preparing a research protocol to investigate the therapeutic potential of psilocybin in the treatment in depression, it became difficult to rationalize embedding psilocybin administration sessions within a course of psychotherapy, as the research grant was necessarily grounded in a biological framework focused on demonstrating "target engagement" of the investigational drug.[5] Operating within a strictly biological framework leaves little room for psychological or spiritual mechanisms of action, which some team members felt could be discredited as "voodoo" or "psychobabble" by grant reviewers.

The drive to conduct clinical trials with psychedelics with utmost scientific rigor is commendable, given the risk of discrediting the entire "psychedelic renaissance" with sloppy science or bad outcomes. However, this cannot come at the expense of losing sight of what distinguishes psychedelics and the psychedelic healing paradigm as distinct from a pharmacology-first treatment model. Adherence to a strict biological paradigm risks promoting a "magic bullet" model of treatment, in which the medicine is given and allowed to do its work without need for further intervention. This has largely been the story of ketamine, a dissociative anesthetic drug with some psychedelic properties, that has recently been popularized in mainstream psychiatry as a rapid-acting antidepressant (Sanacora & Schatzberg, 2014). Characterized in the existent psychiatric literature almost exclusively through its

---

[5]"Target engagement" refers to verification that the intervention has had the predicted effect on the target (National Institute of Mental Health, 2013). This has recently become a requirement to receive grant money from the National Institute of Mental Health (NIMH).

neurobiologic properties, there has been little discussion of potential psychological or spiritual mechanisms of action, and ketamine's dissociative or psychedelic effects have been seen as side effects of the medication. One result of this is that ketamine treatment, unlike psilocybin- or MDMA-*assisted* treatment, has not been paired with psychotherapy, and there is minimal debriefing of the subjective experience. A concerning consequence of this has been a dramatic increase in ketamine providers throughout the United States administering the infusions without any form of integration and without formal training in supporting patients through non-ordinary states of consciousness.

Whether ketamine therapy would yield improved outcomes for mental illnesses if other ontologic understandings were brought to bear on its use, for instance, by capitalizing on its subjective effects or integrating it with psychotherapy, is a question still under investigation (Wilkinson et al., 2017). My argument is that psychedelic science should aim to develop a diverse knowledge base that enables practitioners to effectively draw on different understandings of how these medicines work in a tailored fashion in order to achieve maximal therapeutic benefits for patients.

Methodological Issues Current political, economic, and philosophical determinants will continue to pull psychedelic research and treatment in a biological direction. As I have been arguing, it is critical in this early and resurgent time for psychedelic science that researchers aim to integrate different types of knowledge and design treatment protocols that reflect complex multidimensional understandings of how psychedelic substances and plants bring about healing. This is crucial because treatment guidelines are generally based on evidence produced in clinical trials, and so the models that are designed and tested now will inform future guidelines for the use of these medicines in clinical practice.

However, there are significant challenges in applying the scientific method and typical clinical trial methodology to the study of psychedelics and the broader psychedelic healing paradigm. The primary set of limitations, in my experience, relates to the concept of scientific reductionism, or the tendency to isolate individual variables and characterize their specific (biological) effects, rather than looking at systems as a whole. As Michael Pollan points out in his critique of nutritional science, this reductionist approach "means ignoring complex interactions and contexts, as well as the fact that the whole may be more than, or just different from, the sum of its parts" (Pollan, 2007).

This becomes a practical problem when the Federal Drug Administration's process of rescheduling a substance from Schedule I to II requires that researchers demonstrate that the substance alone is responsible for therapeutic efficacy, in comparison to a placebo. In the context of studying psychedelics, the reductionist tendency does not allow for the study of complex interactions between the physical or biological properties of a medicine like ayahuasca and the metaphysical healing components that are complementary to its use, such as music, dieting, praying, being in nature, and other aspects of shamanism. Such "setting" variables either need to be eliminated, controlled for in placebo condition, or be seen as confounding variables.

In other words, contemporary clinical trial design cannot account for the complex interactions that occur between psychedelic medicines and set and setting variables.

Beyond efficacy studies that isolate the substance as the primary variable, the field of psychedelic science therefore needs to conduct studies on set and setting variables in order to answer important questions, such as: What factors make a person more or less likely to have a favorable or poor outcome to psychedelic-assisted therapy? In what setting and with whom should a person ingest a medicine like ayahuasca to achieve a given effect or outcome? Should a shaman or therapist (s) be present, and should they also ingest the medicine? Does it matter if the therapists have personal experience with the medicine being given or if they have the ability to adjust the music during a dosing session? Only through further interdisciplinary research and intercultural dialogue can we answer these difficult questions about therapeutic approach.

Another methodological problem related to reductionism is the historical tendency of biomedical science to isolate and study single molecular compounds as medicines, rather than looking at combined effects of multiple chemical compounds. The presence of multiple active compounds occurring in differing concentrations in different plant strains (e.g., marijuana) or preparations (e.g., ayahuasca), a phenomenon known as the "entourage effect" (Ben-Shabat et al., 1998), poses significant challenges for a scientific method trying to determine simple cause-and-effect relationships. However, as proponents of whole-plant cannabis or ayahuasca would suggest, the entourage effect is an understudied phenomenon of nature whose secrets hold great therapeutic potential. Fortunately, Sidarta Ribeiro (2018) discusses this important topic in greater depth in this volume. Further research into understanding the entourage effect will critically help psychedelic scientists select particular strains or preparations of plant medicines for testing in future clinical trials.

Lastly, I will only briefly mention the more widely discussed problem of blinding psychedelics in placebo-controlled trials, given their profound and unmistakable subjective effects. This issue is examined more closely in this volume by Katherine Hendy (2018), in her discussion of clinical trials conducted by the Multidisciplinary Association for Psychedelic Studies (MAPS) with MDMA.

A key point to be made before leaving this discussion is that the methodological challenges highlighted above are limitations of the scientific method, not problems inherent to plants, molecules, or complex healing practices. Psychedelic scientists are tasked with the challenge of adapting scientific tools and methods, or creating new ones when necessary, in order to adequately study these phenomenon, rather than packaging them into artificial units that are more conveniently studied by existing scientific methods. I believe that overcoming these challenges of integration represents a significant opportunity for the field of psychedelic science to contribute to the sciences as a whole and to impact the way we study, conceptualize, and treat mental illness.

Ethical Issues An in-depth discussion of the ethical issues surrounding the expansion of plant medicines outside of their original ethnocultural and ecological contexts is beyond the scope of this chapter (please see Labate & Cavnar, 2014; Labate, Cavnar, & Gearin, 2016 for more detailed discussions). However, I would like to briefly acknowledge a number of risks inherent to the work of integrating plant medicines into more mainstream medicine, as they will inform certain design elements of a model clinic.

First is the risk of appropriation of indigenous knowledge. Bringing indigenous plants and knowledge into the gaze of Western biomedicine will undoubtedly involve changing the way the medicines are used and selectively including and excluding bits of indigenous knowledge and practice. At the II World Ayahuasca Conference in Acre, Brazil, held in October 2016, dozens of delegates from ayahuasca-using indigenous communities urged ayahuasca researchers and practitioners to respect their traditions, include them in contemporary discussions about ayahuasca use, and speak out against inappropriate uses of ayahuasca, including its commercialization (World Ayahuasca Conference, 2016). I imagine that some stakeholders will find certain forms of ayahuasca research to be upsetting, incorrect, or unjust.

The second set of ethical concerns relates to the general tenet to do no harm to patients. Treating someone with psychedelic plants and medicines, although shown to be rather safe in well-controlled settings, carries certain inherent risks to physical and psychological health (Barrett, Bradstreet, Leoutsakos, Johnson, & Griffiths, 2016; Halpern, Sherwood, Hudson, Yurgelun-Todd, & Pope Jr., 2005; Halpern, Sherwood, Passie, Blackwell, & Ruttenber, 2008; Johnson, Richards, & Griffiths, 2008; Nichols, 2016). This is especially the case when working with people suffering from significant medical or psychiatric illnesses and may require discontinuation of pharmaceutical medications before undergoing treatment. There may also be unforeseen risks to their social health through stigmatization by family, friends, or co-workers. Thus, the use of these medicines must not be taken lightly, and significant preparation and training must be ensured.

Lastly, engaging in this kind of work carries with it a high degree of social responsibility. Psychedelics currently occupy a tenuous space in society. Legally, they are considered Schedule I illegal drugs in the Unites States, meaning they have "no currently accepted medical use and a high potential for abuse" (United States Drug Enforcement Administration, n.d.). Yet, the use of these substances is widespread globally among diverse groups of people who believe their use to be beneficial. Psychedelic science is currently one of the primary mediators between governments, policymakers, and the public on the regulation of these substances. Thus, we must proceed with caution and integrity in order to avoid further prohibition or criminalization of their use and barriers to their scientific investigation. This would jeopardize the immense potential held in current and future research and therapeutic development.

Theory and Practice of a Model Clinic: Overview

Keeping in mind the various theoretical, methodological, and ethical challenges posed above, I will next turn to the task of envisioning a setting where the multidimensional model of psychedelic healing outlined earlier could both be put into clinical practice and studied in a manner that promotes paradigm integration and critical reflexivity. In light of the limitations of the reductionist mode of clinical trial research, which focuses on the substance or medication as the primary object of inquiry, the model clinic proposed here would endeavor to implement and test a *model of care* based on the psychedelic healing paradigm. In similar fashion to how the Millennium Villages Project was established to serve as a proof of concept that a holistic, intersectoral approach to sustainable development was both feasible and effective for addressing extreme poverty (Millenium Villages Project, n.d.), a model psychedelic healing clinic would serve as proof of concept that a holistic, interdisciplinary approach to mental health, including proper use of psychedelic substances and plants, is feasible and effective for treating psychiatric, substance use, and related disorders. In setting a precedent and generating evidence for a new model of practice, this project would seek to impact thought leaders and policymakers in the health sector and related fields.

In order to achieve the clinic's mission as outlined above, it would need to have the capacity to engage in the following essential interrelated activities: clinical practice, research, knowledge sharing, policy and advocacy, and funding generation. These activities are interrelated as they would generally inform or depend on one another (for instance, research would inform and be informed by clinical practice as well as other forms of knowledge sharing). Given the various aspects of the clinic's mission, the diverse staff and stakeholders that would be involved, and the need to navigate the numerous challenges described above, it would be important for the clinic to have an overarching ethos or unifying theoretical orientation. To fulfill this need, I propose "critical paradigm integration" as a central concept, in order to reflect a few basic tenets that would guide the clinic's activities:

1. Multimodality and interdisciplinary collaboration
2. Knowledge generation and dissemination across paradigms
3. Reflexivity, transparency, and openness

Each aspect of the clinic's mission will now be described in more detail.

Clinical Approach Based on Multimodality and Interdisciplinarity

A clinical approach based on multimodality and interdisciplinary collaboration is one that flexibly and creatively combines theoretical, diagnostic, and therapeutic approaches from different traditions and paradigms with the aims of achieving deep understandings of patients' suffering and delivering safe, effective treatments. Note that in the proposed psychedelic healing model, the actual administration of psychedelic substances and plants is only one potential component of a multifaceted approach to healing. In other words, it is a "psychedelically informed" model of care, rather than one based entirely on the utilization of psychedelics.

The first way in which multimodality applies is in the process of clinical formulation or the way a clinician conceptualizes a person's problem or situation. Multimodal formulation would entail understanding patients from multiple perspectives by involving practitioners with different theoretical perspectives and orientations. Thus, the clinic would seek to recruit a team of clinicians whose backgrounds encompass psychiatry and Western medicine, different psychological schools (e.g., cognitive-behavioral, psychodynamic, transpersonal, existential, trauma-centered), forms of complementary and alternative medicine (naturopathic, holistic, traditional Chinese, Ayurvedic), indigenous shamanism, and other philosophical, spiritual, and ecological perspectives.

Bringing such collective wisdom to bear on a given person's problems could be accomplished in different ways. Two possibilities are team-based interviewing, in which a collection of practitioners interviews a patient altogether, or using a sequential stratified approach. The latter would entail an initial intake assessment with a therapist trained in the psychedelic healing model who then refers the person for additional assessments as indicated or requested by the client.

One way of integrating different clinical perspectives and ontologic understandings into a coherent therapeutic narrative would be to utilize a narrative approach (Lewis, 2011), in which clinicians and patients work collaboratively to create an "illness narrative" (Kleinman, 1988), or a shared understanding of what the problem (s) are, how they came to be, and, ultimately, how various treatments can address them. Adopting such a narrative approach should help set out an arc or trajectory back to a state of health and wellness. Similar results could be attained using other heuristics, such as a medicine wheel.

Based on a shared narrative understanding, clinicians can work with patients to formulate a customized, multimodal treatment plan that matches their understandings, beliefs, expectations, and desires, in order to maximize overall therapeutic benefits via enhanced placebo effects, treatment alliance, and ease of integration of the therapeutic experience back into their daily life. Consistent with the psychedelic model of healing outlined earlier, treatment options would target various domains or dimensions of the person's existence, drawing on different ontologies of psychedelics and plant medicines as organizing principles. For instance, some patients may feel more comfortable with biological and psychological explanations of their suffering and thus be better served by more conventional clinical interventions, while others may be seeking spiritual, emotional, and energetic healing that explicitly differs from conventional treatments received previously. The types of interventions that could be offered include:

1. Lifestyle change: nutritional counseling, implementation of exercise programs and mindfulness and meditation practices, and nature exposure.

2. Psychotherapy with or without the assistance of psychedelic substances and plants:

A full discussion of the principles of psychedelic psychotherapy is beyond the scope of this chapter. However, as described above, clinicians would be trained in a variety of psychotherapeutic modalities that could be tailored to a patient's needs and preferences. As a general orientation, psychotherapy offered would be in line with both existing and emerging principles of psychedelic psychotherapy (e.g., W. A. Richards, 2015), which aim to help people face, accept, and cope with their difficulties and existential situations, rather than avoid them. Psychedelic psychotherapy should also seek to foster a sense of connectedness to one's self, to others, and to one's natural and social environments. Psychotherapeutic modalities that have affinity with this psychedelic approach include acceptance and commitment therapy (ACT), mindfulness-based therapy, logotherapy, and psychodynamic psychotherapy, among others.

When the use of a psychedelic is clinically indicated, ideally, the clinic would be able to facilitate psychedelic-assisted therapies using different medicines as well as different session formats. Drug selection would be based largely on available evidence and clinical formulation. Psychedelic sessions could be either individual- and/or group-based and take place in different contexts; some could occur more in a clinical context, utilizing principles of both "psychedelic" and "psycholytic" therapy paradigms (Abramson, 1967; Grof, 1994; Sherwood & Stolaroff, 1962). Alternatively, sessions could be conducted in a ceremonial context, led by shamans or other qualified personnel with extensive experience working with psychedelic plants as therapeutics. Such ceremonies would be contextualized within the broader treatment plan and involve preparation and integration processes before and after. As mentioned above, integration would be understood as therapeutic practices that help ensure therapeutic gains made during a psychedelic experience or retreat are integrated into a person's everyday life.

Although recent clinical trials with psilocybin, MDMA, and ayahuasca have all been implemented in highly clinical settings, I believe it is critical to incorporate ceremonial context in this proposed model for several reasons. First, I would argue that the elements involved in the ceremonial use of psychedelics, such as music, prayer, intention setting, shamanic and energetic healing, and group process, open up the possibility for healing in different and perhaps deeper ways than in a clinical context. Thus, it is in line with the psychedelic healing paradigm described above which targets multidimensional healing. Second, I believe it is important to generate an evidence base around the ceremonial use of psychedelic medicines in order to legitimize this as an important and novel therapeutic modality and also to legitimize and protect indigenous uses of these plants.[6] As the ceremonial use of plant medicines opens up an important space for

---

[6]This kind of work is being conducted by the Nierika Intercultural Medicine Institute (Nierika, n.d.).

collaboration and dialogue with indigenous healers, its inclusion also helps address the ethical issue of respecting indigenous knowledge and practices.

3. Group and family therapies: Various forms of group therapy may be useful in their own right and as part of the psychedelic psychotherapy process. Groups and the inclusion of family members may help create a sense of community among participants of healing retreats and could facilitate preparation and integration of psychedelic experiences.

4. Medicines: Treatment would include management of pharmaceutical, naturopathic, and herbal medicine regimens, including initiation and discontinuation of appropriate treatments.

5. Other interventions and therapeutic modalities may include but are not limited to acupuncture; art, music, and nature therapy; and forms of social, economic, and political engagement and empowerment.

In order to facilitate the implementation of these various therapeutic modalities, the clinic would be structured as a hybrid outpatient and residential facility that would allow for typical outpatient clinic visits but also multiday or 1–2 week retreats. It would have clinical spaces for group and family therapy, as well as indoor and outdoor spaces for meetings and ceremonies. It would have sufficient access to natural elements to facilitate therapeutic experiences in nature and would also utilize principles of "biophilic design" to incorporate natural elements into the aesthetic of the clinic in a manner that is mindful of the way physical spaces, materials, and light impact consciousness (Kellert, Heerwagen, & Mador, 2011; Ryan, Browning, Clancy, Andrews, & Kallianpurkar, 2014).

Lastly, it is worth noting here that the kind of clinic envisioned here would not currently be possible in most countries due to the legal status of psychedelic substances and plants. A more limited form of this clinic could be implemented in contexts where psychedelics are illegal by conducting clinical work exclusively through research protocols. Funding in this case would be limited to research grants and private donations. In a legal context, funding sources could be more varied, including sliding scale payments and eventually insurance reimbursement, as the evidence base for psychedelic-assisted therapies develops and they are shown to be cost-effective.

Knowledge Generation and Dissemination Across Paradigms

Like the clinical approach proposed, the clinic's modes of generating and sharing knowledge would also utilize an interdisciplinary approach in order to facilitate paradigm integration, or the bringing together of divergent perspectives and types of knowledge. Both research and other knowledge sharing practices, such as meetings, seminars, and trainings, would be guided by core values of reflexivity, transparency, and openness.

Research Agenda Focused on Paradigm Integration The clinic's research agenda would span the basic, clinical, and social sciences. As highlighted above, the clinic's central aim is to implement and study an integrative treatment model based on the psychedelic model of healing. Thus, the primary research objective of the clinic would be to conduct outcomes-oriented clinical research aiming to demonstrate the effectiveness of the model. Many holistic clinics currently exist throughout the world that are utilizing plant medicines, yet only a handful of observational research studies have been published on the outcomes of their work, or on the efficacy of plant medicines, like ayahuasca and ibogaine, in general (Brown & Alper, 2017; Fábregas et al., 2010; Halpern et al., 2008; Labate & Cavnar, 2013; Palhano-Fontes, Barreto, Onias, & Andrade, 2017; Thomas, Lucas, Capler, Tupper, & Martin, 2013). To be clear, the outcomes research proposed here would center the model of care as the object of study, as opposed to the substance, which is the primary variable in conventional clinical trials. This would allow the full range of healing modalities complementary to the use of psychedelic substances and plants to be utilized without them being seen as confounding variables. Treatment outcomes, such as reductions in depression, anxiety, or substance use, could initially be assessed in an observational fashion as treatments are provided to individual patients and then, eventually, in a more controlled, prospective experimental fashion. The latter would involve randomizing patients with similar baseline characteristics to either the psychedelic model of care or conventional psychiatric care.

While this form of outcomes research is not oriented toward the rescheduling of psychedelic substances or plants,[7] it would set a precedent for how the substances could be used therapeutically as dissemination occurs and also demonstrate proof of concept that the psychedelic healing paradigm is effective in its own right or in comparison to standard treatments. This would have important social justice implications, as it could pave the way for governments or insurance companies to pay for these treatments in legal contexts, thus increasing access. Amounting evidence of the safety and efficacy of these treatments may also strengthen the argument for decriminalization and regulation of the substances and plants in religious, spiritual, or recreational contexts.

While treating patients and collecting outcomes data, the clinic could simultaneously collect real-time data on treatment variables and set and setting variables. Treatment variables would include the composition of a plant medicine (the relative amounts of various alkaloids in an ayahuasca preparation), dose administered, and frequency of dosing, as well as the type and frequency of psychotherapy provided. Set variables include demographic information, personality characteristics, and baseline mental health profiles. Setting variables would account for the context and complementary practices used alongside psychedelic therapy, such as use of music, preparatory diet, individual versus group administration, and clinical versus

---

[7]Rescheduling of a substance requires demonstrating therapeutic efficacy through large-scale, randomized, placebo-controlled clinical trials in which the substance itself is isolated as the variable that leads to changes in therapeutic outcomes while controlling for all other variables.

ceremonial context. Retrospective analysis of these variables would help elucidate which aspects of treatment were correlated with therapeutic outcomes in different patient populations. This would importantly allow for the targeting of specific therapeutic practices to particular patient profiles and overall refinement of the treatment model. This data could also inform prospective, randomized studies to increase the quality of evidence behind psychedelic therapy, paving the way for wider dissemination of the model.

As a clinic founded on paradigm integration, quantitative empirical research would not be the only means of evaluating and refining the treatment model. Qualitative and participatory forms of research, such as semi-structured interviews with patients, clinic staff, and other stakeholders, would provide a complementary means of understanding the subjective experience of treatments, thus shedding light on their effectiveness, mechanisms, and areas for improvement. Similarly, incorporation of social sciences, such as medical anthropology and science and technology studies (STS), would generate critical feedback on the clinic's operations and practices, including how they are situated in broader theoretical, cultural, and political contexts. Both these forms of research would inform revisions to treatment protocols in a reflexive manner.

Lastly, the clinic would aim to engage in other forms of scientific research that further its mission of paradigm integration. This would include research that seeks to elucidate how plant medicines, psychedelics, and other complementary practices, such as yoga, meditation, and sound therapy, exert their therapeutic effects through complex interactions between biology, psychology, and spirituality. For instance, Robin Carhart-Harris has demonstrated how psychedelic-induced changes in brain connectivity correlate to specific subjective mystical-type experiences (Carhart-Harris et al., 2012). Undergoing such mystical-type experiences has been shown to correlate with therapeutic benefit in a number of recent clinical trials with psilocybin (Bogenschutz et al., 2015; Garcia-Romeu, Griffiths, & Johnson, 2014; Griffiths et al., 2011). Pursuing this kind of research, likely in collaboration with an academic institution, would help further our understanding of the neurobiology of consciousness and non-ordinary states. Grounding psychedelic and mystical-type experiences in neurobiology would help facilitate acceptance of spiritual and energetic "mechanisms of action" in the field of psychiatry and have the important implication of opening the neurobiology of consciousness as a legitimate treatment target.

Knowledge Sharing and Policy Engagement Beyond having a research mission based largely on the principles of Western empirical science, a model clinic would also seek to engage in other modes and traditions of knowledge generation and sharing. Specifically, the clinic would function as a center for critical dialogue on the intersection of psychiatry, traditional medicine, and other forms of healing. Embedding space for critical dialogue and dispute resolution processes would be essential, as the novel but complex work of integrating healing paradigms would undoubtedly involve significant differences of opinion, ethical dilemmas, and critiques from different stakeholders. By functioning as a place where health workers, shamans, academics, policymakers, and other stakeholders could gather for meetings, debates, conferences, seminars, trainings, and perhaps medicine ceremonies as well, the clinic would be able to (a) rethink its design, practices, and protocols based on feedback and critique; (b) engage in best practice sharing, collaboration, and consultation with other clinics engaged in similar work; (c) advance understandings of the uses of psychedelics and plant medicines more generally; and (d) envision how the principles of psychedelic healing can be translated into nonclinical domains, such as education, environmental science, and social policy.

This last point highlights the responsibility of a clinic whose practice is grounded in the use of psychedelic plants to protect the cultures and ecological environments on which their existence depends. As a result, the clinic's final aspect of its mission would be to engage in policy and public education work promoting indigenous rights, environmental justice, and drug policy reform.

Conclusion

This chapter has sought to outline a path toward a more holistic model of mental health treatment that is premised on interdisciplinary and intercultural perspectives and healing practices. It began by highlighting some of the shortcomings of current psychiatric practice and describing ways that a psychedelic healing paradigm can improve the current state of affairs in this field. Psychedelic substances and plants are critical tools that point us toward a more integrated and holistic way of conceptualizing human suffering and, accordingly, its treatment. Their lessons argue against narrow approaches or those based on fear, avoidance, and passivity. Rather, they help bring into focus our profound and nearly incomprehensible existential condition as impermanent beings intimately connected with all other forms of life, matter, and energy. Alleviating the many forms of suffering that result from the human condition is no easy task; it requires us to draw on many forms of wisdom and knowledge and apply them creatively, often in novel ways, with the courage to face into the unknown.

The model clinic proposed here would bring together different healing modalities and modes of knowledge generation in order to better elucidate the interconnections between various domains of human existence. It would aim to apply such insights in clinical practices that endeavor to bring about deep healing. Through processes of treatment integration and knowledge generation and dissemination, the healing benefits may extend beyond individuals to families, communities, nations, and perhaps, the planet as a whole.

References

Abramson, H. A. (1967). *The use of LSD in psychotherapy and alcoholism.* Indianapolis, IN: Bobbs-Merrill.

Auer, P. (2013). *Code-switching in conversation.* New York, NY: Routledge.

Barrett, F. S., Bradstreet, M. P., Leoutsakos, J. M. S., Johnson, M. W., & Griffiths, R. R. (2016). The challenging experience questionnaire: Characterization of challenging experiences with psilocybin mushrooms. *Journal of Psychopharmacology, 30*(12), 1279–1295. https://doi.org/10.1177/0269881116678781.

Ben-Shabat, S., Fride, E., Sheskin, T., Tamiri, T., Rhee, M. H., Vogel, Z., . . . Mechoulam, R. (1998). An entourage effect: Inactive endogenous fatty acid glycerol esters enhance 2-arachidonoyl-glycerol cannabinoid activity. *European Journal of Pharmacology, 353*(1), 23–31.

Bogenschutz, M. P., Forcehimes, A. A., Pommy, J. A., Wilcox, C. E., Barbosa, P., & Strassman, R. J. (2015). Psilocybin-assisted treatment for alcohol dependence: A proof-of-concept study. *Journal of Psychopharmacology, 29*(3), 289–299. https://doi.org/10.1177/0269881114565144.

Bracken, P., Thomas, P., Timimi, S., Asen, E., Behr, G., Beuster, C., . . . Yeomans, D. (2012). Psychiatry beyond the current paradigm. *The British Journal of Psychiatry, 201*(6), 430–434. https://doi.org/10.1192/bjp.bp.112.109447.

Brown, T. K., & Alper, K. (2017). Treatment of opioid use disorder with ibogaine: Detoxification and drug use outcomes. *The American Journal of Drug and Alcohol Abuse, 44*(1), 1–13. https://doi.org/10.1080/00952990.2017.1320802.

Carhart-Harris, R. L., Erritzoe, D., Williams, T., Stone, J. M., Reed, L. J., Colasanti, A., . . . Nutt, D. J. (2012). Neural correlates of the psychedelic state as determined by fMRI studies with psilocybin. *Proceedings of the National Academy of Sciences, 109*(6), 2138–2143. https://doi.org/10.1073/pnas.1119598109.

Carhart-Harris, R. L., Muthukumaraswamy, S., Roseman, L., Kaelen, M., Droog, W., Murphy, K., . . . Nutt, D. J. (2016). Neural correlates of the LSD experience revealed by multimodal neuroimaging. *Proceedings of the National Academy of Sciences, 113*(17), 4853–4858. https://doi.org/10.1073/pnas.1518377113.

Carlat, D. (2010). *Unhinged.* New York, NY: Simon and Schuster.

Domínguez-Clavé, E., Soler, J., Elices, M., Pascual, J. C., Álvarez, E., la Fuente Revenga, de, M., . . . Riba, J. (2016). Ayahuasca: Pharmacology, neuroscience and therapeutic potential. *Brain Research Bulletin, 126*(Part 1), 89–101. https://doi.org/10.1016/j.brainresbull.2016.03.002.

El-Seedi, H. R., Smet, P. A. G. M. D., Beck, O., Possnert, G., & Bruhn, J. G. (2005). Prehistoric peyote use: Alkaloid analysis and radiocarbon dating of archaeological specimens of Lophophora from Texas. *Journal of Ethnopharmacology, 101*(1–3), 238–242. https://doi.org/10.1016/j.jep.2005.04.022.

Engel, G. L. (1980). The clinical application of the biopsychosocial model. *American Journal of Psychiatry, 137*(5), 535–544.

Fábregas, J. M., González, D., Fondevila, S., Cutchet, M., Fernández, X., Barbosa, P. C. R., . . . Bouso, J. C. (2010). Assessment of addiction severity among ritual users of ayahuasca. *Drug and Alcohol Dependence, 111*(3), 257–261. https://doi.org/10.1016/j.drugalcdep.2010.03.024.

Garcia-Romeu, A., Griffiths, R. R., & Johnson, M. W. (2014). Psilocybin-occasioned mystical experiences in the treatment of tobacco addiction. *Current Drug Abuse Reviews, 7*(3), 157–164.

Goff, D. C., Falkai, P., Fleischhacker, W. W., Girgis, R. R., Kahn, R. M., Uchida, H., . . . Lieberman, J. A. (2017). The long-term effects of antipsychotic medication on clinical course in schizophrenia. *American Journal of Psychiatry, 174*(9), 840–849. https://doi.org/10.1176/appi.ajp.2017.16091016.

Griffiths, R. R., Johnson, M. W., Carducci, M. A., Umbricht, A., Richards, W. A., Richards, B. D., . . . Klinedinst, M. A. (2016). Psilocybin produces substantial and sustained decreases in depression and anxiety in patients with life-threatening cancer: A randomized double-blind trial. *Journal of Psychopharmacology, 30*(12), 1181–1197. https://doi.org/10.1177/0269881116675513.

Griffiths, R. R., Johnson, M. W., Richards, W. A., Richards, B. D., McCann, U., & Jesse, R. (2011). Psilocybin occasioned mystical-type experiences: Immediate and persisting dose-related effects. *Psychopharmacology, 218*(4), 649–665. https://doi.org/10.1007/s00213-011-2358-5.

Grof, S. (1994). *LSD psychotherapy*. Alameda, CA: Hunter House.

Halpern, J. H., Sherwood, A. R., Hudson, J. I., Yurgelun-Todd, D., & Pope, H. G., Jr. (2005). Psychological and cognitive effects of long-term peyote use among Native Americans. *Biological Psychiatry, 58*(8), 624–631. https://doi.org/10.1016/j.biopsych.2005.06.038.

Halpern, J. H., Sherwood, A. R., Passie, T., Blackwell, K. C., & Ruttenber, A. J. (2008). Evidence of health and safety in American members of a religion who use a hallucinogenic sacrament. *Medical Science Monitor: International Medical Journal of Experimental and Clinical Research, 14*(8), SR15–SR22.

Hendy, K. (2018). The placebo paradox. In B. C. Labate & C. Cavnar (Eds.), *Plant medicines, healing and psychedelic science: Cultural perspectives*. Heidelberg: Springer.

Johnson, M. W., Garcia-Romeu, A., & Griffiths, R. R. (2016). Long-term follow-up of psilocybin-facilitated smoking cessation. *The American Journal of Drug and Alcohol Abuse*, 1–6. https://doi.org/10.3109/00952990.2016.1170135.

Johnson, M., Richards, W., & Griffiths, R. (2008). Human hallucinogen research: Guidelines for safety. *Journal of Psychopharmacology, 22*(6), 603–620. https://doi.org/10.1177/0269881108093587.

Kellert, S. R., Heerwagen, J., & Mador, M. (2011). *Biophilic design*. San Francisco, CA: Wiley.

Kleinman, A. (1988). *The illness narratives*. New York, NY: Basic Books.

Labate, B. C., & Cavnar, C. (2013). *The therapeutic use of ayahuasca*. New York, NY: Springer. https://doi.org/10.1007/978-3-642-40426-9.

Labate, B. C., & Cavnar, C. (2014). *Ayahuasca shamanism in the Amazon and beyond*. New York, NY: Oxford University Press.

Labate, B. C., Cavnar, C., & Gearin, A. K. (2016). *The world ayahuasca diaspora*. New York, NY: Routledge.

Leary, T., Metzner, R., & Alpert, R. (1995). *The psychedelic experience*. New York, NY: Citadel Press.

Lewis, B. (2011). *Narrative psychiatry*. Baltimore, MD: JHU Press.

Luna, L. E. (1984). The concept of plants as teachers among four mestizo shamans of Iquitos, northeastern Peru. *Journal of Ethnopharmacology, 11*(2), 135–156.

Millenium Villages Project. (n.d.). *Millennium villages |Overview*. Retrieved from http://millenniumvillages.org/about/overview/

Moynihan, R., & Cassels, A. (2006). *Selling sickness*. New York, NY: Nation Books.

National Institute of Mental Health. (2013, December 7). *NIMH's new focus in clinical trials*. Retrieved from https://www.nimh.nih.gov/funding/grant-writing-and-application-process/concept-clearances/2013/nimhs-new-focus-in-clinical-trials.shtml

Nichols, D. E. (2016). Psychedelics. *Pharmacological Reviews, 68*(2), 264–355. https://doi.org/10.1124/pr.115.011478.

Nierika. (n.d.). *The Nierika Intercultural Medicine Institute*. Retrieved from http://nierika.info/english/medicine-institute/

Olfson, M., & Marcus, S. C. (2010). National trends in outpatient psychotherapy. *American Journal of Psychiatry, 167*(12), 1456–1463. https://doi.org/10.1176/appi.ajp.2010.10040570.

Palhano-Fontes, F., Barreto, D., Onias, H., & Andrade, K. C. (2017). Rapid antidepressant effects of the psychedelic ayahuasca in treatment-resistant depression: A randomised placebo-controlled trial. *Biorxiv*, 103531. https://doi.org/10.1101/103531.

Pollan, M. (2007, January 28). *Unhappy meals*. Retrieved from http://michaelpollan.com/articles-archive/unhappy-meals/

Ribeiro, S. (2018). Whole organisms or pure compounds? Entourage effect versus drug specificity. In B. C. Labate & C. Cavnar (Eds.), *Plant medicines, healing and psychedelic science: Cultural perspectives*. Heidelberg: Springer.

Richards, W. A. (2015). *Sacred knowledge*. New York, NY: Columbia University Press. https://doi. org/10.7312/rich17406.

Ross, S., Bossis, A., Guss, J., Agin-Liebes, G., Malone, T., Cohen, B., . . . Schmidt, B. L. (2016). Rapid and sustained symptom reduction following psilocybin treatment for anxiety and depression in patients with life-threatening cancer: A randomized controlled trial. *Journal of Psychopharmacology, 30*(12), 1165–1180. https://doi.org/10.1177/0269881116675512.

Ryan, C. O., Browning, W. D., Clancy, J. O., Andrews, S. L., & Kallianpurkar, N. B. (2014). Biophilic design patterns: Emerging nature-based parameters for health and well-being in the built environment. *International Journal of Architectural Research: ArchNet-IJAR, 8*(2), 62–76.

Samara, M. T., Dold, M., Gianatsi, M., Nikolakopoulou, A., Helfer, B., Salanti, G., & Leucht, S. (2016). Efficacy, acceptability, and tolerability of antipsychotics in treatment-resistant schizophrenia. *JAMA Psychiatry, 73*(3), 199–112. https://doi.org/10.1001/jamapsychiatry. 2015.2955.

Sanacora, G., & Schatzberg, A. F. (2014). Ketamine: Promising path or false prophecy in the development of novel therapeutics for mood disorders? *Neuropsychopharmacology, 40*(2), 259–267. https://doi.org/10.1038/npp.2014.261.

Sherwood, J. N., & Stolaroff, M. J. (1962). The psychedelic experience: A new concept in psychotherapy. *Journal of Neuropsychiatry, 4*, 69–80. https://doi.org/10.1080/02791072. 1968.10524522.

Tafur, J. (2017). *The fellowship of the river: A medical doctor's exploration into traditional Amazonian plant medicine*. Phoenix, AZ: Espiritu Books.

Thomas, G., Lucas, P., Capler, N. R., Tupper, K. W., & Martin, G. (2013). Ayahuasca-assisted therapy for addiction: Results from a preliminary observational study in Canada. *Current Drug Abuse Reviews, 6*(1), 30–42.

Tindle, H. A., Davis, R. B., & Phillips, R. S. (2005). Trends in use of complementary and alternative medicine by US adults: 1997–2002. *Therapies in Health, 11*(1), 42–49.

Torres, C. M. (1995). Archaeological evidence for the antiquity of psychoactive plant use in the Central Andes. *Annuli Dei Musei Civici Roverero, 11*, 391–326.

Tupper, K. W., & Labate, B. C. (2014). Ayahuasca, psychedelic studies and health sciences: The politics of knowledge and inquiry into an Amazonian plant brew. *Current Drug Abuse Reviews, 7*(2), 71–80.

United States Drug Enforcement Administration. (n.d.). *Drug scheduling*. Retrieved from https:// www.dea.gov/druginfo/ds.shtml

Warden, D., Rush, A. J., Trivedi, M. H., Fava, M., & Wisniewski, S. R. (2007). The STAR* D Project results: A comprehensive review of findings. *Current Psychiatry Reports, 9*(6), 449–459.

Wilkinson, S. T., Wright, D., Fasula, M. K., Fenton, L., Griepp, M., Ostroff, R. B., & Sanacora, G. (2017). Cognitive behavior therapy may sustain antidepressant effects of intravenous ketamine in treatment-resistant depression. *Psychotherapy and Psychosomatics, 86*(3), 162–167. https://doi.org/10.1159/000457960.

World Ayahuasca Conference. (2016). *Open letter from the Indigenous people of Acre, Brazil*. Retrieved from http://www.ayaconference.com/index.php/conclusoes?lang=en

Chapter 8
Whole Organisms or Pure Compounds? Entourage Effect Versus Drug Specificity

Sidarta Ribeiro

Abstract As the therapeutic use of sacred plants and fungi becomes increasingly accepted by Western medicine, a tug of war has been taking place between those who advocate the traditional consumption of whole organisms and those who defend exclusively the utilization of purified compounds. The attempt to reduce organisms to single active principles is challenged by the sheer complexity of traditional medicine. Ayahuasca, for example, is a concoction of at least two plant species containing multiple psychoactive substances with complex interactions. Similarly, cannabis contains dozens of psychoactive substances whose specific combinations in different strains correspond to different types of therapeutic and cognitive effects. The "entourage effect" refers to the synergistic effects of the multiple compounds present in whole organisms, which may potentiate clinical efficacy while attenuating side effects. In opposition to this view, mainstream pharmacology is adamant about the need to use purified substances, presumably more specific and safe. In this chapter, I will review the evidence on both sides to discuss the scientific, economic, and political implications of this controversy. The evidence indicates that it is time to embrace the therapeutic complexity of psychedelics.

As Western medicine discovers the medicinal properties of whole organisms deemed sacred by traditional cultures, a fierce debate has been set between proponents of the use of purified chemicals versus supporters of long-established ritual uses of plants, fungi, and animals. As a professional neuroscientist with an interest in psychedelic medicines, it is clear to me that the attempt to reduce organisms to single active principles is challenged by the sheer complexity of traditional medicine. Ayahuasca, for example, is a concoction of at least two plant species containing multiple psychoactive substances with a plethora of interactions (Dos Santos et al., 2012; Mckenna, Towers, & Abbott, 1984). Similarly, cannabis contains dozens of psychoactive substances whose specific combinations in different strains correspond to

S. Ribeiro (✉)
Brain Institute, Federal University of Rio Grande do Norte, Natal, RN, Brazil
e-mail: sidartaribeiro@neuro.ufrn.br

© Springer International Publishing AG, part of Springer Nature 2018
B. C. Labate, C. Cavnar (eds.), *Plant Medicines, Healing and Psychedelic Science*,
https://doi.org/10.1007/978-3-319-76720-8_8

distinct types of therapeutic and cognitive effects (Mechoulam, Hanus, Pertwee, & Howlett, 2014). Is there a scientific basis for believing that single molecules are more useful for medicinal purposes than mixtures?

Pharmacopeia of a Single Plant: The Case of Cannabis

Much as the hundreds of dog breeds coevolved with humans in a genetic race for the satisfaction of quite specific human needs (Kekecs et al., 2016; Parker et al., 2017), cannabis coevolved with humans so as to satisfy a wide variety of therapeutic, recreational, and religious needs (Guy, Whittle, & Robson, 2004; Pollan, 2001). There are over 700 strains of cannabis (Gloss, 2015; Sawler et al., 2015), each with characteristic concentrations of hundreds of substances of therapeutic interest, such as cannabinoids, terpenes, and phenols (Andre, Hausman, & Guerriero, 2016; Formukong, Evans, & Evans, 1988; Gertsch, Pertwee, & Di Marzo, 2010). Dozens of cannabinoids have medicinal properties (Izzo, Borrelli, Capasso, Di Marzo, & Mechoulam, 2009; Radwan et al., 2008). Tetrahydrocannabinol (THC), until recently the most studied cannabinoid of cannabis, possesses enormous therapeutic potential, with preliminary or advanced empirical evidence regarding a wide range of diseases, such as multiple sclerosis (Rekand, 2014; Zettl, Rommer, Hipp, & Patejdl, 2016), ischemia (Zani, Braida, Capurro, & Sala, 2007), Alzheimer's disease (Aso, Sanchez-Pla, Vegas-Lozano, Maldonado, & Ferrer, 2015; Cao et al., 2014; Yu et al., 2016), lateral amyotrophic sclerosis (Weber, Goldman, & Truniger, 2010), anorexia (Lewis & Brett, 2010; Verty et al., 2011), Parkinson's disease (van Vliet, Vanwersch, Jongsma, Olivier, & Philippens, 2008), diabetes (Gallant, Odei-Addo, Frost, & Levendal, 2009), cystic fibrosis (Bregman & Fride, 2011), chronic and neuropathic pain (Cannabis-based Medicines, 2003; Johnson et al., 2010; Johnson, Lossignol, Burnell-Nugent, & Fallon, 2013), and epilepsy (Maccarrone, Maldonado, Casas, Henze, & Centonze, 2017). Another very promising recent advance occurred in cancer; we now know that cannabinoids are useful in onco-therapy, not only to alleviate anxiety, pain, lack of appetite, and sleep due to chemotherapy or radiotherapy (Abrams, 2016) but also for their potent antitumor properties (Guzman, 2003; Huff & Chan, 2000; Ladin, Soliman, Griffin, & Van Dross, 2016; Lombard, Nagarkatti, & Nagarkatti, 2005).

A major recent breakthrough revealed THC as a contender for holding the biggest promise of cognitive restoration for the aging human population. The study showed that chronic THC treatment reverses cognitive decline in older mice, restoring learning ability to the levels of young animals (Bilkei-Gorzo et al., 2017). THC treatment also restored synaptic plasticity to the levels typical of young animals, with a concomitant rescue of plasticity-related mRNA and protein levels and increase in the density of dendritic spines (Bilkei-Gorzo et al., 2017). The study showed further that adolescent mice are cognitively impaired after the same treatment, due to excessive plasticity. While it becomes increasingly clear why the early and excessive use of cannabis is ill-advised (Farnsworth, 1976; Schmits & Quertemont, 2013), cannabis strives to supplant the cane as the elder's best friend.

Part of the resistance to cannabis as medicine relates to its great potential to replace or substantially change current therapies. Patients with epilepsy, Parkinson's disease, neuropathic pains, and several other illnesses treatable by cannabis are often refractory to medications presently available for medical prescription (Ohtsuka, Yoshinaga, & Kobayashi, 2000). This problem is clinically addressed by increasing medication doses, leading to higher risks of side effects, which may include cardiac or respiratory arrest (Hookana et al., 2016). In contrast, cannabinoid medications are very safe to use, since there are no cannabinoid receptors in neurovegetative centers (Hu & Mackie, 2015; Moldrich & Wenger, 2000; Tsou, Brown, Sanudo-Pena, Mackie, & Walker, 1998).

The main psychological deficit acutely caused by cannabis intake is an impairment of working memory (Fadda, Robinson, Fratta, Pertwee, & Riedel, 2004). Interestingly, the scientific basis for the use of cannabis to treat a variety of diseases related to excess or inadequate neuronal synchronization, such as epilepsy, Parkinson's disease, Tourette syndrome, and chronic and neuropathic pain, is probably related to the same biological property that impairs working memory in a dose-dependent manner: the capacity of cannabinoids to desynchronize neuronal activity (Robbe et al., 2006). Working memory impairment is mostly related to THC and can be avoided by mixing it with other cannabinoids and terpenes (Cannabis-based medicines, 2003; Johnson et al., 2013; Koehler, 2014; Maccarone et al., 2017; Patti, 2016; Rekand, 2014; Sastre-Garriga, Vila, Clissold, & Montalban, 2011; Zettl et al., 2016), as typically for *in natura* cannabis (Russo, 2011). The antidepressant effects of cannabis (de Mello Schier et al., 2014; Jiang et al., 2005), as well as its use to mitigate the consequences of stroke (Bravo-Ferrer et al., 2017), are likely related to its role in the induction of neurogenesis (Avraham et al., 2014; Jin et al., 2004; Xapelli et al., 2013).

Plants United, Entourage of Molecules

The understanding of the medicinal use of whole organisms is greatly illuminated by the notion of *entourage effect*, a term coined by chemists Raphael Mechoulam and Simon Ben-Shabat to refer to the cooperative effects of the multiple compounds present in whole organisms that may potentiate clinical efficacy while attenuating side effects (Ben-Shabat et al., 1998). One clear example of such entourage effect is the additive effect of cannabidiol (CBD) and THC, two main constituents of cannabis, in the enhancement of radiotherapy for the treatment of glioma (Scott, Dalgleish, & Liu, 2014). Cooperative effects also link cannabinoids to the perfumed organic compounds called terpenes. Chemically similar to cannabinoids and abundant in cannabis, these substances can facilitate the passage of chemicals through the blood-brain barrier and counterbalance memory deficits induced by THC (Russo, 2011).

From the psychiatric point of view, CBD and THC have very different and, in fact, complementary effects (Fadda et al., 2004; Morgan, Freeman, Schafer, & Curran, 2010; Morgan, Schafer, Freeman, & Curran, 2010), with relaxation and sedation following CBD intake and excitation following THC intake. CBD is anxiolytic and antipsychotic, while THC is anxiogenic and pro-psychotic (Fakhoury, 2016; Sherif, Radhakrishnan, D'Souza, & Ranganathan, 2016; Zuardi et al., 2012). In isolation and at high doses, these substances may have negative health effects, especially for people in key populations (Di Forti et al., 2009). On the other hand, the presence of both compounds in cannabis results in a buffered effect that is anything but unsafe from the patient's perspective (Silva, Balbino, & Weiber, 2015).

Did Science Finally Catch Up with the Traditional Shamans?

Is cannabis beneficial? Is cannabis dangerous? Should we legalize cannabis? The absurdity of these questions can be exposed by performing an apt substitution: Are dogs beneficial? Are dogs dangerous? Should we legalize dogs? We must not forget that the traditional use of whole organisms such as cannabis coevolved with the plant itself (McPartland & Guy, 2004; Pollan, 2001). Cannabis was probably used in the first rope, cloth, paper, and medicine. The Ebers Papyrus of Ancient Egypt (~1550 BC) contains a prescription of cannabis for inflammation (Dawson, 1934). We now know that the plant contains several anti-inflammatory substances (de Lago, Moreno-Martet, Cabranes, Ramos, & Fernandez-Ruiz, 2012; Fabisiak & Fichna, 2017; Liu, Fowler, & Dalgleish, 2010; Molina-Holgado et al., 2003; Nagarkatti, Pandey, Rieder, Hegde, & Nagarkatti, 2009; Zurier, 2003). The "Siberian Ice Lady," a beautifully tattooed mummy from the fifth century BC, discovered in 1993 in the Russian Altai Mountains near the borders of China, Mongolia, and Kazakhstan, was found with a pouch of cannabis at the rich burial site. The mummy also had a primary tumor in her right breast, with signs of metastasis (Letyagin, Savelov, & Polosmak, 2014). Could the "Siberian Ice Lady" have used cannabis to treat cancer? In the past 17 years, biomedical research has shown that cannabinoids have antitumoral effects in breast cancer and a variety of other cancer types, including glioma, lung, colon, liver, skin, prostate, thyroid, and pancreatic cancer (Ladin et al., 2016).

The artificial selection of cannabis, performed widely in central Asia in the past 6000 years both north and south of the Himalayas, led to strains characterized by cannabinoid mixtures, rather than strains dominated by a single cannabinoid (Elsohly & Slade, 2005; Fetterman & Turner, 1972). We know now that an extract of the entire plant, with similar amounts of THC and CBD ("Sativex"), is more effective in reducing pain and spasms of multiple sclerosis than the pure synthetic compound, Dronabinol ("Marinol"), analogous to THC (Keating, 2017). If purified compounds were indeed always best for therapy, single-compound strains should have been favored over time. Yet, the opposite happens to be true. Traditional shamans use whole plants and have advocated for this sort of medicine as a major root of their practice (Labate & Cavnar, 2014a). We should listen to our ancestors here.

"Purified Compounds Only" Is Snake Oil

What is best for medicinal use, whole organisms or isolated active principles? Mainstream pharmacology is adamant about the need to use purified substances for medical treatment, because these are presumably more specific and safe (Zuardi, Crippa, & Hallak, 2010). This position is defended fiercely in the media and also in academic publications, as if there was much more clinical knowledge accumulated about the effects of the purified compounds than about the effects of whole organisms; however, this is often not the case. The traditional use of whole organisms has centuries and, in some cases, millennia of cultural experience, while purified compounds only recently started to be investigated. As a useful analogy, consider that to say that the use of purified cannabinoids is medically safer than the use of cannabis *in natura* is similar to the fallacy of considering cesarean delivery scientifically superior to natural childbirth. Rimonabant, an anti-obesity medicine based on an antagonist of a cannabinoid receptor, is the most infamous example of the potential dangers of a single compound; it was removed from the market in 2008 due to the association with suicide cases (Rimonabant, 2009; Topol et al., 2010). The whole cannabis plant, however, with various proportions of THC, CBD, and many other cannabinoids, is clinically safe for people outside key populations and can even be used in these populations provided that adequate, specific strains of cannabis are used. For example, CBD-rich cannabis is safe for psychotic patients and can be used as psychiatric treatment (Zuardi et al., 2012). In the case of ayahuasca, compound combination is advantageous not because of safety issues but due to the fact that the N-N-dimethyltryptamine (DMT) contained in the plant *Psychotria viridis* is entirely degraded by the monoamine oxidases (MAO) present in the gastrointestinal tract in the absence of pharmacological protection (Buckholtz & Boggan, 1977). Indeed, the DMT contained in ayahuasca would be innocuous if the brew did not include another plant, the liana *Banisteriopsis caapi*, which is rich in inhibitors of MAO and therefore allows the psychedelic experience to occur. These substances by themselves increase the levels of dopamine and other neurotransmitters (Iurlo et al., 2001) and induce the formation of new neurons (Dakic et al., 2016). An argument favoring isolated compounds can perhaps be made for the use of psilocybin rather than whole mushrooms, although there is no symbolic equivalency between these forms of use; the rich cultural context of mushroom consumption comprises an important part of the setting that is absent in the case of ingesting a purified compound.

One cornerstone of the mesmerizing argument favoring purified compounds is the notion that their biological action is equally "pure" and, therefore, "specific," two very loaded words. Much of the credibility that psychiatrists have in the public debate, whether it is about the pharmacological treatment of mental illness or about drug policy, stems from the well-publicized specificity of the single compounds sold as psychiatric drugs. It may be surprising to most readers that the opposite happens to be true: Single molecules often bind to multiple receptors in the brain (Rickli, Moning, Hoener, & Liechti, 2016; U'Prichard, 1980), at various dose-dependent affinities (Hamblin, Leff, & Creese, 1984) and with complex long-distance (allosteric) molecular interactions (Price et al., 2005; Solt, Ruesch, Forman, Davies, & Raines, 2007). The simple is simply not simple.

Time to Debunk the Prohibition Myths

Facing the inquisition, Galileo Galilei was forced, in 1663, to deny the notion that it is the Earth that moves around the Sun, not the other way around. Galileo is said to have muttered *Eppur si muove* ("And yet it moves") in an act of resistance to ecclesiastical irrationalism. This dire situation has parallels today in the deadlock in the public debate regarding the medical use of cannabinoid and serotonergic psychedelics.

The risks associated with these substances—in particular, cannabis and THC—have been used as an intellectual "straw man" in the public debate. Many of the substances sold in pharmacy are acutely dangerous at high doses, which is not the case with cannabis. To justify the prohibition of cannabis based on the existence of key populations at risk for cannabis use is to ignore that every substance has risks. To give a familiar example, it is not because there are people intolerant to lactose that milk should be banned. The way to deal with lactose intolerance is to inform consumers properly and to market lactose-free milk.

The prohibition paradigm feeds from a great degree of media-induced moral panic targeting specific illicit drugs (Forsyth, 2001), in disagreement with the scientific evidence regarding harm potential (Nutt, King, Phillips, & Independent Scientific Committee on Drugs, 2010). The fallacious arguments used to bar whole organisms from the repertoire of official medical treatment often take the form of inadequate biological analogies, such as: "The purified compounds of snake venom are medicinal, but as a whole snake venom kills." This proposition does not survive inspection. The first drug derived from snake venom was an inhibitor of the angiotensin-converting enzyme, a toxin found in the venom of the Brazilian pit viper *Bothrops jararaca* (Ferreira, 1965; Rocha e Silva, 1963), and basis of synthetic compounds used worldwide to control high blood pressure, treat chronic heart failure, and prevent cardiovascular risk (Flather et al., 2000). Later snake-derived drugs include a modified version of an antiplatelet toxin produced by the rattlesnake *Sistrurus miliarius barbouri*, used broadly to treat heart attacks and prevent blood clotting (Phillips & Scarborough, 1997). Both kinds of drugs are dangerous at high doses (Attaya, Kanthi, Aster, & McCrae, 2009; Augenstein, Kulig, & Rumack, 1988; Coons, Barcelona, Freedy, & Hagerty, 2005; Dawson et al., 1990; Parakh, Naik, Rohatgi, Bhat, & Parakh, 2009; Park, Purnell, & Mirchandani, 1990), so it is disingenuous to sustain that whole venoms are lethal but purified compounds are not.

The real motivation underlying the venom fallacy is the conflict of interest of the medical establishment, in bed with Big Pharma. Where will the profits come from, when medicine can be grown at home and used in small, infrequent doses? And yet, how will it be possible to block patients from accessing the life-transforming psychedelic medicine at very low cost?

The healthcare regulation of traditional medicine based on whole organisms must consider regional differences and social inequality. Currently, the illicit drug market is conducted through retail locations in poor neighborhoods and communities. Regulation in the context of legalization must be oriented to mitigate regional imbalances, to encourage harm reduction, and to promote the social inclusion of those who now live from the illicit market but are usually excluded from the debate on their regulation. Whole organisms offer hope in the treatment of substance abuse (Winkelman, 2014), as documented preliminarily for the use of cannabis to treat crack addiction (Labigalini Jr, Rodrigues, & Da Silveira, 1999) and for the use of ayahuasca to treat alcohol, tobacco, and cocaine abuse (2014; Thomas, Lucas, Capler, Tupper, & Martin, 2013).

And Yet It Moves: The Psychedelic Renaissance Is On

The year 2017 will be remembered as a landmark of the "psychedelic renaissance"; the terrible barriers that have been imposed for decades on the research and the therapeutic use of psychedelic substances—cannabis, ayahuasca, LSD, psilocybin, MDMA, DMT, and many others—are being lifted. In April, researchers from around the world gathered in Oakland for 3 days of intense exchange of knowledge at Psychedelic Science 2017, a meeting promoted by the Multidisciplinary Association for Psychedelic Studies (MAPS) and the Beckley Foundation. The first time I attended a MAPS congress, it was its 25th anniversary conference, the *Cartographie Psychedelica* in 2011. The bulk of the audience seemed composed of characters from J. R. Tolkien's *The Lord of the Rings*. The California hippie-chic mixed with few but quite serious scientists in an atmosphere of celebration of the interest of science in psychedelia. The congress attracted about 1100 people, and most of the interest seemed to fall on pure compounds of medicinal interest, although ayahuasca had its own track.

The following MAPS congress I attended, Psychedelic Science 2013, had about 2000 people and a noticeable change in composition. Scientists invaded Tolkien's arena, merging with the mythological beings of Middle-Earth in equal proportions. Anthropologist Beatriz Labate organized a crowded track of presentations on aya-huasca, marking the heightened public interest regarding traditional medicines that bring with them as complex cultural package, with a use setting of its own (Labate & Cavnar, 2013, 2014a, 2014b).

Psychedelic Science 2017 grew like a tsunami. There were over 3000 partici-pants, lots of renowned scientists, multiple events of scientific and artistic relevance, international press, and closed hotel rooms for documentary recording. The beings of Tolkien practically disappeared, although some still were present, undercover in plain clothes. The main difference of the 2017 congress compared to previous ones was the conspicuous arrival of foundations and companies interested in funding research on the use of psychedelics to treat anxiety, depression, post-traumatic stress syndrome, and even cancer. Importantly, the ayahuasca session grew into an entire track ("Plant Medicine") dedicated to whole organisms in general.

The meeting was remarkable for bringing up and coming mainstream, traditional, and syncretic contemporary medicine, together with hardcore science performed by leading researchers in cell and molecular biology, biochemistry, neurophysiology, psychology, and psychiatry. Thomas Insel, the 14-year director of the National Institute of Mental Health (NIMH), who resigned in 2015 to join Verily Life Sciences (Google's spin-off) and now heads the neuroscience company "Mindstrong", publicly acknowledged the immense therapeutic potential of psychedelics. Major advances in basic psychedelic research were presented. For instance, pharmacologist David Nichols, from Chapel Hill University, reported groundbreaking results on lysergic acid diethylamide (LSD), featured on *Cell*'s cover, demonstrating that the molecular structure of the serotonin receptor locks LSD in its binding site (Wacker et al., 2017). In principle, this mechanism explains the delayed, and yet intense, long-lasting effects of LSD, even at tiny doses. This likely relates to the trendy habit of microdosing LSD, by which people seek cognitive and emotional enhancement without unintended side effects. Microdosing (including the use of whole plants or concoctions with low concentrations of psychedelic compounds) should be understood vis-à-vis the fact that most drug effects correlate with dose according to inverted-U curves, and therefore the use of low doses keeps effects on the rising side of the dose-response curve.

Also remarkable were the experimental results shown by molecular and cell biologist Stevens Rehen, from the D'Or Institute for Research and Teaching and Federal University of Rio de Janeiro, who showed that 5-methoxy-N,N-dimethyltryptamine (5-MeO-DMT), a psychedelic substance present in ayahuasca, in the indigenous snuff *Yopo,* and in the Sonoran desert toad *Bufo alvarius* (Barceloux, 2012), can induce neurogenesis (Dakic et al., 2016) and synaptic plasticity (Dakic et al., 2017).

Major advances in translational psychedelic research were also featured. The research presented by neuroscientist Draulio de Araujo was one of the biggest highlights. With his team from the Federal University of Rio Grande do Norte, Araujo obtained excellent evidence that ayahuasca is quite useful in the effective care of treatment-resistant major depression in a randomized, placebo-controlled clinical trial (Palhano-Fontes et al., 2017). In contrast with regular antidepressants that take weeks to act, ayahuasca quickly attenuates depressive symptoms (Osorio et al., 2015), with a significant effect 40 min after ingestion (Sanches et al., 2016). Importantly, when compared to placebo, this effect persists for at least 7 days (Palhano-Fontes et al., 2017), substantially more than the effect obtained with the single-molecule ketamine, at present ayahuasca's direct clinical competitor for fast yet durable antidepressant effect (Romeo, Choucha, Fossati, & Rotge, 2015; Zarate Jr et al., 2006). Preliminary results from the Araujo group indicate that the antidepressant effect is proportional to the degree of perceptual alteration (Palhano-Fontes, 2017), which is known to involve major activation of visual cortical areas (de Araujo et al., 2012). In the author's own words, "the more intense the psychedelic experience, the stronger is the antidepressant effect" (Palhano-Fontes, 2017).

Prohibition: What Is to Be Done?

The core issue at stake is the fact that the phyto-therapeutic approach to psychedelic medicine is successful in multiple countries, and quite scalable, due to the low cost of home-growing whole organisms. The therapeutic use of cannabis is currently legal in Austria, Belgium, Canada, Chile, Colombia, the Czech Republic, Finland, Israel, the Netherlands, Spain, the United Kingdom, Uruguay and several US states. Ayahuasca is currently legal in multiple countries (Labate & Cavnar, 2014a, 2014b).

Phyto-therapeutic medicine is feasible because doses can be kept within controlled ranges and because knowing the precise dose is often not essential for effective therapeutics. After all, few would defend the notion that taking vitamin pills provides better nutrition than eating fresh fruit and vegetables. Purified compounds are much more expensive to make and necessarily reach the final consumer at much higher prices than whole organisms. The clinical use of purified compounds for subjects with low socioeconomic status is further hampered by Big Pharma patent rights and marketing strategies. Still, in recent years, the large margin of profit for the commercialization of purified compounds has motivated a strong corporative push for the adoption of purified compounds as the gold standard for medical practice involving psychedelic substances. In the case of medical marijuana, cannabis *in natura* versus isolated cannabinoids is a billion-dollar question.

To make safe use of any substance, it is necessary to understand its use in three different dimensions of the experience: substance (dose, interaction), set (body and mind), and setting (social context). Prohibition compromises the three dimensions altogether. With regard to the substance, it increases the chances of dose uncertainty, contamination, and degradation. With respect to the set, it hinders free dialogue about key populations. With regard to the setting, it promotes violence, paranoia, marginalization, and stigmatization. Prohibition is the heaviest of all drugs, and the ban on psychedelic drugs leads to unregulated iatrogenic use without harm reduction, nor scientific control, decreasing the protection of the society.

In view of current scientific knowledge (Abrams, 2016; Ben Amar, 2006; Fasinu, Phillips, ElSohly, & Walker, 2016; Ladin et al., 2016; Rosenberg, Tsien, Whalley, & Devinsky, 2015; Sznitman & Lewis, 2015), it is of paramount importance for medicine and research to legalize the use, possession, planting, cultivation, harvesting, manipulation, manufacture, distribution, marketing, import, export, and prescription of *Cannabis sativa L.* and other varieties of cannabis, as well as products obtained from these plants. The same applies to ayahuasca, peyote, mushrooms, toads, and various other psychedelic organisms (Labate & Cavnar, 2014a, 2014b). Whole organisms must be legalized and regulated to protect people at risk and respect users. These measures will give doctors, patients, and researchers maximum therapeutic options and the widest range of tools while at the same time reducing costs, offering access options according to each patient profile or type of research, avoiding dependence on foreign products, and preventing patients from buying medicine from the illicit market of questionable quality and with active principles in unknown concentrations. These measures will also promote production by patient associations and promote the self-care of patients who carry out their own cultivation.

We are living in the era of psychedelic renaissance. Science finally caught up with the knowledge, wisdom, and curiosity of healers and psychonauts, and the new medicine of the future may come from ancient medicine invented by Amazonian *pajés* and Siberian shamans of the past. New questions are becoming as widespread as new answers. Now is the prime time to discuss the potential advantages and disadvantages of therapeutics based on whole organisms versus purified compounds, a debate with major economic, social, and philosophical implications for the future of human health.

References

Abrams, D. I. (2016). Integrating cannabis into clinical cancer care. *Current Oncology, 23*(2), S8–S14. https://doi.org/10.3747/co.23.3099

Andre, C. M., Hausman, J. F., & Guerriero, G. (2016). *Cannabis sativa*: The plant of the thousand and one molecules. *Frontiers in Plant Science, 7*, 19. https://doi.org/10.3389/fpls.2016.00019

Aso, E., Sanchez-Pla, A., Vegas-Lozano, E., Maldonado, R., & Ferrer, I. (2015). Cannabis-based medicine reduces multiple pathological processes in AbetaPP/PS1 mice. *Journal of Alzheimer's Disease, 43*(3), 977–991. https://doi.org/10.3233/JAD-141014

Attaya, S., Kanthi, Y., Aster, R., & McCrae, K. (2009). Acute profound thrombocytopenia with second exposure to eptifibatide associated with a strong antibody reaction. *Platelets, 20*(1), 64–67. https://doi.org/10.1080/09537100802592676

Augenstein, W. L., Kulig, K. W., & Rumack, B. H. (1988). Captopril overdose resulting in hypotension. *JAMA, 259*(22), 3302–3305.

Avraham, H. K., Jiang, S., Fu, Y., Rockenstein, E., Makriyannis, A., Zvonok, A., . . . Avraham, S. (2014). The cannabinoid CB(2) receptor agonist AM1241 enhances neurogenesis in GFAP/Gp120 transgenic mice displaying deficits in neurogenesis. *British Journal of Pharmacology, 171*(2), 468–479. https://doi.org/10.1111/bph.12478

Barceloux, D. G. (2012). *Medical toxicology of drug abuse: Synthesized chemicals and psychoactive plants*. Hoboken, NJ: Wiley.

Ben Amar, M. (2006). Cannabinoids in medicine: A review of their therapeutic potential. *Journal of Ethnopharmacology, 105*(1–2), 1–25. https://doi.org/10.1016/j.jep.2006.02.001

Ben-Shabat, S., Fride, E., Sheskin, T., Tamiri, T., Rhee, M. H., Vogel, Z., . . . Mechoulam, R. (1998). An entourage effect: Inactive endogenous fatty acid glycerol esters enhance 2-arachidonoyl-glycerol cannabinoid activity. *European Journal of Pharmacology, 353*(1), 23–31.

Bilkei-Gorzo, A., Albayram, O., Draffehn, A., Michel, K., Piyanova, A., Oppenheimer, H., . . . Zimmer, A. (2017). A chronic low dose of Delta9-tetrahydrocannabinol (THC) restores cognitive function in old mice. *Nature Medicine, 23*(6), 782–787. https://doi.org/10.1038/nm.4311

Bravo-Ferrer, I., Cuartero, M. I., Zarruk, J. G., Pradillo, J. M., Hurtado, O., Romera, V. G., . . . Moro, M. A. (2017). Cannabinoid type-2 receptor drives neurogenesis and improves functional outcome after stroke. *Stroke, 48*(1), 204–212. https://doi.org/10.1161/STROKEAHA.116.014793

Bregman, T., & Fride, E. (2011). Treatment with tetrahydrocannabinol (THC) prevents infertility in male cystic fibrosis mice. *Journal of Basic and Clinical Physiology and Pharmacology, 22* (1–2), 29–32. https://doi.org/10.1515/jbcpp.2011.004

Buckholtz, N. S., & Boggan, W. O. (1977). Monoamine oxidase inhibition in brain and liver produced by beta-carbolines: Structure-activity relationships and substrate specificity. *Biochemical Pharmacology, 26*(21), 1991–1996.

Cannabis-based medicines--GW pharmaceuticals: High CBD, high THC, medicinal cannabis--GW pharmaceuticals, THC:CBD. (2003). *Drugs R D, 4*(5), 306–309.

Cao, C., Li, Y., Liu, H., Bai, G., Mayl, J., Lin, X., . . . Cai, J. (2014). The potential therapeutic effects of THC on Alzheimer's disease. *Journal of Alzheimer's Disease, 42*(3), 973–984. https://doi.org/10.3233/JAD-140093

Coons, J. C., Barcelona, R. A., Freedy, T., & Hagerty, M. F. (2005). Eptifibatide-associated acute, profound thrombocytopenia. *Annals of Pharmacotherapy, 39*(2), 368–372. https://doi.org/10.1345/aph.1E244

Dakic, V., Maciel, R. M., Drummond, H., Nascimento, J. M., Trindade, P., & Rehen, S. K. (2016). Harmine stimulates proliferation of human neural progenitors. *PeerJ, 4*, e2727. https://doi.org/10.7717/peerj.2727

Dakic, V., Nascimento, J. M., Sartore, R. C., Maciel, R. M., de Araujo, D. B., Ribeiro, S., . . . Rehen, S. K. (2017). Short term changes in the proteome of human cerebral organoids induced by 5-methoxy-N,N-dimethyltryptamine. *BioRxiv*. https://doi.org/10.1101/108159

Dawson, W. (1934). Studies in the Egyptian medical texts: III. *The Journal of Egyptian Archaeology, 20*(1/2), 41–46.

Dawson, A. H., Harvey, D., Smith, A. J., Taylor, M., Whyte, I. M., Johnson, C. I., . . . Roberts, M. J. (1990). Lisinopril overdose. *Lancet, 335*(8687), 487–488.

de Araujo, D. B., Ribeiro, S., Cecchi, G. A., Carvalho, F. M., Sanchez, T. A., Pinto, J. P., . . . Santos, A. C. (2012). Seeing with the eyes shut: Neural basis of enhanced imagery following ayahuasca ingestion. *Human Brain Mapping, 33*(11), 2550–2560. https://doi.org/10.1002/hbm.21381

de Lago, E., Moreno-Martet, M., Cabranes, A., Ramos, J. A., & Fernandez-Ruiz, J. (2012). Cannabinoids ameliorate disease progression in a model of multiple sclerosis in mice, acting preferentially through CB1 receptor-mediated anti-inflammatory effects. *Neuropharmacology, 62*(7), 2299–2308. https://doi.org/10.1016/j.neuropharm.2012.01.030

de Mello Schier, A. R., de Oliveira Ribeiro, N. P., Coutinho, D. S., Machado, S., Arias-Carrion, O., Crippa, J. A., . . . Silva, A. C. (2014). Antidepressant-like and anxiolytic-like effects of cannabidiol: A chemical compound of *Cannabis sativa*. *CNS & Neurological Disorders-Drug Targets, 13*(6), 953–960.

Di Forti, M., Morgan, C., Dazzan, P., Pariante, C., Mondelli, V., Marques, T. R., . . . Murray, R. M. (2009). High-potency cannabis and the risk of psychosis. *The British Journal of Psychiatry, 195* (6), 488–491. https://doi.org/10.1192/bjp.bp.109.064220

Dos Santos, R. G., Grasa, E., Valle, M., Ballester, M. R., Bouso, J. C., Nomdedeu, J. F., . . . Riba, J. (2012). Pharmacology of ayahuasca administered in two repeated doses. *Psychopharmacology (Berl), 219*(4), 1039–1053. https://doi.org/10.1007/s00213-011-2434-x

Elsohly, M. A., & Slade, D. (2005). Chemical constituents of marijuana: The complex mixture of natural cannabinoids. *Life Sciences, 78*(5), 539–548. https://doi.org/10.1016/j.lfs.2005.09.011

Fabisiak, A., & Fichna, J. (2017). Cannabinoids as gastrointestinal anti-inflammatory drugs. *Neurogastroenterology & Motility, 29*(3). https://doi.org/10.1111/nmo.13038

Fadda, P., Robinson, L., Fratta, W., Pertwee, R. G., & Riedel, G. (2004). Differential effects of THC- or CBD-rich cannabis extracts on working memory in rats. *Neuropharmacology, 47*(8), 1170–1179. https://doi.org/10.1016/j.neuropharm.2004.08.009

Fakhoury, M. (2016). Could cannabidiol be used as an alternative to antipsychotics? *Journal of Psychiatric Research, 80*, 14–21. https://doi.org/10.1016/j.jpsychires.2016.05.013

Farnsworth, D. L. (1976). What is the evidence for an amotivational syndrome in cannabis users? *Annals of the New York Academy of Sciences, 282*(1), 1.

Fasinu, P. S., Phillips, S., ElSohly, M. A., & Walker, L. A. (2016). Current status and prospects for cannabidiol preparations as new therapeutic agents. *Pharmacotherapy, 36*(7), 781–796. https://doi.org/10.1002/phar.1780

Ferreira, S. H. (1965). A bradykinin-potentiating factor (bpf) present in the venom of bothrops jararaca. *British Journal of Pharmacology and Chemotherapy, 24*(1), 163–169. https://doi.org/10.1111/j.1476-5381.1965.tb02091.x

Fetterman, P. S., & Turner, C. E. (1972). Constituents of *Cannabis sativa* L. I. Propyl homologs of cannabinoids from an Indian variant. *Journal of Pharmaceutical Sciences, 61*(9), 1476–1477.

Flather, M. D., Yusuf, S., Kober, L., Pfeffer, M., Hall, A., Murray, G., . . . Braunwald, E. (2000). Long-term ACE-inhibitor therapy in patients with heart failure or left-ventricular dysfunction: A systematic overview of data from individual patients. ACE-Inhibitor Myocardial Infarction Collaborative Group. *Lancet, 355*(9215), 1575–1581.

Formukong, E. A., Evans, A. T., & Evans, F. J. (1988). Analgesic and antiinflammatory activity of constituents of *Cannabis sativa* L. *Inflammation, 12*(4), 361–371.

Forsyth, A. J. M. (2001). Distorted? A quantitative exploration of drug fatality reports in the popular press. *The International Journal of Drug Policy, 12*(5–6), 435–453. https://doi.org/10.1016/S0955-3959(01)00092-5

Gallant, M., Odei-Addo, F., Frost, C. L., & Levendal, R. A. (2009). Biological effects of THC and a lipophilic cannabis extract on normal and insulin resistant 3T3-L1 adipocytes. *Phytomedicine, 16*(10), 942–949. https://doi.org/10.1016/j.phymed.2009.02.013

Gertsch, J., Pertwee, R. G., & Di Marzo, V. (2010). Phytocannabinoids beyond the Cannabis plant – do they exist? *British Journal of Pharmacology, 160*(3), 523–529. https://doi.org/10.1111/j.1476-5381.2010.00745.x

Gloss, D. (2015). An overview of products and bias in research. *Neurotherapeutics, 12*(4), 731–734. https://doi.org/10.1007/s13311-015-0370-x

Guy, G. W., Whittle, B. A., & Robson, P. (2004). *The medicinal uses of cannabis and cannabinoids*. Chicago, IL: Pharmaceutical Press.

Guzman, M. (2003). Cannabinoids: Potential anticancer agents. *Nature Reviews Cancer, 3*(10), 745–755. https://doi.org/10.1038/nrc1188

Hamblin, M. W., Leff, S. E., & Creese, I. (1984). Interactions of agonists with D-2 dopamine receptors: Evidence for a single receptor population existing in multiple agonist affinity-states in rat striatal membranes. *Biochemical Pharmacology, 33*(6), 877–887.

Hookana, E., Ansakorpi, H., Kortelainen, M. L., Junttila, M. J., Kaikkonen, K. S., Perkiomaki, J., & Huikuri, H. V. (2016). Antiepileptic medications and the risk for sudden cardiac death caused by an acute coronary event: A prospective case-control study. *Annals of Medicine, 48*(1–2), 111–117. https://doi.org/10.3109/07853890.2016.1140225

Hu, S. S., & Mackie, K. (2015). Distribution of the endocannabinoid system in the central nervous system. *Handbook of Experimental Pharmacology, 231*, 59–93. https://doi.org/10.1007/978-3-319-20825-1_3

Huff, J., & Chan, P. (2000). Antitumor effects of THC. *Environmental Health Perspectives, 108*(10), A442–A443.

Iurlo, M., Leone, G., Schilstrom, B., Linner, L., Nomikos, G., Hertel, P., . . . Svensson, H. (2001). Effects of harmine on dopamine output and metabolism in rat striatum: Role of monoamine oxidase-A inhibition. *Psychopharmacology (Berl), 159*(1), 98–104. https://doi.org/10.1007/s002130100879

Izzo, A. A., Borrelli, F., Capasso, R., Di Marzo, V., & Mechoulam, R. (2009). Non-psychotropic plant cannabinoids: New therapeutic opportunities from an ancient herb. *Trends in Pharmacological Sciences, 30*(10), 515–527. https://doi.org/10.1016/j.tips.2009.07.006

Jiang, W., Zhang, Y., Xiao, L., Van Cleemput, J., Ji, S. P., Bai, G., & Zhang, X. (2005). Cannabinoids promote embryonic and adult hippocampus neurogenesis and produce anxiolytic- and antidepressant-like effects. *The Journal of Clinical Investigation, 115*(11), 3104–3116. https://doi.org/10.1172/JCI25509

Jin, K., Xie, L., Kim, S. H., Parmentier-Batteur, S., Sun, Y., Mao, X. O., . . . Greenberg, D. (2004). Defective adult neurogenesis in CB1 cannabinoid receptor knockout mice. *Molecular Pharmacology, 66*(2), 204–208. https://doi.org/10.1124/mol.66.2.204

Johnson, J. R., Burnell-Nugent, M., Lossignol, D., Ganae-Motan, E. D., Potts, R., & Fallon, M. T. (2010). Multicenter, double-blind, randomized, placebo-controlled, parallel-group study of the efficacy, safety, and tolerability of THC:CBD extract and THC extract in patients with intractable cancer-related pain. *Journal of Pain and Symptom Management, 39*(2), 167–179. https://doi.org/10.1016/j.jpainsymman.2009.06.008

Johnson, J. R., Lossignol, D., Burnell-Nugent, M., & Fallon, M. T. (2013). An open-label extension study to investigate the long-term safety and tolerability of THC/CBD oromucosal spray and oromucosal THC spray in patients with terminal cancer-related pain refractory to strong opioid analgesics. *Journal of Pain and Symptom Management, 46*(2), 207–218. https://doi.org/10.1016/j.jpainsymman.2012.07.014

Keating, G. M. (2017). Delta-9-Tetrahydrocannabinol/Cannabidiol oromucosal spray (Sativex(R)): A review in multiple sclerosis-related spasticity. *Drugs, 77*(5), 563–574. https://doi.org/10.1007/s40265-017-0720-6

Kekecs, Z., Szollosi, A., Palfi, B., Szaszi, B., Kovacs, K. J., Dienes, Z., & Aczel, B. (2016). Commentary: Oxytocin-gaze positive loop and the coevolution of human-dog bonds. *Frontiers in Neuroscience, 10*, 155. https://doi.org/10.3389/fnins.2016.00155

Koehler, J. (2014). Who benefits most from THC:CBD spray? Learning from clinical experience. *European Neurology, 71*(Suppl 1), 10–15. https://doi.org/10.1159/000357743

Labate, B. C., & Cavnar, C. (2013). *The therapeutic use of ayahuasca.* New York, NY: Springer.

Labate, B. C., & Cavnar, C. (2014a). *Ayahuasca shamanism in the Amazon and beyond.* New York, NY: Oxford University Press.

Labate, B. C., & Cavnar, C. (2014b). *Prohibition, religious freedom, and human rights: Regulating traditional drug use.* New York, NY: Springer.

Labigalini, E., Jr., Rodrigues, L. R., & Da Silveira, D. X. (1999). Therapeutic use of cannabis by crack addicts in Brazil. *Journal of Psychoactive Drugs, 31*(4), 451–455. https://doi.org/10.1080/02791072.1999.10471776

Ladin, D. A., Soliman, E., Griffin, L., & Van Dross, R. (2016). Preclinical and clinical assessment of cannabinoids as anti-cancer agents. *Frontiers in Pharmacology, 7*, 361. https://doi.org/10.3389/fphar.2016.00361

Letyagin, A. Y., Savelov, A. A., & Polosmak, A. A. (2014). High field magnetic resonance imaging of a mummy from Ak-Alakha-3 mound 1, Ukok plateau, Gorny Altai: Findings and interpretations. *Archaeology Ethnology & Anthropology of Eurasia, 42*(4), 83–91.

Lewis, D. Y., & Brett, R. R. (2010). Activity-based anorexia in C57/BL6 mice: Effects of the phytocannabinoid, Delta9-tetrahydrocannabinol (THC) and the anandamide analogue, OMDM-2. *European Neuropsychopharmacology, 20*(9), 622–631. https://doi.org/10.1016/j.euroneuro.2010.04.002

Liu, W. M., Fowler, D. W., & Dalgleish, A. G. (2010). Cannabis-derived substances in cancer therapy--an emerging anti-inflammatory role for the cannabinoids. *Current Clinical Pharmacology, 5*(4), 281–287.

Lombard, C., Nagarkatti, M., & Nagarkatti, P. S. (2005). Targeting cannabinoid receptors to treat leukemia: Role of cross-talk between extrinsic and intrinsic pathways in Delta9-tetrahydrocannabinol (THC)-induced apoptosis of Jurkat cells. *Leukemia Research, 29*(8), 915–922. https://doi.org/10.1016/j.leukres.2005.01.014

Maccarrone, M., Maldonado, R., Casas, M., Henze, T., & Centonze, D. (2017). Cannabinoids therapeutic use: What is our current understanding following the introduction of THC, THC:CBD oromucosal spray and others? *Expert Review of Clinical Pharmacology, 10*(4), 443–455. https://doi.org/10.1080/17512433.2017.1292849

Mckenna, D. J., Towers, G. H. N., & Abbott, F. (1984). Monoamine-oxidase inhibitors in South-American hallucinogenic plants: Tryptamine and beta-carboline constituents of ayahuasca. *Journal of Ethnopharmacology, 10*, 195–223.

McPartland, J. M., & Guy, G. W. (2004). The evolution of Cannabis and coevolution with the cannabinoid receptor—a hypothesis. In G. Guy, B. A. Whittle, & P. Robson (Eds.), *The medicinal use of cannabis and cannabinoids* (pp. 71–101). Grayslake, IL: Pharmaceutical Press.

Mechoulam, R., Hanus, L. O., Pertwee, R., & Howlett, A. C. (2014). Early phytocannabinoid chemistry to endocannabinoids and beyond. *Nature Reviews Neuroscience, 15*(11), 757–764. https://doi.org/10.1038/nrn3811

Moldrich, G., & Wenger, T. (2000). Localization of the CB1 cannabinoid receptor in the rat brain. An immunohistochemical study. *Peptides, 21*(11), 1735–1742.

Molina-Holgado, F., Pinteaux, E., Moore, J. D., Molina-Holgado, E., Guaza, C., Gibson, R. M., & Rothwell, N. J. (2003). Endogenous interleukin-1 receptor antagonist mediates anti-inflammatory and neuroprotective actions of cannabinoids in neurons and glia. *Journal of Neuroscience, 23*(16), 6470–6474.

Morgan, C. J., Freeman, T. P., Schafer, G. L., & Curran, H. V. (2010). Cannabidiol attenuates the appetitive effects of Delta 9-tetrahydrocannabinol in humans smoking their chosen cannabis. *Neuropsychopharmacology, 35*(9), 1879–1885. https://doi.org/10.1038/npp.2010.58

Morgan, C. J., Schafer, G., Freeman, T. P., & Curran, H. V. (2010). Impact of cannabidiol on the acute memory and psychotomimetic effects of smoked cannabis: naturalistic study: Naturalistic study [corrected]. *The British Journal of Psychiatry, 197*(4), 285–290. https://doi.org/10.1192/bjp.bp.110.077503

Nagarkatti, P., Pandey, R., Rieder, S. A., Hegde, V. L., & Nagarkatti, M. (2009). Cannabinoids as novel anti-inflammatory drugs. *Future Medicinal Chemistry, 1*(7), 1333–1349. https://doi.org/10.4155/fmc.09.93

Nutt, D. J., King, L. A., Phillips, L. D., & Independent Scientific Committee on Drugs. (2010). Drug harms in the UK: A multicriteria decision analysis. *Lancet, 376*(9752), 1558–1565. https://doi.org/10.1016/S0140-6736(10)61462-6

Ohtsuka, Y., Yoshinaga, H., & Kobayashi, K. (2000). Refractory childhood epilepsy and factors related to refractoriness. *Epilepsia, 41*(Suppl 9), 14–17.

Osorio, L., Sanches, R. F., Macedo, L. R., Santos, R. G., Maia-de-Oliveira, J. P., Wichert-Ana, L., ... Hallak, J. E. (2015). Antidepressant effects of a single dose of ayahuasca in patients with recurrent depression: A preliminary report. *Revista Brasileira de Psiquiatria, 37*(1), 13–20. https://doi.org/10.1590/1516-4446-2014-1496

Palhano-Fontes, F. (2017). *Os efeitos antidepressivos da ayahuasca, suas bases neurais e relação com a experiência psicodélica* [The antidepressant effects of ayahuasca, its neural bases and relation with the psychedelic experience] (Doctoral dissertation). Federal University of Rio Grande do Norte, Natal. Retrieved from https://repositorio.ufrn.br/jspui/handle/123456789/24156

Palhano-Fontes, F., Barreto, D., Onias, H., Andrade, K. C., Novaes, M., Pessoa, J., ... de Araujo, D. B. (2017). Rapid antidepressant effects of the psychedelic ayahuasca in treatment-resistant depression: A randomised placebo-controlled trial. *BioRxiv*. https://doi.org/10.1101/103531

Parakh, S., Naik, N., Rohatgi, N., Bhat, U., & Parakh, K. (2009). Eptifibatide overdose. *International Journal of Cardiology, 131*(3), 430–432. https://doi.org/10.1016/j.ijcard.2007.07.132

Park, H., Purnell, G. V., & Mirchandani, H. G. (1990). Suicide by captopril overdose. *Journal of Toxicology: Clinical Toxicology, 28*(3), 379–382.

Parker, H. G., Dreger, D. L., Rimbault, M., Davis, B. W., Mullen, A. B., Carpintero-Ramirez, G., & Ostrander, E. A. (2017). Genomic analyses reveal the influence of geographic origin, migration, and hybridization on modern dog breed development. *Cell Reports, 19*(4), 697–708. https://doi.org/10.1016/j.celrep.2017.03.079

Patti, F. (2016). Health authorities data collection of THC:CBD oromucosal spray (L'Agenzia Italiana del Farmaco Web Registry): Figures after 1.5 years. *European Neurology, 75*(Suppl 1), 9–12. https://doi.org/10.1159/000444236

Phillips, D. R., & Scarborough, R. M. (1997). Clinical pharmacology of eptifibatide. *American Journal of Cardiology, 80*(4A), 11B–20B.

Pollan, M. (2001). *The botany of desire: A plant's eye view of the world* (1st ed.). New York, NY: Random House.

Price, M. R., Baillie, G. L., Thomas, A., Stevenson, L. A., Easson, M., Goodwin, R., . . . Ross, R. A. (2005). Allosteric modulation of the cannabinoid CB1 receptor. *Molecular Pharmacology, 68* (5), 1484–1495. https://doi.org/10.1124/mol.105.016162

Radwan, M. M., Elsohly, M. A., Slade, D., Ahmed, S. A., Wilson, L., El-Alfy, A. T., . . . Ross, S. A. (2008). Non-cannabinoid constituents from a high potency *Cannabis sativa* variety. *Phytochemistry, 69*(14), 2627–2633. https://doi.org/10.1016/j.phytochem.2008.07.010

Rekand, T. (2014). THC:CBD spray and MS spasticity symptoms: Data from latest studies. *European Neurology, 71*(*Suppl 1*), 4–9. https://doi.org/10.1159/000357742

Rickli, A., Moning, O. D., Hoener, M. C., & Liechti, M. E. (2016). Receptor interaction profiles of novel psychoactive tryptamines compared with classic hallucinogens. *European Neuropsychopharmacology, 26*(8), 1327–1337. https://doi.org/10.1016/j.euroneuro.2016.05.001

Rimonabant: Depression and suicide. (2009). Prescrire International, *18*(99), 24.

Robbe, D., Montgomery, S. M., Thome, A., Rueda-Orozco, P. E., McNaughton, B. L., & Buzsaki, G. (2006). Cannabinoids reveal importance of spike timing coordination in hippocampal function. *Nature Neuroscience, 9*(12), 1526–1533. https://doi.org/10.1038/nn1801

Rocha e Silva, M. (1963). The physiological significance of bradykinin. *Annals of the New York Academy of Sciences, 104*, 190–210.

Romeo, B., Choucha, W., Fossati, P., & Rotge, J. Y. (2015). Meta-analysis of short- and mid-term efficacy of ketamine in unipolar and bipolar depression. *Psychiatry Research, 230*(2), 682–688. https://doi.org/10.1016/j.psychres.2015.10.032

Rosenberg, E. C., Tsien, R. W., Whalley, B. J., & Devinsky, O. (2015). Cannabinoids and epilepsy. *Neurotherapeutics, 12*(4), 747–768. https://doi.org/10.1007/s13311-015-0375-5

Russo, E. B. (2011). Taming THC: Potential cannabis synergy and phytocannabinoid-terpenoid entourage effects. *British Journal of Pharmacology, 163*(7), 1344–1364. https://doi.org/10.1111/j.1476-5381.2011.01238.x

Sanches, R. F., de Lima Osorio, F., Dos Santos, R. G., Macedo, L. R., Maia-de-Oliveira, J. P., Wichert-Ana, L., . . . Hallak, J. E. (2016). Antidepressant effects of a single dose of ayahuasca in patients with recurrent depression: A SPECT study. *Journal of Clinical Psychopharmacology, 36*(1), 77–81. https://doi.org/10.1097/JCP.0000000000000436

Sastre-Garriga, J., Vila, C., Clissold, S., & Montalban, X. (2011). THC and CBD oromucosal spray (Sativex(R)) in the management of spasticity associated with multiple sclerosis. *Expert Review of Neurotherapeutics, 11*(5), 627–637. https://doi.org/10.1586/ern.11.47

Sawler, J., Stout, J. M., Gardner, K. M., Hudson, D., Vidmar, J., Butler, L., . . . Myles, S. (2015). The genetic structure of marijuana and hemp. *PLoS One, 10*(8), e0133292. https://doi.org/10.1371/journal.pone.0133292

Schmits, E., & Quertemont, E. (2013). Les drogues dites "douces": Cannibas et syndrome amotivationnel [So called "soft" drugs: cannabis and the amotivational syndrome]. *Revue Médicale de Liège, 68*(5–6), 281–286.

Scott, K. A., Dalgleish, A. G., & Liu, W. M. (2014). The combination of cannabidiol and Delta9-tetrahydrocannabinol enhances the anticancer effects of radiation in an orthotopic murine glioma model. *Molecular Cancer Therapeutics, 13*(12), 2955–2967. https://doi.org/10.1158/1535-7163.MCT-14-0402

Sherif, M., Radhakrishnan, R., D'Souza, D. C., & Ranganathan, M. (2016). Human laboratory studies on Cannabinoids and psychosis. *Biological Psychiatry, 79*(7), 526–538. https://doi.org/10.1016/j.biopsych.2016.01.011

Silva, T. B., Balbino, C. Q., & Weiber, A. F. (2015). The relationship between cannabidiol and psychosis: A review. *Annals of Clinical Psychiatry, 27*(2), 134–141.

Solt, K., Ruesch, D., Forman, S. A., Davies, P. A., & Raines, D. E. (2007). Differential effects of serotonin and dopamine on human 5-HT3A receptor kinetics: Interpretation within an allosteric kinetic model. *Journal of Neuroscience, 27*(48), 13151–13160. https://doi.org/10.1523/ JNEUROSCI.3772-07.2007

Sznitman, S. R., & Lewis, N. (2015). Is cannabis an illicit drug or a medicine? A quantitative framing analysis of Israeli newspaper coverage. *International Journal of Drug Policy, 26*(5), 446–452. https://doi.org/10.1016/j.drugpo.2015.01.010

Thomas, G., Lucas, P., Capler, N. R., Tupper, K. W., & Martin, G. (2013). Ayahuasca-assisted therapy for addiction: Results from a preliminary observational study in Canada. *Current Drug Abuse Reviews, 6*(1), 30–42.

Topol, E. J., Bousser, M. G., Fox, K. A., Creager, M. A., Despres, J. P., Easton, J. D., ... Investigators, C. (2010). Rimonabant for prevention of cardiovascular events (CRESCENDO): A randomised, multicentre, placebo-controlled trial. *Lancet, 376*(9740), 517–523. https://doi. org/10.1016/S0140-6736(10)60935-X

Tsou, K., Brown, S., Sanudo-Pena, M. C., Mackie, K., & Walker, J. M. (1998). Immunohisto-chemical distribution of cannabinoid CB1 receptors in the rat central nervous system. *Neuroscience, 83*(2), 393–411.

U'Prichard, D. C. (1980). Multiple CNS receptor interactions of ergot alkaloids: Affinity and intrinsic activity analysis in in vitro binding systems. *Advances in Biochemical Psychopharmacology, 23*, 103–115.

van Vliet, S. A., Vanwersch, R. A., Jongsma, M. J., Olivier, B., & Philippens, I. H. (2008). Therapeutic effects of Delta9-THC and modafinil in a marmoset Parkinson model. *European Neuropsychopharmacology, 18*(5), 383–389. https://doi.org/10.1016/j.euroneuro.2007.11.003

Verty, A. N., Evetts, M. J., Crouch, G. J., McGregor, I. S., Stefanidis, A., & Oldfield, B. J. (2011). The cannabinoid receptor agonist THC attenuates weight loss in a rodent model of activity-based anorexia. *Neuropsychopharmacology, 36*(7), 1349–1358. https://doi.org/10.1038/npp. 2011.19

Wacker, D., Wang, S., McCorvy, J. D., Betz, R. M., Venkatakrishnan, A. J., Levit, A., ... Roth, B. L. (2017). Crystal structure of an LSD-bound human serotonin receptor. *Cell, 168*(3), 377–389. e312. https://doi.org/10.1016/j.cell.2016.12.033

Weber, M., Goldman, B., & Truniger, S. (2010). Tetrahydrocannabinol (THC) for cramps in amyotrophic lateral sclerosis: A randomised, double-blind crossover trial. *Journal of Neurology, Neurosurgery & Psychiatry, 81*(10), 1135–1140. https://doi.org/10.1136/jnnp.2009.200642

Winkelman, M. (2014). Psychedelics as medicines for substance abuse rehabilitation: Evaluating treatments with LSD, peyote, ibogaine and ayahuasca. *Current Drug Abuse Reviews, 7*(2), 101–116.

Xapelli, S., Agasse, F., Sarda-Arroyo, L., Bernardino, L., Santos, T., Ribeiro, F. F., ... Malva, J. O. (2013). Activation of type 1 cannabinoid receptor (CB1R) promotes neurogenesis in murine subventricular zone cell cultures. *PLoS One, 8*(5), e63529. https://doi.org/10.1371/journal.pone. 0063529

Yu, Y. Z., Liu, S., Wang, H. C., Shi, D. Y., Xu, Q., Zhou, X. W., ... Huang, P. T. (2016). A novel recombinant 6Abeta15-THc-C chimeric vaccine (rCV02) mitigates Alzheimer's disease-like pathology, cognitive decline and synaptic loss in aged 3 x Tg-AD mice. *Scientific Reports, 6*, 27175. https://doi.org/10.1038/srep27175

Zani, A., Braida, D., Capurro, V., & Sala, M. (2007). Delta9-tetrahydrocannabinol (THC) and AM 404 protect against cerebral ischaemia in gerbils through a mechanism involving cannabinoid and opioid receptors. *British Journal of Pharmacology, 152*(8), 1301–1311. https://doi.org/10. 1038/sj.bjp.0707514

Zarate, C. A., Jr., Singh, J. B., Carlson, P. J., Brutsche, N. E., Ameli, R., Luckenbaugh, D. A., ... Manji, H. K. (2006). A randomized trial of an N-methyl-D-aspartate antagonist in treatment-resistant major depression. *Archives of General Psychiatry, 63*(8), 856–864. https://doi.org/10. 1001/archpsyc.63.8.856

Zettl, U. K., Rommer, P., Hipp, P., & Patejdl, R. (2016). Evidence for the efficacy and effectiveness of THC-CBD oromucosal spray in symptom management of patients with spasticity due to multiple sclerosis. *Therapeutic Advances in Neurological Disorders, 9*(1), 9–30. https://doi.org/10.1177/1756285615612659

Zuardi, A. W., Crippa, J. A., & Hallak, J. E. (2010). *Cannabis sativa*: A planta que pode produzir efeitos indesejáveis e também tratá-los [*Cannabis sativa*: The plant that can induce unwanted effects and also treat them]. *Revista Brasileira de Psiquiatria, 32*(Suppl 1), S1–S2.

Zuardi, A. W., Crippa, J. A., Hallak, J. E., Bhattacharyya, S., Atakan, Z., Martin-Santos, R., . . . Guimaraes, F. S. (2012). A critical review of the antipsychotic effects of cannabidiol: 30 years of a translational investigation. *Current Pharmaceutical Design, 18*(32), 5131–5140.

Zurier, R. B. (2003). Prospects for cannabinoids as anti-inflammatory agents. *Journal of Cellular Biochemistry, 88*(3), 462–466. https://doi.org/10.1002/jcb.10291

Chapter 9
Placebo Problems: Boundary Work in the Psychedelic Science Renaissance

Katherine Hendy

Abstract The revitalization of clinical trials with psychedelics has produced an array of studies investigating different combinations of therapeutic substances and diagnoses. In addition to the bureaucratic negotiations to gain approval for this research, this new wave of studies is also negotiating a new methodological landscape of clinical research. Mid-twentieth century research with drugs like LSD and psilocybin involved both case studies and double-blind studies. However, today, placebo-controlled randomized controlled trials (RCTs) are the institutional standard for research with psychopharmaceuticals. Because psychedelic therapy seeks to induce a radical change in consciousness—to make a subject feel different from her everyday self—blinding these studies using placebo controls has emerged as a methodological sticking point. However, this chapter argues, it is also a rich site for interrogating boundary work around science and psychedelics. While anthropologists have examined placebos as examples of the power of symbolic healing within Western medicine, or as ethically fraught territory of nontreatment, this chapter examines placebos as a research technique around which the scientific status of a study is negotiated. While psychedelic therapy challenges the model of pharmaceutical intervention used in psychiatry today, it must do so while also working within psychopharmacology's evidentiary norms.

In 2001, the Food and Drug Administration approved a new Investigational New Drug Application (IND) for MDMA. Better known by the name "ecstasy," MDMA might have been new to clinical trials, but it was in fact an old pharmaceutical product. First synthesized and patented at the beginning of the twentieth century by Merck pharmaceuticals, the drug was largely ignored until the 1970s,[1] when it was

---

[1]MDMA was incorporated into the US military's Edgewater experiments with psychedelic substances to find a truth serum to be used in interrogations. However, MDMA was only administered to animals and never to humans in these experiments.

K. Hendy (✉)
Department of Comparative Studies, The Ohio State University, Columbus, OH, USA
e-mail: hendy.13@osu.edu

© Springer International Publishing AG, part of Springer Nature 2018
B. C. Labate, C. Cavnar (eds.), *Plant Medicines, Healing and Psychedelic Science*,
https://doi.org/10.1007/978-3-319-76720-8_9

incorporated into the practice of psychedelic therapists, who found that the drug produced states of openness, empathy, and trust that were conductive to therapy (Holland, 2001). In 1985, the US Drug Enforcement Agency (DEA) used its enhanced emergency scheduling powers, granted as part of President Reagan's efforts in the war on drugs, to classify MDMA a Schedule I substance. Schedule I exerts the tightest level of regulatory control over a drug. Substances in this category are deemed to have a high probability for abuse and no therapeutic application. Thus, the therapeutic use of MDMA became illegal in the United States.

The sponsor of the IND was the Multidisciplinary Association for Psychedelic Studies (MAPS), a nonprofit organization founded in the wake of the scheduling of MDMA. The approval of the IND was a critical step in launching a clinical trial program to undo the Schedule I restriction by demonstrating that MDMA was both safe and therapeutic and thus could be prescribed and administered in controlled settings. While MAPS' mission is quite broad—to promote education and research on the therapeutic use of psychedelics and marijuana—the development of MDMA as a prescription pharmaceutical has been the focus of its clinical program. MAPS is based out of Santa Cruz, California; however, like pharmaceutical companies, it sponsors studies taking place all around the world.

In the first MDMA-assisted therapy pilot study, lactose was used as the placebo control, and the results were positive—the majority of subjects enrolled saw improvements in their symptoms (Mithoefer, Wagner, Mithoefer, Jerome, & Doblin, 2011). The FDA and the private institutional review board (IRB) that reviewed the study protocol had no problem with the use of the inert placebo for the pilot study. And in fact, the lactose had a significant advantage: using a placebo without any physiological or psychoactive effects meant that one could easily tell if MDMA caused any adverse events.

Problems arose when MAPS' researchers went to publish the results of their first study. How, reviewers from one journal asked, could the study be considered blind, when MDMA had such robust effects compared to lactose? Could the therapists really have been blinded? Wouldn't the subjects themselves have known what their treatment condition was? MAPS had administered a "Belief of Condition Assignment" in their data collection to both the study subjects and therapists. The Belief of Condition Assignment simply asked what each individual thought had been administered during the experimental sessions: MDMA or placebo? Nineteen of twenty subjects correctly guess their treatment condition, and the therapists themselves guessed correctly 100% of the time (though, there was some level of uncertainty for both populations). In the wake of these critiques, MAPS began experimenting with lower, subtherapeutic doses of MDMA as the control; these low doses were called the "active placebo." The goal was to find a dose that would confuse the therapists and subjects, but that would not work therapeutically.

This chapter contends that these studies are notable, not only because of the unusual substance they are working with but also because of the negotiations around blinding and placebo controls being used in the studies. As this chapter will explore, the development of psychedelic therapy at midcentury corresponded with the rise of psychopharmaceutical treatments and the institutionalization of the randomized controlled trial (RCT). While psychedelics initially promised to bridge the gap between psychotherapy and pharmaceuticals, recent historical scholarship has shown that they were waylaid by their inability to fit into the new institutional norms for pharmaceutical research that required blinding both the study subjects and researchers. This chapter explores contemporary debates about blinding and placebos as negotiations over including psychedelic therapy in the institutional and scientific norms for pharmaceutical research.

Drawing from medical anthropology and science and technology studies, this chapter makes two intersecting arguments about the work of the placebo. Medical anthropologists have argued that the placebo problematizes the Cartesian dualism of mind and body in biomedicine. However, the placebo effect has usually been framed as working only on the mind and body of the person being treated. This chapter argues, first, that as a research technique, placebos also must have effects on the investigators themselves—specifically, they must be fooled. Second, drawing from science studies, this chapter contends that methodological negotiations around placebos in the psychedelic renaissance are a critical site for tracking credibility struggles around psychedelics and thus are a key site for investigating the politics of psychedelic research.

An Anthropologist in the Trial

Anthropology is a diverse discipline that is loosely and, at times, contentiously held together by the question of what it means to be human. Social anthropology—my particular field—attempts to address this question by studying contemporary human societies. Early social anthropologists traveled all over the world to live in small villages and tribes in order to ethnographically document the diverse social structures of human societies. The rule of thumb was that the anthropologist should live in a given village or tribe for at least a year so that they could witness the entire cycle of the seasons.

Today, social anthropology has widened its scope considerably. No longer simply content to examine villages or tribes, anthropologists now use those same ethnographic methods—sometimes called "deep hanging out"—to study a variety of modern social forms (Geertz, 1998). In other words, the goal is to learn about how modern society works by spending time participating in its production. While anthropologists are still interested in kinship, economics, and religion, they are also interested in thinking about science, biomedicine, and bureaucracy. As such, anthropologists spend time with computer hackers, neurobiologists, NGOs, or any number of other social groups.

For my study, I spent time with clinical researchers. Over 18 months, I worked with the researchers coordinating the MDMA-assisted therapy trials. During those years, MAPS' offices were located in a converted single-family house on a busy thoroughfare in Santa Cruz, California. There was a small yard with a lovely picnic table where staff took coffee and smoke breaks amid the smells of the Mexican restaurant next door. A tiny parking fit five very strategically arranged cars. The clinical department, which generally consisted of the Lead Clinical Research Associate supervising various interns like myself, worked out of a small room on the second floor, notable only for its fireproof cabinets for the study documents.

Drugs do not pass through the Santa Cruz office; neither do patients. Those fall under the purview of the study sites. Documents, documents, and more documents are what pass through the office. Clinical trials produce an incredible amount of paperwork: protocols, informed consents (ICFs), standard operating procedures (SOPs), case report forms (CRFs), and source records—to name a few.

My goal was to follow the day-to-day practices of clinical research through which therapeutic efficacy and safety are established for regulatory agencies, in order to understand exactly how the facts about a drug are made tangible in the context of clinical research. Over the course of 18 months of fieldwork, I attended weekly teleconferences, visited study sites, helped to review and draft study documents, monitored studies, and reviewed databases. Thus, I followed the seasons of clinical research: I participated and watched as protocols were drafted, submitted to regulatory agencies, and amended; studies initiated, monitored, and closed out; data was cleaned; and databases were locked. Much of my fieldwork—like much of clinical research—took place around a speakerphone or hunched in front of a computer screen.

This study employs methods and perspectives from both anthropology and the social studies of science. The social studies of science is an interdisciplinary field that examines how science works. Drawing from history, philosophy, sociology, and anthropology, the field examines the social field in which knowledge claims are produced. Rather than seeing science as a value-free and politically neutral territory, science studies scholars hold that scientific practices are actually a key site of negotiations over values and politics. In other words, even if the methodologies employed in scientific practice are objective, the actual workings of science are never without values or political contestation. Rick Doblin, the president and founder of MAPS, is often quoted as saying that MAPS is promoting science over politics, wherein politics is a reference to the drug war in the United States. However, as this chapter points out, even the struggle to do science, or to have research recognized as scientific, is a political act.

In the next section, I discuss the historical convergence of psychedelics, psychiatry, and clinical trials at mid-twentieth century in the United States. Just as substances like LSD and psilocybin were emerging as therapeutic agents, placebos and double-blinds were becoming the institutionalized norms of pharmaceutical research. As recent historical scholarship has demonstrated, these new methodological standards played a critical role in slowing down psychedelic research. Thus, contemporary negotiations around placebos and blinding are a critical site for examining the inclusion of psychedelic research under the heading of science.

Psychedelics, Psychiatry, and the Institutionalization of the Randomized Controlled Trial (RCT)

The twenty-first century has witnessed a resurgence of research on the therapeutic use of psychedelic substances such as psilocybin, LSD, ketamine, ibogaine, cannabis, and ayahuasca. While the array of substances held together as "psychedelic" is quite diverse (and there is debate on the boundaries of the category), many of the studies are reviving a set of therapeutic techniques developed midcentury in North America and Europe by psychiatrists.

The intertwining of psychedelics and psychiatry dates back to the 1950s, when LSD, then a novel pharmaceutical, was distributed by Sandoz pharmaceuticals to researchers throughout North America and Europe. By 1966, over 2000 articles had been published on psychedelics in medical journals (Dyck, 2010). Researchers studied LSD and psilocybin, also a Sandoz product, as treatments for a range of psychiatric disorders: most notably, alcoholism and schizophrenia. Two forms of therapy emerged during this period: psychedelic and psycholytic therapy. Humphry Osmond and Abram Hoffer in Saskatchewan, Canada, developed psychedelic therapy, which involved a single large dose of a psychedelic in conjunction with psychotherapy. In contrast, psycholytic therapy, which was developed in the United Kingdom by Ronald Sandison, used small doses of LSD in conjunction with psychoanalysis (Sandison, 1954). The large dose technique of psychedelic therapy was supposed to induce a new perspective on one's life, while the smaller doses of psycholytic therapy were supposed to induce a dreamlike experience during which material from the unconscious could surface.

These emergent techniques seemed to bridge the gap between the rising interest in pharmaceuticals and psychiatry (Dyck, 2010). Intertwined with this timeline, the discipline of psychiatry was shifting toward biologically based pharmaceutical treatments (Healy, 2002; Starr, 1982). A pharmaceutical needed to intervene in a particular disease—or what Charles Rosenberg has termed the logic of "disease specificity" (Rosenberg, 2002). In order for psychiatry to make this jump into specific treatments, the diseases themselves needed to become objects of diagnostic precision (Kirk & Kutchins, 1992). Gradually, the individuated psychodynamic model of diagnosis and treatment was replaced by institutionalized standards with set diagnostic criteria and corresponding psychometric testing.

Part of what makes the contemporary moment so significant for psychedelics is not simply that they are once again being studied as therapeutic treatments but that they are being studied in double-blind placebo-controlled trials approved by the FDA. Recent historical scholarship by Matthew Oram has argued that research on the therapeutic use of psychedelics slowed down in the 1960s due in part to changes in federal regulation of clinical research (Oram, 2012, 2016). The movement for double-blind placebo-controlled studies had been building over the course of the twentieth century but wasn't required by the FDA until after the thalidomide crisis, in which birth defects were linked to an anti-nausea drug prescribed to pregnant women. According to Oram, research with psychedelics declined due to the institutionalization of controlled studies in clinical research. Psychedelic therapy did not fit easily into the new institutional and methodological standards for research. Researchers posited that the complex relationship between the pharmaceutical and the psychological aspects of the drug made it difficult to study in double-blind placebo-controlled trials.[2] Thus, the fact that psychedelics stopped being developed as pharmaceuticals had just as much to do with the inability of researchers to shift toward the new techniques for pharmaceutical research, as it had to do with the use of these drugs in the counter culture. This line of historical argument shifts the emphasis from the status of psychedelics as "drugs" to their status as "pharmaceuticals." It might be that the recreational use of these drugs was criminalized in response to their widespread use in the counterculture, but halting the development of psychedelics as pharmaceuticals has a more complicated story enmeshed in the institutionalization of the techniques of "regulatory science" (Jasanoff, 1995).

The techniques of the randomized controlled trial (RCT) were themselves long in coming. At the beginning of the twentieth century, the United States did not have any bureaucratic agencies dedicated to monitoring pharmaceuticals. Historian Harry Marks has chronicled the efforts of a group he terms "therapeutic reformers" during the Progressive Era. These reformers were critical to establishing regulatory oversight of the pharmaceutical industry (Marks, 2000). Essential to their project was the institutionalization of the alliance between science and medicine. The reformers championed the use of scientific experiments to evaluate the therapeutic efficacy of a wave of new pharmaceuticals.

Initial reforms focused on creating centralized institutions for evaluating pharmaceutical companies' claims and monitoring the contents of products. It wasn't until the second half of the twentieth century that the RCT was institutionalized as the gold standard of pharmaceutical research. According to Marks, the RCT shifted authority from institutions to methods, as statisticians came to enforce the blinded randomization of subjects. RCTs utilize blinded controls and randomized assignment of subjects to different treatment conditions, all of which remove physicians' judgment from the treatment regimen. Early coordinated studies—the precursor to the contemporary multisite clinical trials—did not have a mechanism preventing physicians from assigning the most promising cases to particular treatment conditions. Researchers in the early twentieth century understood the methodological value of controls and randomization; however, these early studies lacked the social and organizational structure necessary to coordinate and standardize the work of researchers. It was only through the rise in the status of statisticians that these shifts could take place (Marks, 1988).

---

[2]Ido Hartogsohn has argued that the importance of set and setting in the therapeutic use of psychedelics is a parallel phenomenon to the placebo response. They both merit being put under the broad category of meaning response (Hartogsohn, 2016). This argument implies that the very mechanism of action for psychedelics mobilizes the placebo response.

The use of placebo controls and double-blinds in clinical research has been fraught with ethical debate. Initially, some physicians thought that the double-blind violated medical ethics because the treating physician did not know what exactly their patients were being given. These physicians argued that medical care trumped the necessity for scientific objectivity. They held that it was unethical for a physician to be blinded to their patient's treatment condition. This dilemma highlights a central tension between the ethics of scientific objectivity and care shaping clinical research. Even today, debates continue as to whether withholding treatment from subjects assigned to a placebo group is ethical or not. While some believe that withholding care is unethical (Chiodo, Tolle, & Bevan, 2000), others charge that producing the best quality data on pharmaceuticals is the overriding ethical concern (Streiner, 2008).

When MAPS' clinical researchers confronted the issue of blinding and placebos, they were doing so within territory that is itself quite conflicted. In addressing the concerns of journal reviewers, they were confronting two intertwined issues: what did the drug actually do, and how objective were their results? The best way to combat these concerns would be to find a placebo that more closely mimicked MDMA. The harder to tell the placebo apart from MDMA, the more accurately the study results would reflect the "actual" effects of MDMA. To put it another way: the more difficult to tell the two substances apart in the treatment session, the easier it would be to discern differences in efficacy in the data.

This is no small problem, since MDMA is intensely psychoactive. MDMA is not considered a classic psychedelic, like LSD, mescaline, or psilocybin mushrooms. It has been classified by some as an "entactogen"—from a combination of Greek and Latin roots to mean "touching within"—to characterize the intense emotional effects of the drug (Nichols, 1986). However, MDMA is characterized by intense changes to one's affective state, which make masking its presence difficult. It has been reported to reduce feelings of fear and increase feelings of love and empathy.

Subjects have very few encounters with the drug during the study. MAPS is following the treatment model initiated by Osmond and Hoffer: a large dose followed by integrative sessions. In MAPS' protocols, subjects alternate between psychotherapy sessions, which last 60 and 90 min, and experimental sessions, which are eight plus hour sessions in which either a placebo or MDMA is administered. Even though a subject might have over a dozen sessions with the therapists, the "MDMA" will only be administered three times. However, it is blinding the subjects and researchers to what is happening on those three occasions that is the issue for the researchers. How do you blind an experience of non-ordinary consciousness? In order to navigate the contemporary landscape of pharmaceutical research, psychedelic researchers must find novel ways to use placebos and blinds, even when working with substances for which blinding may be impossible. As this chapter argues, the negotiation around blinding and placebos is a key site where researchers must defend the credibility of their studies to the scientific community.

The Problem

We want the dose that fools us without working.

This concise articulation of the problem emanates from Rick Doblin, the president and founder of MAPS. The clinical team was discussing the problem of finding an active placebo dose that could adequately blind the studies of MDMA-assisted therapy for posttraumatic stress disorder (PTSD). The clinical team had been experimenting with using different low doses of MDMA as placebo controls. The goal was to find, as Doblin puts it, the dose that fools without working. The researchers wanted a dose that was high enough to produce some amount of psychoactivity and confusion but not so high as to be therapeutic.[3]

Doblin's quote neatly sets up the paradox around placebos and double-blinds in pharmaceutical research broadly and psychedelic research specifically. Ideally, in clinical research, the placebo group receives only the form—not the content—of the treatment. The placebo group represents all that can be ascertained from the ritual of taking a pill or of being wheeled in and out of an operating room and being put under anesthesia; it controls for both the ritual of the treatment and the ebb and flow of symptoms over time. Some subjects may get better simply because the illness resolves itself or because—as with chronic conditions—symptoms are not stable. Still other subjects may improve because they think they have been treated. Whatever the reason, the placebo control group is supposed to account for everything but the contents of the investigational product. Thus, the effects seen in the placebo group can be subtracted away at the conclusion of a study to reveal what, if any, biochemical effects might be produced by the investigational product.

At the same time, placebos do need to do something: they need to fool the people involved in the study. In other words, placebos may be inactive as therapeutic agents, but they must be effective as research techniques. While anthropologists in particular have focused on the effectiveness of placebos as therapeutic agents, they have often overlooked the question of efficacy of placebos as research techniques. Imbedded in Doblin's statement is a careful calibration between the two mandates of the placebo: similar enough to fool but not so similar that it works. While the clinical trials with MDMA and other psychoactive materials have a specific set of research problems, all placebos in fact must do both: they must "do" enough to fool everyone but not so much that they themselves become active and therapeutic.

Masking the treatment condition has been a site of innovation in contemporary research with psychedelics. A number of different methodologies have been used to balance the need to employ drugs that work precisely by altering the state of

---

[3]In recent years, "microdosing" or "sub-perceptual" dosing has also emerged as a therapeutic use of psychedelics. This technique involves regularly taking a dose of a psychedelic that is so small that it does not produce the robust sensory alterations or ego-boundary loosening of larger doses (Fadiman, 2011). While microdosing more closely mirrors the use of antidepressants as a mood stabilizer and not a therapeutic catalyst, the flexibility of what constitutes a therapeutic dose points to the blurriness around when a drug starts to "work."

consciousness of the person being treated with the need to keep the subjects and therapists from knowing if the drug is present. The Heffter Foundation, another nonprofit investing in research with psychedelics, has been sponsoring clinical studies using psilocybin, the active chemical in psychoactive mushrooms. In a study of mystical experiences, methylphenidate hydrochloride (Ritalin) was used as a placebo (Griffiths, Richards, Mccann, & Jesse, 2006), and in studies of psilocybin to treat anxiety in advanced stage cancer patients, niacin (vitamin B3), which produces flushing, was used as a placebo. In a study of ayahuasca as treatment for depression, the researchers played with one of the commonly expected side effects of the hallucinogenic brew: nausea. Researchers used a placebo that included zinc sulfate, which has emetic properties, in order to mask the real substance (de Fontes, 2017).

MAPS' clinical team considered using Ritalin as a placebo. However, this was eventually rejected, as there was speculation that its amphetamine qualities might increase the anxiety experienced by subjects with PTSD. In subsequent studies, the researchers used different levels of MDMA as the control, varying from 25 to 40 mg and including a "medium" dose of 75 mg. The goal was to find the dose of just enough MDMA that there was confusion but not so much MDMA that there was a therapeutic effect.

When the journal reviewers contested the blinding of the study, they were not contesting the *results* of the study as much as the *source* of treatment efficacy. Independent raters—who were not present for the experimental sessions—administered the psychometric tests used as outcome measures. Thus, at some level, the improvement in symptoms of posttraumatic stress was real; or at least it was documentable. Rather, what was being contested were how much of these documented effects could be attributed to the drug and how much could be attributed to the expectancy of what the drug might do (Rosenthal, 1994). Were the positive effects due to the drug or due to what the participants *expected* from the drug?

Expectancy effect is paradoxically both real and imagined. It works like this: The doctor says they will give you a therapy that may do these particular things. If a subject believes that they have been given that therapy, then they will expect that those effects will manifest. The authority emanating from the doctor endows the substance with efficacy. One of the journal reviewers postulated that the effects attributable to the expectancy effect would quickly fade.

Using an active dose of MDMA led to the next logical question, framed by one of the instigators and therapists, Michael Mithoefer: how often do we have to be wrong for it to work? The Belief of Condition Assignment allowed researchers to assess how well the blind held. It is an unusual step; most clinical studies don't assess how well the study was blinded. Dr. Mithoefer's use of the personal plural pronoun highlights a lacuna in the discussion of placebos. In the next section, I argue that medical anthropologists have critically ignored the placebo as a research technique, and instead focused on the effects of placebos on those being treated. It is not just the study subjects who need to be fooled but also the therapists themselves. As such, the effects of a placebo cannot be narrowly discussed through the idea of when they treat or don't.

The Placebo Effect, Meaning Response, and Ethical Quandaries

Historians and social scientists studying placebos and placebo effects have commented on the variability of the definitions of the phenomena. As Susan Huculak points out, the definition of the two intertwined concepts have "become fraught with interdisciplinary sparring over mind–body dualism, the passive versus active role of the patient and the placebo as a sham versus effective treatment approach" (Huculak, 2013). This chapter argues that social scientists narrowly frame placebos as affecting only those being treated; however, they are meant to produce effects in the researchers as well.

Historian Ann Harington has traced three different arcs of epistemological and moral questions that the placebo has come to answer since the eighteenth century: medical humbug, research confound, and as medically interesting therapeutic phenomena (Harrington, 2006). Initially, placebos were used to expose practices already thought to be fraudulent. However, in the middle of the twentieth century, a second meaning emerged: the placebo effect as universal confound in research design. Ironically, Harrington points out, whereas placebos had previously been used to debunk unorthodox treatments, this new phase universalized the placebo effect such that all treatments were subject to it and all studies had to control for it.

The placebo effect was thus both real and not: it was a confound that needed to be eliminated from the experiment—and thus not the real effect of a drug—but it was also a universal phenomenon. In the 1970s, a third sense of the placebo effect emerged; this time, not as medical humbug, or research confound, but as a robust phenomenon in itself that could yield new treatments. Developments in psychoneuroimmunology and neurobiology lent credibility to the idea that the brain could affect the body: namely, the discovery of endorphins and links between the nervous system and immune system. Neurochemistry gave scientific credence to existing ideas about the power of positive thinking and the potential value of holistic healing. What if treatments didn't have to directly intervene in disease but only had to unleash the power of the body to heal itself?

Serious engagements by medical anthropologists with the placebo effect emerged shortly after the placebo-effect-as-legitimate-therapeutic-phenomena. In particular, medical anthropologists used the placebo effect to make the case for equivalence between the ritual authority granted to traditional healers and those granted to Western biomedical practitioners. Daniel Moerman has framed placebo effects as an example of the "meaning response": physiological and psychological effects generated by the meaning of a treatment (Moerman, 2002). This wave of medical anthropology used the placebo response to critique biomedicine's concept of the individualized body held distinct from mind (Scheper-Hughes & Lock, 1987; Van der Geest & Whyte, 1991).

As medical anthropology has turned toward studying the globalization of the pharmaceutical industry, the ethical and epistemological quandaries of the relationship between RCTs and for-profit medicine have surfaced. Where and for whom placebo controls are considered ethical varies by location, disease, and population. Increasingly, pharmaceutical companies are recruiting subjects from the Global South—in part, because their lack of access to pharmaceutical treatments makes them better research subjects. However, when clinical trials involve vulnerable populations—due to location or type of disease—the ethics of placebo controls becomes murky; or, as Adriana Petryna puts it, ethics becomes a "workable document" (Petryna, 2009).

Science studies scholars have also turned an eye to the questions raised by the entanglement of for-profit pharmaceutical business and scientific methods in determining the safety and efficacy of new biomedical treatments. They have asked critical questions, such as: what are the methodological assumptions of RCTs, and their correlate, evidence-based medicine (EBM)? From what historical and social milieu did these methods and practices emerge? And how are their very standards of proof both productive of new forms of politics and influence and, themselves, the result of a technologies of government (Rose, 2007)? Scholars have pointed out that EBM is not without politics. Ayo Wahlberg and Linsey McGoey have encouraged investigation of the political, regulatory, and commercial contexts in which EBM has become the dominant paradigm. Following Petryna, they call for more work on how scientific models affect the political process downstream (Petryna, 2007; Wahlberg & McGoey, 2007). As they and other scholars have argued, EBM is not simply the transformation of medicine into science. Rather it has been implemented in ways that reflect and create different political possibilities (Jensen, 2007).

While placebo-controlled studies are often framed as methodologically sound, this does not mean that they are not without problem or controversy. Nancy Cartwright points out that the deductive methodology that provides the RCT with a high level of internal validity actually fails when faced with extending conclusions to broader populations. In other words, while the claims generated by an RCT may apply to the group studied, it is actually difficult to expand them to the broader populations for which they are intended to apply (Cartwright, 2007). In fact, there is a constant tension in clinical research between controlling for as many variables as possible and also trying to ensure that the treatment works for a broad population. The emphasis on controlling variables within the clinical trial has led to a pushback to enroll a more diverse population and thus broaden the scope of applicability of RCTs. This political shift has led to what Steven Epstein calls "recruitmentology": "an empirical body of studies scientifically evaluating the efficacy of various social, cultural, psychological, technological, and economic means of convincing people (especially members of 'hard-to-recruit populations') that they want to become, and remain, human subjects" (Epstein, 2008, p. 801).

Despite the attention to the ethical quandaries and methodological suppositions of RCTs, what exactly the placebo does as a research technique has largely gone unnoticed. Notably, Andrew Lakoff has investigated efforts by clinical researchers to eliminate placebo responders in antidepressant trials that struggle to demonstrate efficacy (Lakoff, 2007). He argues that researchers frame the placebo response as either real or artifactual—a result of error in the study design. In the latter case, raters might exaggerate the depression scores in an effort to enroll subjects, or a subject might be enrolled at the peak of their symptoms. In those cases, the change in depression is due to an inflated initial score. Researchers have postulated that, in the case of "real" placebo response, some subjects are more responsive to these hopes and expectations and thus must be eliminated from the trial. In order to eliminate the so-called placebo responders, these studies use a single-blind placebo run-in in which all subjects are given the placebo. This "simulation" of the study allows researchers to identify subjects more likely to be placebo responders. After eliminating these responders from the study, the remaining study population is able to more clearly demonstrate the efficacy of the drug.

The methodological issue for the MDMA trial is distinct from the issue that Lakoff identifies for most psychopharmaceuticals. In the case of antidepressants, the placebo response rate is quite high, which makes demonstrating efficacy of new products difficult. But in the MDMA trials, the problem was the opposite: the worry was that the placebo response was not to the placebo but to the investigational product. It is in this unusual case where placebos fail—rather than work—that the negotiations around blinding reveal the political struggle for psychedelics to be included under the sign of science.

The Boundary-Bridging Work of the Placebo

What if the focus on the mechanism of the placebo was shifted from its work on the body of the subject to the function of the placebo itself in the trial? As I have argued, placebos must work on both the researchers and the subjects. While the subjects must be fooled in order to make sure that expectancy or placebo effect is not clouding the data, the researchers must also be fooled to prevent bias from entering the treatment situation. As Doblin's quote about fooling encapsulates: the placebo is effective as a technique of deception; however, the use of double-blind placebo controls is a relatively recent phenomenon in pharmaceutical research and one that is itself not free from debates over ethics and validity. RCTs are not the only way to produce empirical knowledge about a therapy, but they are the current institutional standard. Thus, the maneuvers around placebos can be framed as a kind of boundary work that is politically necessary to translate the work of psychedelics into pharmaceutical terms.

Thomas Gieryn defined boundary work as a rhetorical move that scientists make to distinguish scientific from nonscientific work. He argued that scientists performed such moves in order to consolidate authority. As a sociologist of science, Gieryn approached science as a social institution and not as a unique empirical form. His argument calls attention to the shifting norms by which the boundary between scientific and nonscientific practices is enacted. "Characteristics of science are examined not as inherent or possibly unique, but as part of ideological efforts by scientists to distinguish their work and it's products from non-scientific efforts" (Gieryn, 1983, pp. 781–782).

In the case of placebo controls, it is less that scientists themselves declared that non-placebo-controlled studies were unscientific and more that a new set of norms for research were institutionalized, which excluded other modes of knowledge production about psychedelics. Research without a double-blind—or that could not be validated by a double-blind—was not institutionally recognized. The contemporary navigation of the placebo controls is an example of the kind of boundary-bridging work that science studies scholars have identified among citizen science groups (Ottinger, 2010). In Gwen Ottinger's study of the epistemological and political battles over the collection of air quality data by citizen scientists, she demonstrates that at times, standards are used by citizen scientists to bridge boundaries between their research and the scientific community. At other moments, standards are used to try and exclude the data collected by citizen scientists. The shifting lines of exclusion and inclusion belie a deeper critique of air quality measurements by citizen scientists, whose use of different techniques of measurement are themselves a response to a different framing of the health issues created by air pollution.

The work of placebos and blinding procedures in the contemporary landscape of psychedelic research is not just about doing good research but also about bridging the boundary between the humanistic and spiritual world of psychedelic therapy and the objective world of pharmaceutical research. When Western psychiatry intertwined with psychedelics mid-twentieth century, it did so through a model of pharmacological therapy that stands in stark contrast to the contemporary world of selective serotonin reuptake inhibitors (SSRIs) and monoamine oxidase inhibitors (MAOIs). Rather than achieve a new neurochemical balance, psychedelic therapy leverages a radical change in consciousness. Thus, at its core, psychedelic therapy challenges the very model of psychopharmacological intervention that is commonly used today. However, even as psychedelic therapy might challenge how drugs can treat anxiety and depression, they are not challenging the methodology by which those knowledge claims are produced. In the next section, I conclude by exploring how even as the search for the active placebo is abandoned, the quest to produce credible, objective data through creative blinding techniques persists.

The Epigraph

In the end, the search for the active placebo has been disregarded. The FDA recently approved the third phase of clinical trials, which will be the basis of the application to approve MDMA as a prescription pharmaceutical. In negotiations with the FDA, MAPS has agreed to return to using lactose as the placebo because of problems with the active placebos. Using MDMA as its own active placebo had an unexpected side effect. Subjects receiving the low dose experienced an uptick in anxiety during the experimental sessions. The clinical team speculated that the subtherapeutic dose might also produce a different affective response, acting like a stimulant that triggered feelings of anxiety in the subjects with PTSD. Not simply less than the full-dose MDMA, the low dose produced a different experience of the drug altogether. So while it improved blinding, the anxiety it produced actually made the full dose of MDMA look better by comparison. Thus, the active placebo proved problematic to both the clinical goal of establishing MDMA's safety and of getting a clearer picture of MDMA's therapeutic effects.

The researchers have returned to where they began but with a different logic. The next phase of studies will use lactose as a placebo, but the design calls for comparing MDMA-assisted therapy to the therapy by itself. The shift in comparison is critical because it negotiates one of the central tensions around the development of MDMA-assisted therapy, which is that the drug works *with* the therapy. The drug requires a specific set of techniques to make it work. What is more, the use of lactose is still critical to sorting out the safety of MDMA. This is of course critical, as safety issues will be incredibly significant in the assessment of MDMA and any other psychedelic medicine. While those interested in my field site have often asked me, if MDMA "works," the more vital question for the political viability of both psychedelic science and medicine is, probably, "Is it safe?"

Perhaps the most critical negotiation has been in the shift to administering the outcome measures. In moving back to the lactose placebo, the researchers are also making changes to address the question of bias by increasing the blinding of the independent raters who administer the outcome measures. While the independent raters have always been blinded to the treatment condition, they have also followed subjects through their enrollment and participation in the study. In current proposals, a randomized pool of raters, who will not know which stage of the study the subjects are in, will administer outcome measures.

What is critical here is that, even though the researchers have returned to the use of lactose, they are also continuing to navigate the institutional norms for pharmaceutical research. Of course, the question remains: What will happen when they go to publish the results? The FDA is just one of the gatekeepers around pharmaceutical research. In order to attain legitimacy for psychedelic research, the studies will need to be validated by peer-reviewed journals—preferably top-tier journals. As the larger psychiatric and medical communities weigh in on these studies, the question remains if the measures taken to ensure objectivity will be enough to persuade the gatekeepers of the validity of psychedelic therapy.

References

Cartwright, N. (2007). Are RCTs the gold standard? *Biosocieties, 2*, 11–20.
Chiodo, G. T., Tolle, S. W., & Bevan, L. (2000). Placebo-controlled trials: Good science or medical neglect? *The Western Journal of Medicine, 172*(4), 271–273.
de Fontes, F. P. X. (2017). *Os efeitos antidepressivos da ayahuasca, suas bases neurais e relação com a experiência psicodélica* [The antidepressant effects of ayahuasca, its neural bases and relation to the psychedelic experience] (Doctoral dissertation). Universidade Federal do Rio Grande do Norte, Natal, Brazil.

Dyck, E. (2010). *Psychedelic psychiatry: LSD from clinic to campus.* Baltimore, MD: Johns Hopkins University Press.

Epstein, S. (2008). The rise of "recruitmentology": Clinical research, racial knowledge, and the politics of inclusion and difference. *Social Studies of Science, 38*(5), 801–832.

Fadiman, J. (2011). *The psychedelic explorer's guide: Safe, therapeutic, and sacred journeys.* Rochester, VT: Park Street Press.

Geertz, C. (1998). Deep hanging out. *New York Review of Books, 45*(16), 69.

Gieryn, T. F. (1983). Boundary-work and the demarcation of science from non-science: Strains and interests in professional ideologies of scientists. *American Sociological Review, 48*(6), 781.

Griffiths, R. R., Richards, W. A., Mccann, U., & Jesse, R. (2006). Psilocybin can occasion mystical-type experiences having substantial and sustained personal meaning and spiritual significance. *Psychopharmacology (Berl), 187*(3), 268–283.

Harrington, A. (2006). The many meanings of the placebo effect: Where they came from, why they matter. *BioSocieties, 1*(2), 181–193.

Hartogsohn, I. (2016). Set and setting, psychedelics and the placebo response: An extra-pharmacological perspective on psychopharmacology. *Journal of Psychopharmacology, 30* (12), 1259–1267. https://doi.org/10.1177/0269881116677852

Healy, D. (2002). *The creation of psychopharmacology.* Cambridge, MA: Harvard University Press.

Holland, J. (Ed.). (2001). *Ecstasy: The complete guide.* Rochester, VT: Park Street Press.

Huculak, S. (2013). Attempting to define placebos and their effects: A keywords approach. *BioSocieties, 8*(2), 164–180.

Jasanoff, S. (1995). Procedural choices in regulatory science. *Technology in Society, 17*(3), 279–293.

Jensen, U. J. (2007). The struggle for clinical authority: Shifting ontologies and the politics of evidence. *BioSocieties, 2*(1), 101–114.

Kirk, S., & Kutchins, H. (1992). *The selling of DSM: The rhetoric of science in psychiatry.* Piscataway, NJ: Transaction Publishers.

Lakoff, A. (2007). The right patients for the drug: Managing the placebo effect in antidepressant trials. *BioSocieties, 2*(1), 57–71.

Marks, H. (1988). Notes from the underground: The social organization of therapeutic research. In R. C. Maulitz & D. E. Long (Eds.), *Grand rounds: One hundred years of internal medicine* (pp. 297–336). Philadelphia, PA: University of Pennsylvania Press. https://doi.org/10.1556/AAlim.2015.0002

Marks, H. (2000). *The progress of experiment: Science and therapeutic reform in the United States, 1900–1990.* Cambridge: Cambridge University Press.

Mithoefer, M. C., Wagner, M. T., Mithoefer, A. T., Jerome, L., & Doblin, R. (2011). The safety and efficacy of ±3,4-methylenedioxymethamphetamine-assisted psychotherapy in subjects with chronic, treatment-resistant posttraumatic stress disorder: The first randomized controlled pilot study. *Journal of Psychopharmacology, 25*(4), 439–452.

Moerman, D. (2002). *Meaning, medicine, and the "placebo effect.".* Cambridge: University of Cambridge Press.

Nichols, D. (1986). Differences between the mechanism of action of MDMA, MBDB, and the classic hallucinogens. Identification of a new therapeutic class: Entactogens. *Journal of Psychoactive Drugs, 18*(4), 305–313.

Oram, M. (2012). Efficacy and enlightenment: LSD psychotherapy and the drug amendments of 1962. *Journal of the History of Medicine and Allied Sciences, 69*(2), 221–260.

Oram, M. (2016). Prohibited or regulated? LSD psychotherapy and the United States Food and Drug Administration. *History of Psychiatry, 27*(3), 290–306.

Ottinger, G. (2010). Buckets of resistance: Standards and the effectiveness of citizen science. *Science, Technology & Human Values, 35*(2), 244–270.

Petryna, A. (2007). Clinical trials offshored: On private sector science and public health. *BioSocieties, 2*(1), 21–40.

Petryna, A. (2009). *When experiments travel: Clinical trials and the global search for human subjects*. Princeton, NJ: Princeton University Press.

Rose, N. (2007). *The politics of life itself: Biomedicine, power and subjectivity in the 21st century*. Princeton, NJ: Princeton University Press.

Rosenberg, C. (2002). The tyranny of diagnosis: Specific entities and individual experience. *The Milbank Quarterly, 80*(2), 237–260.

Rosenthal, R. (1994). Interpersonal expectancy effects: A 30-year perspective. *Current Directions in Psychological Science, 3*(6), 176–179.

Sandison, R. A. (1954). Psychological aspects of the LSD treatment of the neuroses. *The British Journal of Psychiatry, 100*(419), 508–515.

Scheper-Hughes, N., & Lock, M. M. (1987). The mindful body: A prolegomenon to future work in medical anthropology. *Medical Anthropology Quarterly, 1*(1), 6–41.

Starr, P. (1982). *The social transformation of American medicine*. New York City, NY: Basic Books.

Streiner, D. L. (2008). The lesser of 2 evils: The ethics of placebo-controlled trials. *Canadian Journal of Psychiatry, 53*(7), 430–432.

Van der Geest, S., & Whyte, S. (1991). *The context of medicines in developing countries: Studies in pharmaceutical anthropology*. Amsterdam: Het Spinhuis.

Wahlberg, A., & McGoey, L. (2007). An elusive evidence base: The construction and governance of randomized controlled trials. *BioSocieties, 2*(1), 1–10.

Chapter 10
Psychedelic Naturalism and Interspecies Alliance: Views from the Emerging Do-It-Yourself Mycology Movement

Joanna Steinhardt

Abstract Do-it-yourself (DIY) mycology is a movement that has emerged in the last decade in North America. DIY mycologists specialize in easy and accessible methods of mushroom cultivation and mycological experimentation and mobilize a discourse of alliance with the fungal kingdom. They draw primarily on home cultivation methods innovated by *Psilocybe* cultivators in the 1970s and on creative applications popularized by commercial mycologist and psychedelic enthusiast Paul Stamets in the 2000s. As a counterpoint to the newfound visibility and legitimacy of lab-synthesized psilocybin in clinical psychiatry, DIY mycology exemplifies an alternate history of this multispecies engagement. Drawing on ethnographic fieldwork in the San Francisco Bay Area and the Pacific Northwest, this chapter begins with the tacit premise of the psychedelic/entheogenic movement that the use of psychedelics fosters ecological concern. Many DIY mycologists express biocentric ethics and eco-spiritual principles, but interviews revealed a diverse and nuanced relationship to psychedelics. I argue that DIY mycology is best understood as an interspecies (or cross-kingdom) engagement that is part of an emergent ecological ethics and deep ecology worldview, one that subsumes psychedelic experiences as one manifestation of that engagement. DIY mycology exemplifies how the spread of mycological know-how, fascination, and enthusiasm has fostered an engagement with fungi that extends far beyond psychedelics. To understand this engagement, I contextualize it within wider social and cultural shifts, particularly those that reformulated our practical, ethical, and conceptual relationship with the natural world. This movement attests to the existence of multiple means to enact these ethics and to foster meaningful relationality with nonhuman life in contemporary North American society and culture.

J. Steinhardt (✉)
University of California, Humanities and Social Sciences Building (HSSB), Santa Barbara, CA, USA

© Springer International Publishing AG, part of Springer Nature 2018
B. C. Labate, C. Cavnar (eds.), *Plant Medicines, Healing and Psychedelic Science*,
https://doi.org/10.1007/978-3-319-76720-8_10
167

First Encounters

Ben was the first person I met from the Fungal Alliance of the Bay (FAB). When I asked him how he got involved in the group, he explained that he had been on a road trip around California when he stopped at a roadside cafe and found a book called *Mycelium Running* on the bookshelf. "The subtitle said 'How Mushrooms Can Help Save the World.' I flipped through all the pages and I was mesmerized by the pictures and all the information in it. ... I've read it four or five times through."

Ben's first introduction to mycology (the study of fungi) was through taking psychedelic mushrooms, and then learning to grow them, when he was a student in college in Northern California. He and his friends would spend the day in the redwood forests tripping. "Depression is pretty rampant in my family, like, genetically," he told me, "and it was the first time that I saw my mind working in different ways."

When I asked Renée how she got into mushrooms, she told me about living in Olympia, Washington, taking classes in environmental science at Evergreen State College, where she was an undergraduate, and getting involved in Earth First!, the radical environmentalist activist organization. She, too, had discovered *Mycelium Running* and was inspired by its ideas and imagery. She began hunting mushrooms with her friends and learned some easy cultivation techniques.

As she spoke to me about mushrooms, her language became excited and expressive. "I learned about mycorrhizal fungi my freshman year of college and it blew my mind. Just seeing how everything is connected ... how they can clean up oil spills, and how they're part of the healing process, inner and outer, and how they can help create sustainable communities."

Renée and Ben are not alone in the sense of gravity and magic that they ascribe to fungi[1] nor the feelings of wonder and potentiality that the organisms inspire in them. While Renée was living in Olympia, she and a couple of friends started a small organization called the Mycelial Network, whose goal was to teach people basic mycology and cultivation skills. Then, in 2011, after graduating from Evergreen, Renée moved to East Oakland and brought with her the idea of a community-driven collective devoted to applied mycology. That was how FAB got started.[2]

---

[1]What is known as the "mushroom" is in fact the fruit of the fungus (plural: fungi) that lives primarily as an underground network of fine threads called mycelium. Not all fungi produce mushrooms, but all mushrooms are fungi.

[2]Both the Fungal Alliance of the Bay and the Mycelial Network are pseudonyms, as are the names of all of the members of these groups that I mention here.

What is DIY Mycology?

In 2014, I began fieldwork with FAB as part of my dissertation research. FAB was modeled on the Mycelial Network, founded in Olympia, a small college town in the northwest corner of Washington known as a center for radical environmentalism and punk rock. Animated by the local culture, the goal of the Mycelial Network was to teach basic mycology (identification and cultivation) to their friends and the local community. They hosted the first Mycelial Network Convergence in 2012, drawing over 200 people from around North America. Participants taught and learned from each other in self-organized classes, with topics ranging from the uses of medicinal mushrooms to the diversity of lichens. Since then, there have been three more convergences, each drawing a few hundred people. As part of my fieldwork, I also interviewed several members of the Mycelial Network, which is now a small collective scattered around the Pacific Northwest. As for FAB, as of March 2017, the group includes about 39 dues-paying active members, and over 250 listserv subscribers.

Experimentation with applied mycology is becoming more common among amateurs, hobbyists, and self-described citizen scientists, especially biohackers, permaculturalists, and others working at the intersection between ecology and technology. Groups like FAB can now be found around North America in places like Austin (Myco Alliance), Montreal (Champignons Maison), Victoria (DIY Fungi), and Eugene (Fungi for the People). These do-it-yourself (DIY) mycology initiatives are generally loose-knit and collectively run, dedicated to public education and accessibility, and are often driven by radical ecological values, working in partnership with like-minded local groups.[3]

The initial inspiration for both FAB and the Mycelial Network was mycoremediation—the bioremediation of toxins with fungi.[4] The idea was popularized in *Mycelium Running*, the book by mycologist Paul Stamets that inspired Ben, Renée, and many others (Stamets, 2005). It included other mycological applications too, like myco-forestry (forest management through mycological applications), myco-filtration (filtering water with fungi), and medicinal mushrooms. The book is also known for its epic opening chapters that offer a myco-centric history of life on earth, reflections on the "mycelial archetype" (i.e., network and spiral formations), and philosophical proposals about the significance of fungi to the human race. Stamets argues that fungi are sentient (he calls them "Gaia's Internet"), that they

---

[3]These practices are an emergent phenomenon. DIY mycology is not quite a full-fledged movement, although it seems to be taking on the outlines of one. As such, practitioners are not united under one identifiable name. Some call themselves "radical mycologists" or "applied mycologists," but most are unbothered by the question of what their pastime might be called by those outside their social circles. For the sake of consistency, I refer to this practice as do-it-yourself (DIY, pronounced as an acronym, D-I-Y) mycology.

[4]Bioremediation is the use of living organisms to decompose environmental toxins in soil and water. It commonly utilizes microorganisms such as bacteria, but sometimes plants (a practice that is called phytoremediation) and fungi (mycoremediation) are used.

have an ecosystem's best interests in mind, and that, if we as a species are to survive and flourish, we should ally ourselves with the fungal kingdom. The book has an evangelical quality, having the tone of a testimonial at times, but it also has references to peer-reviewed papers, some by Stamets himself, and an extensive bibliography. Overall, it's a compelling and unusual mix of mystical prose, dry scientific explanation, and practical instruction. It's a how-to book in a holistic sense, describing a new way of living with the fungal kingdom.

For FAB, mycoremediation quickly proved too complicated, and they focused their energy elsewhere. One ongoing project is in collaboration with the East Bay Regional Parks, allowing for field experiments in the forested parklands that ring the Bay Area. In one experiment, they're applying a local strain of sulfur shelf (*Laetiporus gilbertsonii*) to accelerate the decomposition of blue-gum eucalyptus (*Eucalyptus globulus*) stumps. Eucalyptus is a notoriously fast-growing and tenacious species that is both ubiquitous and invasive in California and burns long and hot in the wildfires that plague the region. As part of a statewide initiative, the park service is trying to thin its Eucalyptus populations. This myco-forestry method would ideally be an alternative to the application of synthetic pesticides to prevent the rapid resprouting of the trees. FAB has a number of other ongoing projects as well: They partner with a biohacker space in Oakland, host low-cost workshops and events, and table at mycological and science events around town.

FAB is part of a local and regional culture that has been shaped by a history of countercultural and ecological movements, as reflected in members' biographies, vocations, and lifestyles, and the culture of the group itself. Members include a permaculture landscaper, an arborist, a gourmet caterer who specializes in organic and locally produced food, an artisan cheese maker, a computer programmer, and a few teachers. Older members have retired from careers as a carpenter, a baker, and a chemist, respectively. Members share hobbies like organic gardening, beekeeping, beer brewing, making medicinal tinctures, fermenting and pickling, bird watching, and of course, mushroom hunting. Their monthly potluck meetings are packed with what Warren Belasco calls the "counter-cuisine," a mix of natural and seasonal foods made with gourmet ingredients (sometimes called "California cuisine") (Belasco, 2007; Fairfax et al., 2012). The groups' organization is horizontal and nonhierarchical; their meetings are full of joking asides and irreverent humor. The group has a casual atmosphere in this way, their projects driven by personal motivation rather than a sense of obligation and their activities ebbing and flowing along these lines.

One unspoken commonality is participation in the local food movement: that broad collection of practices that position themselves as alternatives to industrial food production. In this vein, almost all members share an interest in horticulture. Younger members in particular are involved in permaculture, the global movement of sustainable agriculture and design principles developed in the late 1970s that incorporates social, ecological, and economic philosophies into its core vision. Older members, on the other hand, voice good-natured skepticism about permaculture; as one of them puts it, "Permaculture really puts the CULT in agriculture."

Along with these ecological values, and as an extension of its DIY ethos, FAB members often describe themselves as citizen scientists and espouse open source science and technology. Their partnership with a local biohacking collective in Oakland reflects this position. Biohacking (also known as DIYBio) is a practice that has emerged in recent years, drawing on computer hacking, the contemporary maker movement, and recent advances in biotechnology. The goal of biohacking is to create spaces outside of academic and corporate settings for public engagement and participation in biology. For FAB, the partnership means access to a professional-grade flow hood and other high-tech lab equipment, storage space, and a platform to advertise the group. In addition, FAB hosts semi-regular low-cost events and pay-what-you-can workshops to help fund their activities and spread mycological knowledge and know-how.

Psychedelia and American Countercultural Ecology

In this chapter, I address a question that has been with me since I first spoke to Ben in the fall of 2014: How do DIY mycologists relate to psychedelic mushrooms, and what can this tell us about how Americans think about and consume psychedelics today? When I began fieldwork, I thought Ben's introduction to mycology would be typical of FAB members, but I found that, although it was common, it wasn't exactly typical. Several DIY mycologists that I interviewed had learned to cultivate mushrooms by growing *Psilocybe cubensis* (the most well-known and easy to cultivate psychedelic mushroom), but their ideas about psychedelics, and their practices related to them, were far from monolithic. Some had tried the mushrooms just once or twice, while others had long histories of use; some saw them as purely recreational, while others used them for explicitly spiritual or therapeutic purposes (or both). A couple were unequivocally dismissive of the idea of truth claims being ascribed to the psychedelic experience—as one FABer put it, the mushrooms just "confuse the brain." There were also three members that had never eaten psychedelic mushrooms. And yet, it was readily apparent that all FABers were gleeful that such mushrooms existed. They loved to joke about them and the altered states they engender as much as they loved to regale each other with stories of the gourmet wild mushrooms they found on their latest forays.

Since their grand entrance onto the American cultural stage, psychedelics have gone through many reversals of fortune. At the time of writing this chapter, it seems that not a month goes by without another mainstream news source reporting on the promise of psilocybin research for depression. Yet, all the mainstream hype about a "psychedelic renaissance" can feel disingenuous: Anyone paying attention knows that psychedelics never went away—they just went underground.[5] After LSD and psilocybin were criminalized in 1970, they disappeared from the public eye but

---

[5] See Jarnow, n.d., on the recurring trope of the "psychedelic renaissance."

remained in the cultural repertoire, especially in subcultures like the Grateful Dead circuit and the rave culture of the 1990s (Jarnow, 2016; Letcher, 2007).

Psychedelics are nonaddictive and usually used infrequently by those who partake of them. They barely register on the National Survey on Drug Use and Health (NSDUH), which defines a user as someone who has used a substance within the last 30 days (Drug Policy Alliance, 2017). Yet, due to their powerful psychological effects, a single use can leave a long-lasting impression. One study tracked "lifetime use" among Americans (i.e., those that have used psychedelics at least once in their lives), based on the 2010 NSDUH survey, and the results were illuminating.[6] The same number of people (around 17%) between the ages of 21 and 49 had used psychedelics as had the so-called baby boomers between the ages of 50 and 64, who came of age in the 1960s and 1970s. And yet the rate of lifetime use was highest (around 20%) among people aged 30–34 (Krebs & Johanson, 2013). In other words, younger Americans today are just as psychedelically "experienced" as young people were in the 1960s and 1970s, the period of American history considered the heart of the psychedelic era.

Psychedelics cast a long shadow across the cultural landscape of the United States. If we look at American pop culture alone, they are usually depicted as a rite of passage or a transformative or revelatory event, sometimes comic, sometimes unexpectedly profound.[7] Of course, this kind of use is lost in the shuffle of surveys meant to measure abuse and dependency. In the case of DIY mycology, the question of participants' relationship to psychedelia has particular historical and cultural resonance. On a practical level, the technical genealogy of DIY mycology is rooted in the psychedelic underground. While the idea of "tinkering" with fungi for targeted, low-tech applications can be traced most recently to *Mycelium Running,* the techniques employed by DIY mycologists originate in the novice experimentations of psychedelic enthusiasts in the 1970s. Paul Stamets is a key figure in this history too, as I'll discuss further on.

DIY mycologists are embedded in a countercultural–ecological milieu in which psychedelics have historically been a significant element. As is well documented, psychedelics were a key component in the counterculture that coalesced around the new environmentalism and the ecological lifestyles of the 1970s that left their marks on California and West Coast culture. At that time, LSD and psilocybin were seen as aids to dropping into one's body, tuning into the universe, becoming one with nature, finding one's authentic self, realizing one's true potential, or simply tackling complex problems (Binkley, 2007; Kirk, 2007; Kripal, 2007; Markoff, 2005; Turner, 2006). FABers and other DIY mycologists participate in hobbies, lifestyles, and vocations that emerged out of these ecological movements. In other words, their

---

[6]The data pool was 57,873 individuals aged 12 and older. The substances they tracked were LSD, psilocybin, peyote, and mescaline.

[7]See, for example, the use of psilocybin mushrooms in American sitcoms like *Silicon Valley* or *This is Us* and in the movie *Boyhood.*

relationships to psychedelic mushrooms and mushroom in general take place in a world that has already been shaped by psychedelics.

Although it's recurrently treated as a breakthrough or dawning cultural revolution, modern American psychedelia is a social and cultural phenomenon with historical depth, one that has undergone its own evolution and ramifications. My inquiry here is set against the background of an interrelated suite of narratives and popular theories about psychedelics that have circulated in the contemporary cultural landscape for some time. Most prominent among them is the notion of an inherent link between the psychedelic experience and ecological concern. This is often part and parcel of a discourse on the redemptive dimensions of these substances, one that is best illustrated by the discourse of entheogens.[8]

Advocates of entheogens often imply (and sometimes state explicitly) that part of the promise of these substances is that they allow users to experience oneness with the natural world, thereby instilling a sense of responsibility and care toward our threatened environment. For example, in an introduction to the special issue of the Multidisciplinary Association for Psychedelic Science (MAPS) bulletin on psychedelics and ecology, psychologists Stanley Kripper and David Luke wrote, "at the very least the consumption of psychedelic substances leads to an increasing concern for Nature and ecological issues" (Krippner & Luke, 2009). Countless psychedelic thinkers, many of them referenced in the piece, have elaborated this idea at length; among them is Paul Stamets.

With his message of universal patterns, mystical depth, and Gaian consciousness and his tone that is both revelatory and evangelical, it doesn't seem surprising that Stamets got his start as an expert in psilocybin mushrooms. For the most part, though, he's an expert at glossing his abiding fascination with the psychoactive mushrooms in texts meant for a general audience. In asserting that fungi are sentient, as he does in *Mycelium Running*, Stamets evokes a kind of neoshamanic vision of communication that in turn alludes to an entheogenic/psychedelic model. Stamets's own biography charts what would seem to be an archetypal psychedelic narrative in which intense use of psychedelic mushrooms reveals insights and intuitive knowledge about the fungi themselves. Of course, the author most closely associated with this scenario is Terence McKenna, the folk philosopher of psychedelia who published several texts in his lifetime that he described as "straight transcription" from "the mushroom" (Deus Ex McKenna, 2011). What's notable about Paul Stamets, who was friends with McKenna, is the way he sublimates this narrative and its epistemological models into his texts as he weaves his assertions, and their implications, with the conventions of contemporary scientific scholarship.

---

[8]Entheogen is a neologism meaning "God/divine-generating" (Ruck, Bigwood, Staples, Ott, & Wasson, 1979). It was coined in the late 1970s by several ethnobotanists that had been researching psychotropic plants and fungus since the 1950s, including R. Gordon Wasson, the banker-turned-mycologist credited with "discovering" psilocybin-active mushrooms in Southern Mexico. The term was meant as a clarification and re-branding of "psychedelics," whose public image had been sullied by countercultural excesses.

In questioning the causal relationship between psychedelics and ecological concern, I take my cue from Nicolas Langlitz, Andy Letcher, and others that seek to historicize and problematize the meaning we ascribe to the psychedelic experience (Langlitz, 2012; Letcher, 2013; Shortall, 2014).[9] In this chapter, I attempt to historicize and contextualize the meaning of psychedelic mushrooms among DIY mycologists. As I show below, along with their diverse relationship to psychedelics, FABers share an ethical system that views nonhuman life as essentially valuable and, in varying degrees, vital in ways continuous with human consciousness. Members told me they believed in "panpsychism," the Gaia theory, and biocentricism, while some expressed respect and awe at the "web of life." But not all those who expressed these ideas cited psychedelics as being part of their personal evolution. In this chapter, drawing on historical and ethnographic material, I hope to add some perspective and complexity and helpfully destabilize the tacit link between psychedelics and ecology that is so often at the core of the redemptive hope projected onto these substances.

The History of DIY Mycology, Part 1: Psilocybin and Ecology

The goal of groups like FAB is not only to use fungi to restore ecosystems but to make mycological knowledge and know-how more accessible to everyone, to inspire people to learn about fungi and its many beneficial applications and give people tools to experiment with and implement fungal applications on their own. DIY mycologists are informed by an ethos of openness and accessibility that combines the countercultural ecology of the 1970s with the hacker and open source movements of the 1980s and 1990s—and, as I'll show below, intertwines with psychedelia in its technical methodology and its cultural values and practices (Kelty, 2008; Kirk, 2007). Paul Stamets's career is one thread that takes us through much of this history.

The first technically accurate manual for growing psychedelic mushrooms was *Psilocybin*, by Terence and Dennis McKenna, writing under the pseudonyms O. T. Oss and O. N. Oeric, published in 1976. It came out about 20 years after R. Gordon Wasson's article in *Life* magazine that described psychoactive mushrooms to mainstream audiences, leading to a steady flow of hippies into Southern Mexico in search of the "magic mushrooms."[10] Although there were a few other pamphlets published before this book, the McKennas' was the first that relied on practical microbiological skills that might, if followed carefully, result in actual mushrooms. The book focused

---

[9]I use the phrase "the psychedelic experience," with the troublesome definite article, to refer to this particular discursive formation as it's circulated over the last 50 years. I do not mean to imply a universal phenomenon.

[10]See Letcher (2007), for this history in depth; Feinberg (2003), for a view of this history from the Mazatec perspective. Also see Feinberg in this volume to revisit this history alongside contemporary practices in the southern Mexican town where Wasson's article took place.

on inconspicuous indoor methods for growing *P. cubensis*. It included a now-famous introduction by Terence McKenna that, speaking in the voice of the mushroom, claimed to usher in a new era of cosmic fungal intelligence (Oss & Oeric, 1976). Mycologist Steven Pollock also published his book *Magic Mushroom Cultivation* around this time, which included outdoor methods. Unfortunately, the book went out of his print after Pollock's murder in 1981 (Morris, 2013).

Paul Stamets learned to cultivate using these books and then, after studying mycology at Evergreen State College, published his first book, a field guide to psilocybin-active species called *Psilocybe Mushrooms and Their Allies* (later renamed *Psilocybin Mushrooms of the World*) (Stamets, 1996, 2014).[11] Stamets then made a name for himself with two cultivation manuals: the first, *The Mushroom Cultivator* (1983) picked up where these earlier manuals left off but was written for a general audience and included a wider range of species. About half were psychoactive *Psilocybes* and the rest were culinary and medicinal mushrooms. As the first book to break down the most obscure aspects of fungal biology and the tricks of cultivation for a general audience, *The Mushroom Cultivator* quickly became the bible of cultivation. *Psilocybes* were interspersed between culinary and medicinal species, minimally described within the highly technical text, normalized within the rapidly growing repertoire of popular mycological knowledge.

Stamets's second book, *Growing Gourmet and Medicinal Mushrooms* (1993), included more historical, philosophical, and hypothetical exposition, as well as a range of creative applications. *Psilocybes* are described more elaborately but still carefully elided with tongue-in-cheek references. This obfuscation makes sense, of course (the mushrooms are illegal after all and could undermine his legitimacy), but any reader paying attention would understand that many of the methods could be applied to these mushrooms too, as many readers did.

The success of these books, and the mycological know-how they helped to foster, is interwoven with several trends that emerged in the 1970s. I've already mentioned the "counter-cuisine"; this was interwoven with the rise of natural medicine, organic agriculture, homesteading,[12] and the revival of preindustrial food practices (pickling, beer brewing, bread baking), all of which reflected a changing relationship to the natural world, especially, in how Americans produced, thought about, and consumed food. Americans developed new tastes, in both senses of the word, and as the countercultural palate grew more exotic and earthy, new markets, industries, and vocations opened up to cater to these tastes. Hippies began foraging—that is, gathering wild plants, fruits, and mushrooms—as a back-to-the-land practice (following Euell Gibbon's cult classic, *Stalking the Wild Asparagus*), while Alice Waters developed what would come to be called "California cuisine." Wild

---

[11]*Psilocybe* is the genus that contains the vast majority of psilocybin-active species.

[12]Homesteading is the practice of simple subsistence living on the land around one's home. It was one component of the back-to-the-land movement in the 1970s, inspired primarily by the writing of Helen and Scott Nearing. For a look at the homesteading movement in the 1970s and beyond, including its particularly American history, see *At Home in Nature: Modern Homesteading and Spiritual Practice in America*, by Rebecca Kneale Gould (University of California Press, 2005).

mushrooms began to appear in the American diet, while macrobiotic cooking and East Asian cuisines brought other "exotic" mushrooms to the dinner table. All of this meant that someone who figured out how to hunt or grow mushrooms could make a modest income selling them.

This shift in tastes corresponded to a new genre of books that catered to this readership, following in the wake of the *Whole Earth Catalog*'s phenomenal success in the late 1960s and early 1970s. Most of these were published by an emerging West Coast publishing industry. Natural food cookbooks taught people how to cook these new foods, various instructional manuals taught DIY and homesteading practices (everything from cheese making to home births), and lifestyle books taught readers how to live in ways that were "natural," "authentic," and "holistic" (Belasco, 2007; Binkley, 2007; Fairfax et al., 2012; Kaiser & McCray, 2016; Paxson, 2013).

Stamets's career reflects this history. His first book combined countercultural interests in foraging and psychedelics. His second book picked up on the DIY and homesteading trend, offering itself as a tool of both the amateur home cultivator and the aspiring small-scale mushroom farmer (and, however tacitly, the illicit cultivator of *Psilocybes*). By the late 1980s, he began to focus on gourmet and medicinal mushrooms, as new markets were opening up for natural medicine and organic mushroom farmers. In general, he wrote for readers who are living ecological lifestyles. All of his books, including *Mycelium Running*, are clearly written with spacious organic gardens in mind. He's also been involved in permaculture since the 1990s; his second book has a chapter called "the Stametsian Model for permaculture with a mycological twist." The company he founded in 1980, Fungi Perfecti, still specializes in mycological products catering to the markets opened up by these ecological values and lifestyles. Besides his books, they sell soil augmentation with mycorrhizal fungi, in-house medicinal mushroom tinctures, and much more.

These trends were the gradual result of the ecology movement that coalesced in the 1970s, growing out of the counterculture and the new wave of environmentalism, producing many offshoots, in various sectors of society. The practices that were popularized through this new literature inculcated a new orientation, both practical and philosophical, to the natural world, one in which fungi are especially significant. With the spread of organic agriculture in both farms and gardens, people became familiarized with the microbial worlds of compost and soil ecology and, along with them, the essential roles of mycorrhizal and endophytic fungi (Ingram, 2007). Paul Stamets played a central role in translating and popularizing the significance of mushrooms and mycology within this web of practices.

These countercultural ecological practices, particularly in the realms of food production, were characterized by a desire to live in balance with the natural world, in closer rhythm with the cycles of life and death, among humans and other life forms. In her ethnography of artisan cheesemakers, Heather Paxson has called this a post-Pasteurian orientation that sees nonhuman agency not as an unruly force that must be put in order—the paradigmatic modern relationship to nature—but rather as forces with whom we can collaborate in mutually beneficial endeavors (Paxson, 2013). This orientation is part of a shift in the position of science and technology vis-á-vis the natural world among countercultural ecologists: Rather than seeing science and technology as opposed to "nature," they sought to subsume it within an ecological worldview (Kirk, 2007).

I see American countercultural ecology as a contemporary variation on an older lineage of ecological thought that can be traced back through Leopold, Muir, Thoreau, and Humboldt— thinkers who, though embedded in the scientific enterprise, expressed a profound ambivalence toward aspects of industrial modernity and scientific materialism and proposed alternative perspectives, from vitalism to biocentrism (Worster, 1985). Countercultural ecology draws on the multivalence of ecology as both a holistic philosophy of interconnectedness and as a scientific understanding of the material world, weaving this thread of ecological thought with the countercultural concerns of social, political, and personal transformation. Paul Stamets is very much in line with this particular American lineage of ecological thinkers and designers.

The History of DIY Mycology, Part 2: The Internet

Around the same time, a vast rhizomorphic web known as the Internet was also growing. Websites like Shroomery and Mycotopia were founded in the mid-1990s, with forums focused on *Psilocybe* cultivation, allowing people to swap information, troubleshoot their failures, and crowdsource solutions. A number of ingenious, jury-rigged techniques came out of these communities and have since become part of home cultivation "best practices." The most famous of these is the PF Tek.

Psylocybe Fanaticus (his real name was Robert McPherson) was part of a flourishing industry that exploited a loophole in the criminalization of psychedelic mushrooms that made possession of *Psilocybes* spores legal in some US states. In 1994, as part of his business selling *Psilocybe* spores to would-be cultivators, Fanaticus published online a method for growing *P. cubensis* with a simplified, streamlined recipe that had no need for sterilization (Letcher, 2007; Yachaj, 2001). He named it the PF Tek—the first initials after his nom de guerre and "tek" being cultivator slang for "technique." Within just a few years, the PF Tek was the go-to method for growing *P. cubensis* and still is today. It's been improved upon with some tricks and updates (inventions of Shroomery and Mycotopia users), but the basic recipe and concept remain tried and true, easily accessible with a simple Google search.

Amateur mushroom cultivation has come a long way since Oss and Oeric. Shroomery and Mycotopia are still the primary resources for technical instruction and advice. The sites are used by DIY mycologists who consult the countless subthreads on culinary and medicinal species. Since the mid-1990s, there are also numerous instructional videos on YouTube and free downloadable PDFs online as well. In all of this, we can see how psilocybin-active mushrooms were the impetus for the development of modular techniques for small-scale home cultivation that were then borrowed and modified for use with other species. This history explains part of the deep appreciation DIY mycologists today feel for psychedelic mushrooms, in that they epitomize the enthusiasm and populism that drives the practice. What's more, besides the obvious mycelial homology, there's another, less obvious relationship between digital technology and DIY mycology: As documented by historian Fred Turner, the *Whole Earth Catalog* milieu was intertwined with the birth of the Internet, as illustrated in their shared discourse of DIY practice and knowledge sharing (Turner, 2006). This common genealogy reveals an inner logic to this convergence.

In all of these activities, people were becoming familiarized with fungi as a life form and home cultivar as the practice itself became increasingly easy and accessible. What began as an attempt to recreate the modern lab in kitchens and closets was now placed alongside revivalist food practices like brewing and fermenting. Creative outdoor applications converged with organic agriculture and wildcrafting techniques. Last, but not least, *Psilocybe* spores were being spread far and wide, both through the mail and on the clothing of people picking wild *Psilocybes*. These strains have found ample new habitat in the woodchip lawns of American cities and suburbs, making them even more available to human curiosity and engagement.

DIY Mycology and Psychedelic Naturalism

Today, DIY mycologists are engaging with fungi in a landscape that has been shaped by all of these developments. Oscar, a FABer since 2013, articulates well several common themes. Now in his late 20s, Oscar grew up foraging for chanterelles with his parents in Northern California. Today, Oscar is an experimental filmmaker, arborist, and permaculture gardener in Oakland. When I asked him if psychedelics shaped how he related to mushrooms, he said that probably the "fractal imagery," as he put it, had an effect ("understanding that mycelium is a fractal") but, he continued, "As far as how that got me into mushrooms, honestly, it's just food. Like, the psychedelic part was definitely a big part of shaping who I am and the path I chose, but what really kept me with mushrooms is that I'm a food person. And I *really* liked foraging. . ."

> The thing about mushroom foraging is that it keys you into the landscape in a way that other things don't. You start to think about *hydrology*, and *shade*, and *aspect*, and *humidity traps*, and. . . just micro-climate because in order to find the mushrooms, you have to find the micro-climate that will get them to fruit. . . . So through my desire to get a bunch of porcinis [laughing] I had to figure out *what makes a porcini—which is a complicated set of variables*. And all of that built my interest in understanding ecosystems. Which is now something I like to apply [in permaculture].

Later, I asked him what he meant when he said psychedelics were a big part in shaping who he is and his path. He told me that he sees psychedelics as a means to produce a spiritual state, which he understands as an innate propensity of human brains.

> When *I* experienced a spiritual state, what became immediately crystal clear to me is that all organisms are valid and alive and interconnected. And we all share life together. None of us exists in any separate bubble. There are *people*—there is no "me" without the ecosystem. There is no me without trees, or bacteria, or mountains and rivers, and there's no me without the entire. . . framework.

> Having had that, then. . . working with organisms, and thinking about nonhuman life, became very central to me. . . . But also death is part of it and that's okay too. Death is necessary. Mushrooms and death are really close to each other. *And that's really cool*, because they eat the dead. The mushrooms are what *deal* with death in the world. They are like the pallbearers of nature. . . . [Laughing] You know, nature's not all flowers and butterflies. It's also rotting things. [Laughing]

This description expresses beautifully the sense of kinship and connection with all life that can be part of the psychedelic experience. It includes the classic experience of ego-dissolution as the "I" (or "me" in this case) is dissolved into the panorama of existence. This is the quintessential psychedelic experience (and its ideal aftermath) referenced in the entheogenic discourse.

However, Oscar's own story reveals interesting discontinuities in this narrative. While his experiences did instill in him a relational, biocentric ethos, it was not the impetus to study mycology; that was foraging. Psychedelics shaped his vocation and that in turn led him to engage with fungi; but it was fungi themselves, in their vital particularity, that maintained his attention. Then, circling back, he described fungi evocatively as having a privileged position in this web of life as the ultimate soil builders and essential actors in the natural cycle, at the seam between life and death.

Toward the end of our conversation, I asked Oscar how he would describe himself in terms of religion. He thought for a second and then said, "Like, 'psychedelic naturalist'. . . I feel at peace and connected, and like, I'm whole, when we go to the woods." This sentiment is quite common among FABers. Stamets himself described the old growth forests of Washington as his and his wife's church (Stamets, 2008). Oscar, though, avoids explicitly religious language.

It's not a coincidence that foraging takes place in the same forests where Oscar finds spiritual sustenance and retreat, a fact that blurs the common distinction between sites of spirituality and sites of practical (profane) activity. Foraging is an active, inquisitive, and pragmatic practice. It calls for skills of attention and attunement in order to perceive that "complicated set of variables" that allow fungi to thrive. This is what anthropologist Anna Tsing has called, in her work on matsutake foragers, "the arts of noticing" (Tsing, 2015). Food motivated Oscar to look for mushrooms, but the practice itself intrigued and enchanted him. In this way, fungi found their place within his broader interest in "working with [and] thinking about nonhuman life" that grew out of his spiritual psychedelic experience. Although Oscar never refers to foraging as "spiritual," it sits geographically, conceptually, and ethically adjacent to things that are.

Renée, quoted earlier, became interested in mushrooms in college when she learned about mycorrhizal fungi and read *Mycelium Running*. As she said, "It blew my mind, just seeing how everything is connected." She added later, "You asked how I got into the mushroom stuff—it was just that I *fell in love* with mushrooms. I started having dreams about them. It was like a spiritual awakening." When I asked her what that process was like, she said it involved "being out in the woods, and hanging out with mushrooms, and eating mushrooms, and growing mushrooms."

Fred, in his mid-twenties, discovered permaculture in college and became enthralled with the idea of combining sustainable food systems with community building. He referred to himself as "spiritual," which he described as "an understanding that I'm connected to everything. ... That's how I see it. Like, I'm a microorganism living in the earth [the way] there's gut bacteria inside of me." When I asked him if mushrooms played into his spirituality, he mentioned psychedelic mushrooms as "empowering" and told me he had used them to cure himself of a chronic twitch and to quit smoking. Then he added, "and foraging, it's an amazing thing. It's just a really deep connection—I mean that's spirituality to me in a nutshell: it's connection; connection to myself. Connection to community, and to the earth, and obviously, to mushrooms."

For these DIY mycologists, the connectivity of all life is an ecological reality with spiritual, affective, and ethical dimensions. Foraging enacts this connectedness as a kind of purposeful relationality, through attention and attunement to nonhuman life. They access "spirituality" through seemingly mundane activities, like foraging, cultivating, and walking in the woods. In their words, these activities become enchanting and immersive. The revelatory experience of psychedelics is less significant than the profound connectivity of everyday practice in one's engagement with life, human and otherwise.

In fact, they took pains to differentiate their take on fungi from typical psychedelic discourse. For example, Fred expressed skepticism at cultivators that were a little too into "the gospel and the dogma."

> I have known a lot of people that have taken that shit *way* too far. They're like, [dopey voice] "You know, like the mushrooms were like telling me that they don't really like being in plastic..." And it's like, "You know, shut up!" If you observed that they don't do as well in plastic as they do in glass jars, that's one thing, but just because you took a few mushrooms and you're trippin' a little bit...

Sam, a 27-year-old member of the Mycelial Network, dates his interest in mycology to his teenage love of psychedelic mushrooms, but when I asked him if psychedelics influenced his relationship to fungi today, he responded pointedly:

> I'm not guided by psychedelics. It's not like that's my hidden agenda, to get people to start eating psychedelic mushrooms. My agenda is that I want to live in a world that's better, where people have so much more ... you know, respect for themselves and for others and for the planet and for the universe and for the complexity of this fuckin' infinite crazy reality.

As with Oscar, we find an implicit aversion to ritual prescriptions and the imposition of supernatural beliefs (presumably representing the "religion" to their "spirituality" in the sense of "spiritual-not-religious"). To be constrained by "dogma," or merely following "gospel," is to ignore "the complexity of this fuckin' infinite crazy reality"; it's both escapist and pretentious. Empiricism, on the other hand, is both authentic and the doorway to wonder and enchantment in its own right.

Ultimately, it's this commitment to authenticity ("reality") and "respect" that translate into the everyday ethics invested in these practices.

In contrast to common narratives of psychedelic revelation and communion, DIY mycologists construed psychedelics primarily as a form of natural medicine or therapy. Renée's only mention of them is in the reference to "inner and outer" healing. For Ben (quoted at the beginning of this chapter), they are a natural treatment for depression. Fred characterizes them as "empowering." David, the FAB member who told me that they just "confuse the brain," corrected me when I told him I was quoting him in this chapter: "They are good for depression

But not good for divining truth," he told me (quoting my prose back to me). Although David expressed a classically materialist understanding of the natural world, he too had been persuaded by the discourse of psilocybin as a treatment for depression. In short, DIY mycologists have multiple and nuanced understandings of psilocybin-active mushrooms. While the neoshamanic construction circulates, it is treated ambivalently for complicated reasons; in contrast, the practical, therapeutic construction has become more widespread in both spiritual and non-spiritual contexts. What's more, these two constructions—as a means to achieve a spiritual experience on one hand and a means of therapy on the other—are not opposed. Rather, they signal a shift within countercultural ecological discourse.

This shifting discourse reveals the more basic element of power and potentiality that informs both constructions and that DIY mycologists tend to extend to the whole of the fungal kingdom. When I asked Fred specifically if psychedelics motivated his interest in mycology, he said yes, but it was hard to say how, and then he added:

> Understanding that there is such a thing as a psychedelic mushroom is kind of a cornerstone to the unbelievable nature of mushrooms, and fungus, in general. I mean, if you don't know *anything* about them, you at least know that they can kill you or make you trip balls [laughing]. You know?

This recalls Oscar's description of fungi's essential role as "the pallbearers of nature." The ability of fungi to "deal with death" adds another dimension to their mystical character, one that Stamets includes in his more evocative passages of *Mycelium Running*. It also reflects the underlying, and sometimes unnerving, power associated with the organisms, to which Fred alludes: fungi are ecologically critical as the ultimate decomposers,[13] but they can also be deadly in and of themselves, containing some of the most lethal toxins in nature (i.e., amatoxins).

There is gravitas in the fungal kingdom in this proximity to both death and healing. In this sense, fungi epitomize the etymological constellation engendered by the Latin root *potis*, as "power," "potency," and "potential," expressed here as empowerment, capacity, transformation, and resilience. They exemplify what philosopher of science Isabelle Stengers refers to as the *pharmakon*, the thing that can

---

[13]Fungi breakdown the lignin from plants (e.g., in dead trees) and other carbon-based materials, including animal excrement and corpses. This quality of fungal life makes it essential to forest ecosystems. This ability to creatively produce digestive enzymes adapted to the material in their environments is also what makes them promising as remediative organisms.

either kill and heal, depending on the dosage (Stengers, 2015). For DIY mycologists, this ultimate quality of fungi as imperial, cryptic, and magical all at once subsumes the neoshamanic abilities ascribed to some species in the genus *Psilocybe*.

American Biomysticism and the Human–Fungal Alliance

Over the last half century, a love of psychedelic mushrooms has gradually been encompassed by an emergent cross-kingdom relationship between humans and fungi. Historically, psychedelic mushrooms were the gateway to mycological enthusiasm that led to small-scale indoor cultivation and, eventually, imaginative experimental methods that could be understood and implemented by nonexperts. The recuperation of psilocybin by normative medical discourse—in the form of a lab-synthesized compound—as a potential treatment for persistent mood disorders like anxiety and depression can be seen as the most triumphant and visible product of the psychedelic entheogenic movement. But the lineage of underground technical innovations, like the ones recounted here, alongside the broad cultural shifts they were intertwined with, accounts for another, less visible history of the psychoactive *Psilocybe*, one that is more ambivalent, complex, and varied in the practical knowledge and collective fascination it generated. Today, *Psilocybes* occupy just one corner of a broad, multidimensional engagement with the fungal kingdom. From one angle, it looks like domestication; from another, it looks like technological invention. It is this unexpected human–fungal relationship—under-determined, in formation, and invested with potentiality and hope—that is the larger story here.

In the midst of contemporary environmental crisis, our ties—ecological, microbiological, ethical, and spiritual—with other life-forms have come to the fore. Contemporary anthropological discourse reflects this moment with its own turn to multispecies ethnography and post-humanist theorizing. DIY mycology takes on this crisis through attempting to live otherwise with other beings, realizing a biocentric ethics without disavowing science but rather extending a populist, DIY, and open source scientific practice. This builds on the counter modern thread of ecological thought that courses through modern Euro-American history, as expressed in Paul Stamets's work and in related countercultural–ecological practices like permaculture.

In his ethnography of psychedelic researchers, Nicolas Langlitz concludes that, although "natural science and mysticism appear to be antagonistic," in practice, scientific materialism can be compatible with certain kinds of mysticism. He calls this "biomysticism" and explains that "its spiritual focal point is not the extraordinary mental states engendered by hallucinogenic drugs but rather the ordinary existence to which the self-experimenter eventually returns" (Langlitz, 2012, p. 110). DIY mycology typifies a populist, secular biomysticism in which psychedelics are appreciated and revered but are just one of several access points into a casual spirituality of vital connectivity. The singularity of the psychedelic experience is overshadowed by the everyday ethics and practice of how we *live with* other beings. This reality is enriched and propelled by the post-Pasteurian turn and its opening into intersubjective relationality.[14] The rhetoric of alliance is distinguished from the neoshamanic conceit of intuitive communion: Fred's rhetorical rebuke to just "observe" the mushrooms reflects the values of scientific objectivity and empiricism, as well as the arts of noticing that are the essence of successful foraging and cultivation. In this way, the psychedelic experience as a path into an ecologically inspired spirituality is decentered. This history suggests that the link between psychedelics and ecological care is not as natural as it seems, but might just as well be a case of historical propinquity.

References

Belasco, W. (2007). *Appetite for change: How the counterculture took on the food industry*. Ithaca, NY: Cornell University Press.
Binkley, S. (2007). *Getting loose: Lifestyle consumption in the 1970s*. Durham, NC: Duke University Press.
Deus Ex McKenna – Terence McKenna Archive. (2011, July 24). *Terence McKenna – The syntax of psychedelic time – July 1983* [Video file]. Retrieved from https://www.youtube.com/watch?v=I4V-eO_e7Ns
Drug Policy Alliance. (2017). *Psilocybin mushrooms fact sheet*. New York, NY: Drug Policy Alliance.
Fairfax, S. K., Dyble, l. N., Guthey, G. T., Gwin, L., Moore, M., & Sokolove, J. (2012). *California cuisine and just food*. Cambridge, MA: MIT Press.
Feinberg, B. (2003). *The Devil's book of culture: History, mushrooms, and caves in Southern Mexico*. Austin, TX: University of Texas Press.
Ingram, M. (2007). Biology and beyond: The science of "back to nature" farming in the United States. *Annals of the Association of American Geographers, 97*, 298–312.
Jarnow, J. (2016). *Heads: A biography of psychedelic America*. Boston, MA: De Capo Press.
Jarnow, J. (n.d.). Why psychedelic history matters. *Volteface.me*. Retrieved from http://volteface.me/features/psychedelic-history-matters/
Kaiser, D., & McCray, W. P. (2016). *Groovy science: Knowledge, innovation, and American counterculture*. Chicago, IL: University of Chicago Press.
Kelty, C. (2008). *Two bits: The cultural significance of free software*. Durham, NC: Duke University.
Kirk, A. (2007). *Counterculture green: The Whole Earth Catalog and American environmentalism*. Lawrence, KS: University Press of Kansas.
Krebs, T. S., & Johanson, P. (2013) Over 30 million psychedelic users in the United States. *F1000Research, 2*, 98.
Kripal, J. (2007). *Esalen: America and the religion of no religion*. Chicago, IL: University of Chicago Press.
Krippner, S., & Luke, D. (2009). Psychedelics and species connectedness. *MAPS Bulletin Special Issue: Psychedelics and Ecology, 19*(1), 12–15.
Langlitz, N. (2012). *Neuropsychedelia: The revival of hallucinogen research since the decade of the brain*. Berkeley, CA: University of California Press.

[14]See Dev in this volume for a contemporary shamanic perspective on interspecies relationality. Her chapter provides a fruitful juxtaposition to the conditional absorption of modern epistemologies among my North American interlocutors.

Letcher, A. (2007). *Shroom: A cultural history of the magic mushroom*. New York, NY: Harper Perennial.

Letcher, A. (2013). Deceptive cadences: A hermeneutic approach to the problem of meaning and psychedelic experience. In D. Luke & D. King (Eds.), *Breaking convention: Essays on psychedelic consciousness*. Strange Attractor: London, UK.

Markoff, J. (2005). *What the dormouse said: How the sixties counterculture shaped the personal computer industry*. New York, NY: Penguin.

Morris, H. (2013, July). Blood spore: Of murder and mushrooms. *Harper's Magazine*. Retrieved from https://harpers.org/archive/2013/07/blood-spore/

Oss, O. T., & Oeric, O. N. (1976). *Psilocybin: Magic mushroom grower's guide*. Berkeley, CA: And/Or Press.

Paxson, H. (2013). *The life of cheese: Crafting food and value in America*. Berkeley, CA: University of California Press.

Ruck, C. A. P., Bigwood, J., Staples, D., Ott, J., & Wasson, R. G. (1979). Entheogens. *Journal of Psychedelic Drugs, 11*(1–2), 145–146.

Shortall, S. (2014). Psychedelic drugs and the problem of experience. *Past and Present, 222*(Suppl. 9), 187–206.

Stamets, P. (1993). *Growing gourmet and medicinal mushrooms*. New York, NY: Ten Speed Press.

Stamets, P. (1996). *Psilocybin mushrooms of the world: An identification guide*. Berkeley, CA: Ten Speed Press.

Stamets, P. (2005). *Mycelium running: How mushrooms can help save the world*. New York, NY: Ten Speed Press.

Stamets, P. (2008, March). *6 ways mushrooms can save the world* [Video file]. Retrieved from https://www.ted.com/talks/paul_stamets_on_6_ways_mushrooms_can_save_the_world

Stamets, P. (2014, December 1). *Psychoactivity conference – Amsterdam 1999: Psilocybin mushrooms of the world: Powerful allies* [Video file]. Retrieved from https://www.youtube.com/watch?v=A2JzirUelmg

Stengers, I. (2015). *In catastrophic times: Resisting the coming barbarism*. London, UK: Open Humanities Press.

Tsing, A. L. (2015). *The mushroom at the end of the world: On the possibility of life in capitalist ruins*. Princeton, NJ: Princeton University Press.

Turner, F. (2006). *From counterculture to cyberculture: Stewart Brand, the Whole Earth Network, and the rise of digital utopianism*. Chicago, IL: University of Chicago Press.

Worster, D. (1985). *Nature's economy: A history of ecological ideas*. Cambridge, UK: University of Cambridge Press.

Yachaj. (2001). Mushroom cultivation: From falconer to fanaticus and beyond. *The Entheogen Review, 10*(4), 127–139.

Chapter 11
Plant Knowledges: Indigenous Approaches and Interspecies Listening Toward Decolonizing Ayahuasca Research

Laura Dev

Men and women searching for spirituality must plant humility in their hearts.
– Kátia Luiza (Hushahu) Yawanawa, World Ayahuasca Conference (2016)

Abstract The ayahuasca research community is familiar with the concept of plant intelligences; however, they have yet to be adequately accounted for by commonly used research practices. This chapter is a call to examine the ontological and epistemological assumptions that underlie research practices and how these practices and assumptions may reinforce hierarchies of knowledge and animacy. The first part of this chapter describes some absences created by following a "methods as usual" approach when researching ayahuasca, based on ethnographic fieldwork at the World Ayahuasca Conference in 2016 (AYA2016). This highlights the need for researchers to acknowledge the methodological, disciplinary, and identity-based limitations on our abilities to produce and represent certain knowledges. Secondly, this chapter is a call to seriously and humbly engage with Indigenous sciences and epistemologies. This requires an honest reckoning with how research has contributed to colonial appropriation and marginalization of Indigenous knowledges. Indigenous ways of knowing have precedent for collaborating with teacher plants in producing knowledge and have much to contribute to discourse on multispecies perspectives. Lastly, I discuss possibilities for including multispecies sensibilities and Indigenous standpoints in research practices to create more collaborative and decolonial knowledges.

L. Dev (✉)
Department of Environmental Science, Policy, and Management, University of California, Berkeley, CA, USA
e-mail: lauradev@berkeley.edu

© Springer International Publishing AG, part of Springer Nature 2018
B. C. Labate, C. Cavnar (eds.), *Plant Medicines, Healing and Psychedelic Science*,
https://doi.org/10.1007/978-3-319-76720-8_11

185

Introduction

When I first began research in the Ucayali Region of Peru at the beginning of 2015, I intended to study how botanical knowledge was passed down generationally among Shipibo healers. Shipibo healing practices, along with those of several other Indigenous groups, have garnered global attention for their use of ayahuasca. I was under the impression that healers would learn their practices during an apprenticeship period, usually with older family members. However, when I began interviews I was surprised that, though some of them had apprenticed with an elder, when asked who their teachers were and how they learned, most of them began by describing their plant teachers.

Healers learn from plant teachers during quiet periods of deprivation and relative solitude called *dietas* (diets) (as described by, e.g., Jauregui, Clavo, Jovel, and Pardo-de-Santayana (2011)). The dieta is a sensitive time in which the healer develops a relationship with a specific plant spirit that then assists them in learning and healing. Ayahuasca, a strong psychoactive decoction taken ceremonially, is used to open the dieter to the spirit worlds and aid in communicating with and learning from the spirit of the plant they are dieting. Though not all Amazonian peoples use ayahuasca, nor plant diets, many use these practices either together or separately to learn plant knowledges. In many Indigenous histories, the plants used to make ayahuasca, *caapi (Banisteriopsis caapi)* and *chacruna (Psychotria viridis)*, also had some generative role in the making of humans. These stories are told by both people and plants and help to establish an interspecies cosmovision in which both participate.

It was only after I began dieting plants, and cultivating my own direct relationships with teacher plants, that an understanding started to take root in the interspecies connection space between the plants and myself. In this space, I continually realize that plants have their own knowings and produce their own worlds. However, the more I learn how to learn from plants and am exposed to plant worlds, the less I am certain of anything at all. It seems that this form of plant education is more about unknowing than knowing, which presents a puzzling situation when my role as a researcher is ostensibly to produce some knowledge product. This chapter is meant as a compassionate critique for the field of ayahuasca research, to clear some ground for my future self and fellow researchers who may find themselves in a similar sort of existential crisis because of the cognitive dissonance we experience when our own knowings and unknowings do not seem to have a place in the research paradigms we use to produce consumable knowledge.

In this chapter, I first examine the ontological and epistemic assumptions inherent in various knowledge-making practices and discuss how these determine the relationships between knower and known and the types of knowledges produced. Second, I discuss how hegemonic knowledges exclude Indigenous sciences and epistemologies from equal footing in academic matters. I argue the necessity to interrogate our research paradigms and engage seriously with Indigenous epistemologies to avoid complacency in recreating hegemonic knowledges and structural power imbalances. I explore what science and knowledge production might look like if we begin with the premise that other-than-humans can know, act, and produce their own worlds. Finally, I discuss how Indigenous standpoints and multispecies perspectives are important for decolonizing research.

To set up this puzzle, I draw on the second World Ayahuasca Conference (AYA2016, hereafter) that took place in October 2016 in Rio Branco, Brazil, where I documented ways that researchers and other presenters produce knowledge and how they spoke about their relationships with plants. The location and format of the conference itself are evidence of the strides the field of ayahuasca research is taking toward the decolonization of knowledge. Rio Branco, in the state of Acre, is situated centrally to many Indigenous territories and is also the birthplace of the Santo Daime, a Brazilian ayahuasca religion. Indigenous representatives comprised a large portion of the presenters at the conference, though non-Indigenous researchers and practitioners comprised the majority.

Many of the researchers at AYA2016 referenced their own personal relationships with plant spirits or plant beings. However, I observed little academic research that allowed for plant agency or animacy or that accounted for the knowledge that is produced in relationship with these plants. There seems to be a discrepancy between researchers' intersubjective relationships with these plants and the approaches most often used to produce knowledge about them; and I include myself in this critique. Researchers often struggle with their own subjectivities and the subjectivities of their supposed objects of study. This is problematic because, if we limit our knowings to an inanimate and unrelated world, we may lose contact with our own humanity. It is increasingly clear that multispecies assemblages of relations that we are "becoming with" (Haraway, 2008) are precisely what make us human at all. Attending to relations with other species can give us different insights and knowledges than would otherwise be available.

Relating with plants as teachers or healers may be intuitive to some, but to others, the prospect may cause some bodily or intellectual discomfort. Such a perspective clearly challenges some of the naturalized ways that Westerners are accustomed to understanding plants: as inanimate, or at least very low on the animacy hierarchy. Animacy hierarchies constrain and arrange both living and nonliving matter according to some relative ranking of liveliness (Chen, 2012). Disrupting these hierarchies and granting subjectivity to plants may mean unseating oneself from a position of being a privileged knower, and it fundamentally questions human supremacy and Eurocentric hegemonic knowledges. Relating with plants as teachers requires humility, meeting the other subject at one's limits of knowing, and acknowledging that we cannot circumscribe them in our own minds nor with our usual methods.

Absences

Here, I explore what absences are created by leaving out perspectives generated from more intimate, embodied, and personal relationships with plants-as-teachers. I argue that what is at stake is not only who gets to exist in the world, as Donna Haraway (2008) has said, but also whose worlds get to exist, as well as whose knowledges get to count. First, plants are excluded from ontological status as knowing or even animate beings. Second, we limit all that exists to only those things knowable by humans with specific ways of knowing. Lastly, by excluding researchers' personal relationships with plant spirits, we reproduce racialized knowledge hierarchies that continue to place plant spirits in the realm of "Indigenous beliefs" and thereby construct those holding these beliefs as less valid knowers.

Ontological Tensions: Ayahuasca as a Boundary Being

Perhaps at the heart of the challenges posed by ayahuasca to researchers is an ontological tension about the exact nature of ayahuasca. Ayahuasca is ontologically slippery and ambiguous (Tupper & Labate, 2014) and defies simple categorization and objectification for the purposes of study. For context, the variety of themes and discourses that presenters at AYA2016 used to describe ayahuasca are shown in Table 11.1 and range from "creator" or "mother" to a "drug" or "experience." It has varied meanings, names, and stories for different peoples and communities of practice. The uneasiness ayahuasca presents to making clear divisions between being and not-being highlights the need to reconsider who has authority to determine what constitutes life and how these divisions are enforced (Povinelli, 2016).

At this conference, ayahuasca acted similarly to a "boundary object" (Star & Griesemer, 1989) or, as Brian Anderson (2012) suggests, a "boundary experience," for creating shared understandings across different communities of practice. I suggest that viewing ayahuasca as a "boundary being," that is, with its own agency and agenda, is the more appropriate term. Although ayahuasca has different meanings and ontological status for different groups, it serves to connect these disparate communities and creates a "bridge" or "path" (see Table 11.1) for dialogue and translation across social worlds, knowledges, and cultures. Ayahuasca also works to connect plants and humans and facilitates communication and translation across their distinct but partially overlapping worlds (Viveiros de Castro, 2004).

Part of the ontological slipperiness of ayahuasca is that the spirit of ayahuasca, the brew, and the plants used to make ayahuasca are not fully separable. Nor do I believe that it is desirable to construct ayahuasca as coherent or singular, since, as a boundary being, it has meaning and makes meaning in multiple worlds. The ayahuasca experience is well known for challenging Western ontological assumptions, perhaps by providing a new method with which to observe the world(s) (e.g., Tupper & Labate, 2014) and communicate with other-than-human beings. When

Table 11.1 General themes used to speak about ayahuasca by presenters at the second World Ayahuasca Conference, in 2016. Select quotes are shown to demonstrate the variation in language used for each theme. Many quotes were recorded based on live interpretations to English from Portuguese or Spanish

Ontology: What is ayahuasca?	
Commodity	"Ayahuasca is not in the forest, it is in the Internet"; "a source of money"; "it is commercial"; "a big business"
Chemical complex	"A preparation of DMT"; "ayahuasca = harmaline + DMT"; "complex of chemical compounds"
Drug/ Experience	"Short- and long-term effects"; "a drug"; "affects humans"; "a complete sensory experience"; "intoxicating"; "a hazard to human mental health"; "recreational use"; "a hallucinogen"; "a substance that promotes finding oneself"
Story	"Long important story"; "beautiful story"; "very difficult and delicate story"; "prophesy given millions of years ago"
Plant species	"A species in the forest"; "ayahuasca harvested in the wild"; "good to plant the plants"; "medicine that comes from the forest"
Indigenous	"Carries with it the culture of Indigenous people"; "Indigenous heritage"; "traditional medicine"; "science of Indigenous culture"
Sacred	"Sacred"; "sacrament"; "god"; "gift from the gods"; "holy"; "sacred brew"; "our sacred drink"; "holy thing that brings us connection"; "sacred source of strength and knowledge"; "instrument for religion"; "sacred medicine for humanity"
Path/bridge	"Path of light we seek for healing"; "path for dialogues between different kinds of knowledge"; "intercultural bridge"; "open to spirit world"; "with ayahuasca we enter the spiritual world and connect with beings"
Therapy/tool	"Psychotherapeutic tool"; "therapeutic medicine"; "therapy"; "millennial tool"
Medicine/ healing	"The healing of humanity"; "medicine"; "plant medicine"; "medicine for healing"
Entity	"Medicines are alive, not just substances"; "they have spirits"; "it is a living thing"; "she is an entity, an identity"; "has its own agency"; "sentient being in the plant itself"; "plant intelligence"; "all plants have importance and purpose"; "plants are reaching out and awakening us"; "she has freedom"
Teacher	"One of the teachers of the world"; "a book for learning"; "to learn different types of knowledge"; "professor"; "our teacher"; "the greatest master/teacher/ professor"; "learning comes from the plant"
Mother/mother earth	"Mother ayahuasca"; "our mother and teacher"; "mother earth speaking"; "she is simply the earth goddess doing what she needs to do"
Life/creator	"Medicine is life"; "essence of creation"; "*oni* means generator"

researchers develop relationships with ayahuasca, they may be faced with ontological tension around the existence of spirits. As Rachel Harris (2017) describes it, her feeling of tension was exacerbated to the status of an ontological crisis when faced with her interview data showing that 75% of the 81 North Americans she interviewed also reported having a relationship with the spirit of ayahuasca.

An ontological tension (or crisis) can also arise when the ontological understandings of the researcher and the subjects of the study are antagonistic, or conflict with the ontological underpinnings of the research approach itself. In this case, the researcher may be faced with either reevaluating their research paradigm or (re) producing fundamental gaps between their or their informants' actual understanding of the situation and the knowledge they are able to produce. Most often, research produces knowledges that are congruent with what was already assumed to knowably exist (Kuhn, 1962). One's perspective, relationships, and ability to perceive all contribute to our ontological understandings (what we understand to exist) and thereby the worlds we inhabit.

Epistemological Tensions: Ways of Knowing Ayahuasca

Our worlds and our ways of knowing dialectically inform each other. Epistemological assumptions about how we understand the world and communicate knowledge (Crotty, 2003) include theoretical frameworks about what forms of knowledge can be obtained and how we decide what is true and what is false. Ontological understandings and epistemological assumptions together constrain the questions we ask, the methods used, and the interpretation of information. These results in turn influence our understandings of what exists and what we can describe, hence the dialectic, illustrated by the famous quote by the Nobel laureate physicist, Werner Heisenberg (1958), "We have to remember that what we observe is not nature herself, but nature exposed to our method of questioning." In this section, I examine practices and assumptions used to learn about ayahuasca and the types of knowledge that are then able to be produced, with attention to the role of plants in these different approaches to knowledge production. The resulting analysis locates the most common types of research on ayahuasca, based in part on the presentations at AYA2016, with respect to three main epistemological and theoretical frameworks (Table 11.2).

Limitations of Objectivism In the objectivist epistemological framework, there is a fundamental divide between the knower and the known, assuming a singular unified reality exists independently of a knowing subject. Objectivity is one of many potential epistemic virtues (Daston & Galison, 2007) and emphasizes that knowledge should not be influenced by subjective interpretation. A positivist theoretical framework relies on quantification and experimentation to test falsifiable hypotheses. Objectivism and positivism describe the classical approach to science (Gray, 2014) that traditionally excludes nature (and therefore plants) from the social domain. Medical and pharmacological studies (e.g., de Araujo et al., 2012; Riba et al., 2003) generally rely on positivism as an approach that generates high predictability and control. Many ethnobotanical studies also use positivist-based methods, such as creating quantifiable indices of cultural importance, though these are sometimes combined with interpretivist and ethnographic methods (e.g., Tudela-Talavera, La Torre-Cuadros, & Native Community of Vencedor, 2016).

However, science studies scholars have long critiqued objectivity, pointing out that all knowledges are socially situated, and therefore only partial (Haraway, 1991),

Table 11.2 A simplified representation of common epistemological and methodological frameworks used to understand ayahuasca; this table does not encompass all possible approaches. This categorization scheme is not meant to reinforce divisions among disciplines and theoretical frameworks but is still useful for organizing purposes

Epistemologies: How to know ayahuasca?		
Theoretical framework	Types of studies	Approach to knowing ayahuasca
1. Objectivist epistemology: **meaningful reality exists outside of the knowing subject**		
Positivism: Looks for causal relationships through hypothesis testing. Assumes that valid data should be objective, reproducible, and measurable. A deductive and empirical approach 1.	*Ecological and botanical*	Measure plant behaviors, interactions, responses, or physical/chemical properties
	Biomedical, pharmacological, psychological	Measure physical or behavioral responses in humans consuming ayahuasca or its constituents
2. Subjectivist epistemology: **meaning is derived from subjective experiences**		
Positivism: Looks for causal effects and tests hypotheses. Often relies on indices to produce quantifiable data	*Psychotherapeutic and psychological*	Measure psychological effects of consuming ayahuasca on human participants
Interpretivism: Seeks to understand and interpret others' experiences. Focuses on subjective meaning and details		Describe how human participants interpret their experiences with ayahuasca
Relationalism: Understanding is achieved intersubjectively or dialogically between researcher and participant		Understand through interactive dialogue about participants' experiences
3. Constructionist epistemology: **meaning is constructed interactively through social practices**		
Positivism: Assumes that valid data should be objective, reproducible, and measurable	*Ethnobotanical*	Evaluate traditional botanical knowledge and uses for validity and convergence
Interpretivism: Seeks to understand others' ways of making meaning. Focuses on social phenomena and cultural meanings	*Ethnobotanical and Ethnographic*	Describe cultural knowledges, beliefs, practices, and governance around the use of ayahuasca
Relationalism: Understanding is achieved intersubjectively. Centered on relationship building	*Ethnographic*	Attend to intersubjective relationships as a way of understanding the other
	Participatory research	Dialogue with community. Build cross-cultural understanding
4. Indigenous epistemologies: **heterogeneous and self-defined ways of making meaning**		
Relationalism: Understanding is achieved relationally	*Shamanic and animistic*	Engage and communicate directly with plants and/or spirits

and arise out of political and social practices (Latour, 1988). Indeed, according to Sandra Harding (1992), sciences that claim universality and neutrality will produce more distorted knowledges compared to sciences that contextualize their historical and positional standpoints. Despite these critiques, positivist frameworks emphasizing neutrality are still often privileged in academia by funders, publishers, employers, and institutions. The objectivist epistemology, however, is not able to account for the subjectivity of its objects of study and therefore is not designed to produce knowledge about plant subjectivities nor human subjective experiences. Nonetheless, objectivist approaches in botany have been used to show how plants communicate through chemical signaling and thereby establish plant agency. As Dennis McKenna said at AYA2016, the existence of plant intelligences is "not that controversial anymore."

Limitations of Subjectivism A subjectivist epistemology focuses on how individuals make meaning and locates meaningful reality in the subjective experience. For this reason, subjectivism is the most common epistemology used in psychological and psychotherapeutic studies, such as Benny Shanon's (2002) work, *The Antipodes of the Mind*, which seeks to describe and categorize the range of experiences of those who take ayahuasca. According to Shanon, "What is special about Ayahuasca is the extraordinary subjective experiences this brew generates in the mind" (p. 31). Though Shanon describes several types of supernatural beings, the ontological questions that arise from these encounters, he admits, are beyond the scope of the subjectivist epistemology.

Subjectivist studies sometimes reproduce positivist methodologies, for example, by using experimental designs with control groups and converting qualitative data into quantifiable indices (e.g., Barbosa, Cazorla, Giglio, & Strassman, 2009). Positivist frameworks are often uncritically accepted as disciplinary standards in psychology (Breen & Darlaston-Jones, 2008). However, studies using interpretive or relational frameworks that seek more descriptive and qualitative accounts are also prevalent and are sometimes also combined with positivist approaches.

Limitations of Constructionism Presently, I am using a constructionist epistemology, in which meaning is constructed out of practices. This goes along with the ontological understanding that there is no singular objective reality and no one can be truly objective. Therefore, knowledge is understood to be the result of current convention (Roosth & Silbey, 2008). This allows one to use an interpretivist framework to examine the conditions that give rise to differing knowledge claims and to treat knowledge claims equally, whether regarded as true or false. I locate ethnographic studies somewhere between an interpretivist approach, in which the ethnographer seeks to describe the meanings made by their informants, and a relationalist approach, in which meaning is co-constructed between both the ethnographer and the informants (Table 11.2).

Ethnographic studies do have room to view plant teachers and spirits as ontologically valid, as they are seeking to describe the worlds of their informants (e.g., Brabec de Mori, 2012), but they are often interpreted as mere cultural constructs. There is traditionally little ethnographic engagement directly with other-than-human beings, particularly the immaterial kind. Instead, they are described secondhand, through other people who do engage with these beings (Fotiou, 2010).

Researchers *can* engage directly with plant beings and spirits by using autoethnographic methods to analyze their own experiences with respect to the research context (Ellis, Adams, & Bochner, 2010). For example, ethnobotanists like Terence McKenna (1993) and Wade Davis (1996), among others, use autoethnographic writing to tell the stories of their relationships with plants. However, these techniques are not always successful at accounting for plant agency, and there is the danger that including personal stories can come across as gratuitous or sensationalized. More experimental writing practices, as part of the self-reflexive process, can also be used to reflect on social relationships with other-than-human beings and spiritual encounters (e.g., Fotiou, 2010; Harris, 2017). Richard Doyle (2012) uses such methods to recount his experiences with plant intelligences and healing:

> I share my own experience as an invitation to experiment with post normal contemplative science not because I know it to be true—its truth would be the outcome of the process that sorts through my account as well as others like it—but because of an unavoidable perception of its efficacy.. ... I make no claims for the universality of my experience and insist, rather, on its particularity. (Doyle, 2012, p. 31)

Using participant observation as a method—for example, consuming ayahuasca and participating in rituals—is not, by itself, an autoethnographic method for understanding ayahuasca, unless the researcher explicitly includes their own experiences as part of their analysis. Likewise, autoethnography goes beyond the sharing of personal anecdotes and asides, which are perceived as extraneous to knowledge making, and not included in published studies. However, these sharings are important. In the absence of disclosure of the researcher's own process encountering (or not encountering) spirits and plant beings, ethnographic description often relegates these spirits and plant beings to the realm of supernatural Indigenous beliefs. This constructs a philosophical divide between the researcher and the Indigenous "other" that then serves to justify the proposal that researchers, as privileged knowers, may study, categorize, and represent the other (Stengers, 2011), thus reproducing hierarchies of knowledge and knowing.

Moving Beyond Research as Usual

As I have illustrated, the most common research approaches used to produce knowledge about ayahuasca have limited engagement with plant intelligences, if plants are granted any agency, animacy, or intelligence at all. Therefore, knowledge about plants is often limited to what is physically measurable or what is learned in interpretivist studies of (mostly) secondhand accounts of human experiences with plants. These knowledges are perfectly valuable for certain research objectives but do not approach the knowledge or worlds that are produced by plants directly.

Further, when unexamined, certain approaches can reproduce problematic knowledge hierarchies.

At AYA2016, I found that less established researchers, particularly in fields with objectivist approaches, were less likely to mention plants as beings at all. It may be that their ontological paradigms do not incorporate plant beings, or perhaps it can be perceived as professionally risky to deviate from norms of discipline or mention plant spirits or plant agency, unless speaking about someone else's beliefs. Because of the marginalized nature of psychedelic research in general, and the contested legitimacy of the topic of research, ayahuasca researchers in certain fields may be less likely to deviate from methodological norms toward more epistemically vulnerable approaches.

However, nearly across the board, researchers agreed that it is not enough to see these plants as simply their chemical components. At the conference, plants were widely recognized by researchers as having their own agency and knowledges and as being intertwined with Indigenous traditions. Yet, there are few precedents for cross-cultural, interspecies, intercosmic collaboration in producing knowledge and little framework for engaging with plant agencies or plant worlds. Even researchers, like myself, who call for something different and reference the inspirited nature of these plants, are still mired in disciplinary methods that reproduce old paradigms and old hierarchies.

Challenging Scientism: Indigenous and Interspecies Approaches

Here, I explore how both interspecies and Indigenous perspectives are marginalized and how attending to these perspectives can move us toward decolonizing knowledge production. Indigenous sciences and epistemologies have crucial insight to contribute to multispecies scholarship (TallBear, 2011), and interspecies relating can contribute to how we understand ayahuasca and plant knowledges in general. As a White, North American, non-Indigenous researcher myself, I feel it is important to reconnect myself within a web of interspecies relating while still reckoning with how my use of Indigenous methods, and working in Indigenous communities at all, can be done in culturally appropriate and morally engaged ways. It brings up important and difficult questions about whether and how non-Indigenous researchers can engage with Indigenous ways of knowing in ways that do not further colonize them by their inclusion in the academy.

Scientism and the Great Divide

Scientism is the belief that science is better than all other ways of knowing and that "reality" or "truth" is limited to what is verifiable by that one way of knowing. This epistemic supremacy becomes hegemonic when it is naturalized and uncritically accepted even by those whose knowledges it subjugates. Colonial power relations contributed to creating a hegemony out of Eurocentric knowledge systems, based in the mechanistic, positivist science that has marginalized other knowledges and worlds for the last two centuries or so (Escobar, 2007; Mignolo, 2000). In *The Death of Nature*, Carolyn Merchant (1980) describes how the rise of the mechanistic worldview in Europe served to essentially exorcize the knowable, natural world of any life or intelligence beyond the human. Mechanistic science defined nature as its object of inquiry and thereby categorized any phenomena not answerable to scientific questioning, such as spirits and plant beings, as supernatural (outside of nature).

Defining science as beyond the influence of the social or political domains also created what Bruno Latour (2012) calls the "great divide," in which human culture was constructed as fundamentally separate from nonhuman nature (the realm of science), thereby excluding nonhumans from social and political spheres. This created an ontological tension for humans whose worlds included social relations with other-than-humans. These "animists" were constructed as premodern others who could then also be objectified for the purpose of scientific inquiry (Povinelli, 2016; Stengers, 2011). Therefore, separation between humans and nonhumans, which gave rise to human exceptionalism, shares its epistemic roots with the division that subjugated Indigenous knowledges and excluded Indigenous peoples from participation in politics and science (de la Cadena, 2010).

Indigenous knowledges are important for critically interrogating hegemonic knowledge systems (Dei, 2000). Approaching ayahuasca research from both Indigenous perspectives and plant perspectives can provide an orientation for revealing our human-centric and scientistic assumptions that are otherwise made invisible. Through interspecies thinking that privileges Indigenous epistemologies, there is an opportunity to restore the animacy and worldmaking activities of other-than-humans, elevate Indigenous ways of knowing these other-than-humans, and thereby disrupt hegemonic knowledges.

Indigenous Approaches to Knowing and Epistemic Injustice

It is not necessary to explain everything about our knowledge. That can be our own internal knowledge. There are many names for the plant—it is a multicultural matter. Each Indigenous people has their own names and stories. Researchers sometimes generalize all of this diverse knowledge.

– Joaquin Mana (Huni Kuin), World Ayahuasca Conference (2016)

Indigenous sciences are quite heterogeneous; yet perhaps their greatest commonality, and what really allows them to be grouped together in this way, is their exclusion from mainstream knowledge systems and denial of validity based on their identity or practices. This is what Miranda Fricker (2007) calls "epistemic injustice." Indigenous knowledges are expected to be "authentic," often defined by a distance from Western science and worldviews, but are then studied and verified using scientific frameworks. This is highlighted by the somewhat sarcastic quote from Benki Piyako, an Asháninka presenter at AYA2016: "Perhaps through science we will say once and for all whether ayahuasca is sacred or is intoxicating." Power imbalances between researchers and Indigenous communities are reinscribed when one form of knowledge is used to validate another.

Shamanic approaches use certain ways of relating with other-than-human beings, including communicating with plant beings and spirits. Knowledge comes from collaborative, intimate interactions and dialogue with plants as teachers that often arise in intuitions, dreams, and visions. For Shipibo healers, singing, dieting, and consuming ayahuasca are methods for accessing or channeling the knowledge and songs of a plant spirit (Brabec de Mori, 2012). They are then able to use these plant knowledges for healing or other purposes. Note that learning plant knowledges is importantly distinct from learning *about* plants.

Indigenous approaches to knowing can engage with other-than-human subjects more directly than the usual research approaches I discussed earlier. Shipibo healers, for instance, have a long precedence for producing knowledge in collaboration with plants. However, the engagement between Indigenous ways of knowing and non-Indigenous researchers has a record of unequal power relations, exclusion, and appropriation. Indigenous knowledges have historically been denied legitimacy, and Indigenous people have been denied status as valid knowers.

Working With(in) Indigenous Worldviews

How can non-Indigenous researchers engage Indigenous ways of knowing in a manner that is not furthering the colonial project of cultural appropriation nor ignoring or excluding these ways of knowing from what are considered valid knowledge-making practices? I turn to theories and methods developed by Indigenous researchers and scholars who explore what it means to work within Indigenous worldviews to produce knowledge as academic researchers. These perspectives are invaluable to the conversation on the decolonization and democratization of knowledge, as current research conventions are still not ontologically and epistemologically appropriate to accommodate Indigenous worldviews (Botha, 2011). Instead, Indigenous scholarship and knowledge are often subsumed into Western worldviews. We need embodied insights on how to bring together different knowledges and knowledge communities without subsuming one into the other but allowing them to be sovereign, collaborative, and non-hierarchically organized. Anishinaabe scholar Sonya Atalay (2012) offers us the concept of "braiding knowledge" (p. 207) to create better and more complete kinds of science that are more inclusive and multifaceted.

Centering Indigenous ontologies and epistemologies allows for the transformation of research practices and can work toward filling gaps in dominant discourses while also opening up entirely new spaces for inquiry. Martin and Mirraboopa (2003) emphasize that learning and abiding by Indigenous methods for knowing and relating are paramount to conducting culturally respectful research. Within their framework, ways of knowing inform ways of being or relating, including relating with other-than-humans. For TallBear (2014), relationship building also becomes the primary research approach and works toward "softening" the divisions between knower and known that are so problematic in Western research.

Participatory research (e.g., Fals-Borda, 1982; Fortmann, 2008) encompasses several process-oriented relational approaches (e.g., community-based participatory research, learning communities, participatory action research) that rely on dialogue and co-learning between the researcher and the community. With these approaches, community members are active partners in the research, from setting research goals to interpretation, and the knowledge produced is often meant to be put into practice, rather than to be described (Davidson-Hunt & O'Flaherty, 2007). Though not without limitations and potential pitfalls, these approaches are becoming recommended practice for any type of research done in Indigenous communities, as a step toward decolonizing the research process (e.g., National Congress of American Indians Policy Research Center [NCAI] & Montana State University Center for Native Health Partnerships [MSU], 2012). Relational frameworks also morally engage researchers to privilege the lives and futures of the community by allying themselves with Indigenous struggles.

Although I am not aware of much community-based participatory ayahuasca research in partnership with Indigenous communities, several researchers at AYA2016 encouraged these approaches, prioritizing intercultural dialogue over predetermined research goals. Beatriz Labate, an anthropologist who was one of the organizers of AYA2016, and was also the organizer of the Plant Medicine Track at the Psychedelic Science Conference in 2017 (from which this book originated), has been an important player in bringing more diverse voices and perspectives to the table, particularly those from Indigenous practitioners and researchers, as well as from women. Her work has also foregrounded dialogue about cultural considerations with the expansion of the use of ayahuasca (e.g., Labate, 2017; Labate & Cavnar, 2011). The strength and presence of the Indigenous panels at AYA2016 indicate that the field is moving toward including multiple knowledges and ways of knowing, though inequalities are still apparent. These are nonetheless important steps, as leaving absences around the existence of multiple knowledges, even when contested, implies complicity in creating marginalization (Dei, 2000). The next steps are to work out ways to produce knowledges more collectively and collaboratively, led by and in alliance with Indigenous interests.

Incorporating Multispecies Approaches

Despite the challenges of engaging with plant intelligences, it takes only a small amount of ecological knowledge to demonstrate that plants *are* agents and *do* make their own meanings of the world. Plants desire, seek nourishment, and have their own forms of language (Marder, 2013). Perhaps because plants rely on other species for reproduction—the birds and the bees so to speak—and on fungi for nutrient acquisition, plant communication is especially interspecies. Plants communicate with and respond to their environments by creating new chemical expressions. For example, when plants are exposed to grazing or insect predation, they may respond by producing different secondary compounds like tannins (phytophenols), which defend against herbivory (Bryant et al., 1991), or odors that act as signals that are interpreted by insects (Landolt & Phillips, 1997) or other plants (Dicke & Bruin, 2001).

These same secondary compounds are responsible for the toxic, medicinal, and psychoactive effects of plant medicines (Callicott, 2013). Ayahuasca's constituent plants, *B. caapi* and *P. viridis*, for instance, produce molecules that act on animal neuroreceptors. These compounds allow humans to relate with them in direct and embodied ways and are responsible for much of the "psychedelic" experience. Christina Callicott (2013) even theorizes *icaros* (songs associated with ayahuasca) as skillful sonic interpretations of plant phytochemical semiotics (signaling). Richard Doyle (2012) also uses the concept of phytosemiotics as a way of understanding plant intelligence and communication. However, neuroactive chemicals are not necessarily the only way by which humans exchange information with plants when drinking ayahuasca, and I caution against reductionist approaches to plant spirits and trans-species communication with plants.

By centering Indigenous ontologies and epistemologies, we can explore how our research methods change when plant intelligence and animacy are considered a priori knowledge that does not need to be proven, contested, or even understood. To take plant agencies and plant spirits seriously, as I think this conversation demands, again, requires humility, acknowledging that we cannot know these plant beings completely and that part of the other exists beyond knowability. Whether we are using science or other knowledge-making practices, we can only view a facet of an animate other's existence. This acknowledgment alone piques curiosity, invites relating, and grants agency to the other being. What will it reveal to our methods of questioning? How does it wish to be known? How does it know?

This also challenges the usual research frameworks. How can one account for the subjectivity of the supposed object of study, when one is supposed to be the knower, and the other the known, and when the two do not speak the same language? For decades, anthropologists and ethnographers have been working through the role of their research practices in constructing otherness and marginalizing the subjectivities of those whom they seek to study. Multispecies approaches to knowing challenge researchers to extend questions of agency, subjectivity, and relationality to other-than-human beings.

Multispecies studies describe how other-than-human beings participate in social, economic, ecological, and political activities (Kirksey & Helmreich, 2010) and recognize the animacy and worldmaking capabilities of other-than-humans. Eduardo Kohn (2013), for example, uses principles of semiotics to demonstrate how animals, like dogs, monkeys, and walking-stick insects, make and interpret their own significations. He also demonstrates compellingly, through thinking with Indigenous worldviews, how even animal masters—spirit beings who live in the forest and are responsible for certain animals—create signs interpretable by humans and therefore have their own ontological existence. Scholars, including Anna Tsing (2015) and Robin Wall Kimmerer (2015), use economic and ecological narratives to describe interspecies relationships and the entanglements of livelihoods among fungi, plants, and humans. Kimmerer, a Native American (Potawatomi) plant ecologist, reframes ecological experiments as a way of posing questions to plants and listening for their answers. Kimmerer's approach has helped me to recognize that objectification is not always a requisite for scientific inquiry.

One of the reasons why Kim TallBear (2011) argues that interspecies perspectives need Indigenous standpoints is that multispecies ethnographies tend to limit themselves in the types of relations they consider—generally, to material, organismal beings. Indigenous ontologies can extend the web of relationality to both material, non-organismal beings (e.g., rocks, mountains, stars) and immaterial or spirit beings. For example, Karen Martin's aboriginal research framework includes relating with other-than-human entities:

> Methods such as storying and exchanging talk are most often used amongst People but methods for interacting with other Entities (e.g. Animals, Weather, Skies) are equally necessary. This requires fieldwork that immerses the researcher in the contexts of the Entities and to watch, listen, wait, learn and repeat these processes as methods for data collection. (Martin & Mirraboopa, 2003, p. 213)

The process described here is similar to the animist methodological approach outlined by Barrett (2011), which also stresses the importance of embodied, "porous," sensual, multispecies listening. This requires a certain intimacy with other-than-human beings, as a site for the social production of knowledge, and reworking of boundaries (Raffles, 2002). Intimacy is non-hierarchical and emphasizes the importance of specificity of the encounter, of time and space and bodies. However, intimacy has often been portrayed as local and contextual and as lacking the mobility and universality of more quantitative ways of knowing.

Working toward research that engages the many ways that psychoactive plants relate with humans—as teachers, healers, and kin—in addition to their well-worn role as objects of study, can provide different and productive valences to the encounters between plants and researchers. As of now, there are few examples of this type of work, and it is even difficult to imagine research that truly engages with agencies of plants or other species in general. However, my view is that this is a worthwhile aim, even if (and perhaps especially because) we cannot quite see ahead to what it will eventually look like to have a true multispecies collaboration. In the unknown mystery of the encounter lies the creative and transformative potential.

Decolonizing Ayahuasca Research

Unsettling animacy and knowledge hierarchies requires radical decolonization of the ways that we understand the world. Decolonization of research requires drawing explicit connections between power and knowledge relations to address the under-lying roots of these asymmetries (Agrawal, 1995) and critically interrogating research practices and intellectual property. According to Restrepo and Escobar (2005), decolonization of knowledge needs to occur at multiple layers of power relations: epistemic transformation aimed at making other knowledges and worlds visible; social and political transformation, which locates the role of the academy in global colonial power relations; and institutional transformation, which seeks to decolonize expertise by moving through or past borders of discipline and academy.

It is important for all researchers to think through the norms and practices that unevenly determine what knowledges are produced and circulated and how these contribute to reproducing hegemonic knowledges. Ayahuasca research, because of the ontological tensions generated by relating with plants, and its inherent cross-cultural engagements, is a fertile ground for decolonizing work, and the colonial relations around the use of ayahuasca in general require deep examination. I suggest that, through foregrounding Indigenous standpoints and inviting interspecies relat-ing, researchers can make steps toward decolonizing their knowledge-making prac-tices. However, there is danger that adopting Indigenous practices may further a sense of colonial entitlement or fuel settler adoption fantasies (Tuck & Yang, 2012), so I advise continual self-reflection and deep inquiry into the literature on decoloni-zation that I only touch on superficially here.

I would like to follow Shawn Wilson's (2008) reframing of research as a type of academic ritual or ceremony that also involves intercultural and interspecies com-munication. Research, like ritual, is a repeatable and mimetic process, whose structure is taught to initiates. Viewing academic practices as rituals can be useful in situating them in their own cultural context, rather than universalizing them. It is important to understand the rituals we are performing, and to enact them consciously and delicately, in a way that allows for exposure of the hierarchies and social structures that we may reproduce. This includes the relationship between researcher and researched as subject and object relationship. I suggest that, by performing ayahuasca research as a ritual boundary engagement with Indigenous ontologies and epistemologies, and with plant worlds and knowledges, there is a potential for beginning an emancipatory move from a research system that is linked to a long and violent history of colonialism. By focusing on creating direct engagement with plant beings as part of our research endeavors, we also bring ourselves into relation-ship in a felt way within a multispecies ecology of other selves (Kohn, 2013) that have been denied subjectivity since the beginning of the scientific project.

Conclusion

I have argued that research-as-usual creates absences that exclude plant knowledges and marginalize Indigenous ways of knowing. Privileging Indigenous sciences and multispecies perspectives creates the potential for intercultural and interspecies collaboration. To make baby steps toward decolonizing ayahuasca research, it is important to examine how research practices contribute to hierarchies of knowing. This chapter introduces plant intelligences and ayahuasca research into an ongoing conversation that links multispecies perspectives with decolonization of knowledge, but is really only a point of departure for this important topic.

I find myself at the crossroads of the challenges I have highlighted: to write this chapter in a way that does not reproduce hierarchical knowledge systems, while still seeking ground in the academy. I try to honor the knowledges and ways of knowing that I have been learning from my teachers, both humans and plants, while also translating these knowledges into academic dialogues. However, I feel I have inadequately portrayed the wonder, beauty, and enchantment of the worlds and knowledges to which I point, and I recognize the danger that my writing will further colonize and objectify the very ones I seek to honor.

While writing this chapter, I had the opportunity during an ayahuasca ceremony to propose some of the ideas I have written about here to some of the plant beings with whom I have been developing relationships. However, I realized in the moment of the asking, that I should have begun this dialogue long ago, or perhaps it was simply part of the same conversation we have been having all along. Nonetheless, what I gathered is that these ideas excite them. When I then queried that place where I meet the plant worlds, what collaboration in making knowledge would look like for them, the answer I clearly perceived, after only a moment, was "we build life." This of course cannot be denied and, again, made me feel very small and humble at how little I actually know about the ways and motivations of these plant beings, how insignificant my question seemed in comparison with their great works.

Despite human limitations to understanding, it is critical to learn to consult with and listen to intelligences beyond the human. Interspecies collaboration is going to be necessary as human futures become increasingly linked to those of other species (not that they ever were separate). I call ayahuasca a boundary being because of its ability to facilitate listening and dialogue across species and worlds. To be in proper reciprocity, one cannot use this being for human spiritual needs while ignoring the spirit of ayahuasca itself. Attending to plant beings, in my own experience, means loosening my grasp on what constitutes knowledge, sensitizing myself to interspecies listening, and resituating myself in relationship with plants-as-knowers.

References

Agrawal, A. (1995). Dismantling the divide between indigenous and scientific knowledge. *Development and Change, 26*(3), 413–439.

Anderson, B. T. (2012). Ayahuasca as antidepressant? Psychedelics and styles of reasoning in psychiatry. *Anthropology of Consciousness, 23*(1), 44–59.

Atalay, S. (2012). *Community-based archaeology.* Berkeley, CA: University of California Press.

Barbosa, P. C. R., Cazorla, I. M., Giglio, J. S., & Strassman, R. (2009). A six-month prospective evaluation of personality traits, psychiatric symptoms and quality of life in ayahuasca-naïve subjects. *Journal of Psychoactive Drugs, 41*(3), 205–212.

Barrett, M. J. (2011). Doing animist research in academia: A methodological framework. *Canadian Journal of Environmental Education, 16,* 123–141.

Botha, L. (2011). Mixing methods as a process towards indigenous methodologies. *International Journal of Social Research Methodology, 14*(4), 313–325.

Brabec de Mori, B. (2012). About magical singing, sonic perspectives, ambient multinatures, and the conscious experience. *Indiana, 29,* 73–101.

Breen, L., & Darlaston-Jones, D. (2008). Moving beyond the enduring dominance of positivism in psychological research: An Australian perspective. *Presented at the 43rd Australian Psychological Society annual conference,* Hobart, Tasmania.

Bryant, J. P., Provenza, F. D., Pastor, J., Reichardt, P. B., Clausen, T. P., & du Toit, J. T. (1991). Interactions between woody plants and browsing mammals mediated by secondary metabolites. *Annual Review of Ecology and Systematics, 22*(1), 431–446.

Callicott, C. (2013). Interspecies communication in the Western Amazon: Music as a form of conversation between plants and people. *European Journal of Ecospsychology, 4,* 32–43.

Chen, M. Y. (2012). *Animacies: Biopoltics, racial mattering, and queer affect.* Durham NC: Duke University Press.

Crotty, M. (2003). *The foundations of social research: Meaning and perspectives in the research process.* London: Sage.

Daston, L., & Galison, P. (2007). *Objectivity.* Cambridge, MA: MIT Press.

Davidson-Hunt, I. J., & O'Flaherty, R. M. (2007). Researchers, indigenous peoples, and place-based learning communities. *Society & Natural Resources, 20*(4), 291–305.

Davis, W. (1996). *One river: Explorations and discoveries in the Amazon Rainforest.* New York, NY: Simon & Schuster.

de Araujo, D. B., Ribeiro, S., Cecchi, G. A., Carvalho, F. M., Sanchez, T. A., Pinto, J. P., . . . Santos, A. C. (2012). Seeing with the eyes shut: Neural basis of enhanced imagery following ayahuasca ingestion. *Human Brain Mapping, 33*(11), 2550–2560.

de la Cadena, M. (2010). Indigenous cosmopolitics in the Andes: Conceptual reflections beyond "politics". *Cultural Anthropology, 25*(2), 334–370.

Dei, G. J. S. (2000). Rethinking the role of Indigenous knowledges in the academy. *International Journal of Inclusive Education, 4*(2), 111–132.

Dicke, M., & Bruin, J. (2001). Chemical information transfer between plants: Back to the future. *Biochemical Systematics and Ecology, 29*(10), 981–994.

Doyle, R. (2012). Healing with plant intelligence: A report from ayahuasca. *Anthropology of Consciousness, 23*(1), 28–43.

Ellis, C., Adams, T. E., & Bochner, A. P. (2010). Autoethnography: An overview. *Forum Qualitative Sozialforschung/Forum: Qualitative Social Research, 12*(1.) Art 10. Retrieved from http://nbn-resolving.de/urn:nbn:de:0114-fqs1101108

Escobar, A. (2007). Worlds and knowledges otherwise: The Latin American modernity/coloniality research program. *Cultural Studies, 21*(2–3), 179–210.

Fals-Borda, O. (1982). Participatory research and rural social change. *Journal of Rural Cooperation, 10*(1), 25–40.

Fortmann, L. (Ed.). (2008). *Participatory research in conservation and rural livelihoods: Doing science together.* Oxford, UK: Blackwell.

Fotiou, E. (2010). Encounters with sorcery: An ethnographer's account. *Anthropology and Humanism, 35*(2), 192–203.

Fricker, M. (2007). *Epistemic injustice: Power and the ethics of knowing.* Oxford, UK: Oxford University Press.

Gray, D. E. (2014). *Doing research in the real world.* Los Angeles, CA: Sage.

Haraway, D. J. (1991). *Simians, cyborgs, and women: The reinvention of nature.* New York, NY: Routledge.

Haraway, D. (2008). *When species meet, Posthumanities* (Vol. 3). Minneapolis, MN: University of Minnesota Press.

Harding, S. (1992). Rethinking standpoint epistemology: What is "strong objectivity?". *The Centennial Review, 36*(3), 437–470.

Harris, R. (2017). *Listening to ayahuasca: New hope for depression, addiction, PTSD, and anxiety.* Novato, CA: New World Library.

Heisenberg, W. (1958). *Physics and philosophy: The revolution in modern science.* Lectures delivered at University of St. Andrews, Scotland, Winter 1955–56. New York, NY: Harper and Row.

Jauregui, X., Clavo, Z. M., Jovel, E. M., & Pardo-de-Santayana, M. (2011). "Plantas con madre": Plants that teach and guide in the shamanic initiation process in the East-Central Peruvian Amazon. *Journal of Ethnopharmacology, 134*(3), 739–752.

Kimmerer, R. W. (2015). *Braiding sweetgrass: Indigenous wisdom, scientific knowledge and the teachings of plants.* Minneapolis, MN: Milkweed Editions.

Kirksey, S. E., & Helmreich, S. (2010). The emergence of multispecies ethnography. *Cultural Anthropology, 25*(4), 545–576.

Kohn, E. (2013). *How forests think.* Berkeley, CA: University of California Press.

Kuhn, T. (1962). *The structure of scientific revolutions* (Vol. 1). Chicago, IL: University of Chicago Press.

Labate, B. C. (2017). MAPS – Community forums at psychedelic science 2017: A vibrant dialogue between scientists and practitioners. *MAPS Bulletin, 27*(1–Special ed.: Psychedelic Science). Retrieved from http://www.maps.org/news/bulletin/articles/420-bulletin-spring-2017/6614-community-forums-at-psychedelic-science-2017-a-vibrant-dialogue-between-scientists-and-practitioners

Labate, B. C., & Cavnar, C. (2011). The expansion of the field of research on ayahuasca: Some reflections about the ayahuasca track at the 2010 MAPS "Psychedelic Science in the 21st Century" conference. *International Journal of Drug Policy, 22*(2), 174–178.

Landolt, P. J., & Phillips, T. W. (1997). Host plant influences on sex pheromone behavior of phytophagous insects. *Annual Review of Entomology, 42*(1), 371–391.

Latour, B. (1988). *Science in action: How to follow scientists and engineers through society.* Cambridge, MA: Harvard University Press.

Latour, B. (2012). *We have never been modern.* Cambridge, MA: Harvard University Press.

Marder, M. (2013). *Plant-thinking: A philosophy of vegetal life.* New York, NY: Columbia University Press.

Martin, K., & Mirraboopa, B. (2003). Ways of knowing, being and doing: A theoretical framework and methods for indigenous and indigenist re-search. *Journal of Australian Studies, 27*(76), 203–214.

McKenna, T. (1993). *Food of the gods: The search for the original tree of knowledge a radical history of plants, drugs, and human evolution.* New York, NY: Bantam.

Merchant, C. (1980). *The Death of nature: Women, ecology and the scientific revolution.* San Francisco, CA: Harper.

Mignolo, W. (2000). *Local histories/global designs: Coloniality, subaltern knowledges, and border thinking.* Princeton, NJ: Princeton University Press.

National Congress of American Indians Policy Research Center and Montana State University's Center for Native Health Partnerships. (2012). *"Walk softly and listen carefully": Building research relationships with tribal communities.* Bozeman, MT: Authors. Retrieved from http://www.ncai.org/policy-research-center/initiatives/research-regulation

Povinelli, E. A. (2016). *Geontologies: A requiem to late liberalism.* Durham, NC: Duke University Press.

Raffles, H. (2002). Intimate knowledge. *International Social Science Journal, 54*(173), 325–335.

Restrepo, E., & Escobar, A. (2005). "Other anthropologies and anthropology otherwise": Steps to a world anthropologies framework. *Critique of Anthropology, 25*(2), 99–129.

Riba, J., Valle, M., Urbano, G., Yritia, M., Morte, A., & Barbanoj, M. J. (2003). Human pharmacology of ayahuasca: Subjective and cardiovascular effects, monoamine metabolite excretion, and pharmacokinetics. *Journal of Pharmacology and Experimental Therapeutics, 306*(1), 73–83.

Roosth, S., & Silbey, S. (2008). Science and technology studies: From controversies to posthumanist social theory. In B. S. Turner (Ed.), *Blackwell companion to social theory.* Chichester: Blackwell.

Shanon, B. (2002). *The antipodes of the mind: Charting the phenomenology of the ayahuasca experience.* Oxford, UK: Oxford University Press.

Star, S. L., & Griesemer, J. R. (1989). Institutional ecology, 'translations' and boundary objects: Amateurs and professionals in Berkeley's Museum of Vertebrate Zoology, 1907–39. *Social Studies of Science, 19*(3), 387–420.

Stengers, I. (2011). Reclaiming animism. In A. Franke & S. Folie (Eds.), *Animism: Modernity through the looking glass.* Vienna: Generali Foundation.

TallBear, K. (2011, April 24). Why interspecies thinking needs indigenous standpoints. *Cultural Anthropology* website. Retrieved from https://culanth.org/fieldsights/260-why-interspecies-thinking-needs-indigenous-standpoints

TallBear, K. (2014). Standing with and speaking as faith: A feminist-indigenous approach to inquiry. *Journal of Research Practice, 10*(2), 17.

Tsing, A. L. (2015). *The mushroom at the end of the world: On the possibility of life in capitalist ruins.* Princeton, NJ: Princeton University Press.

Tuck, E., & Yang, K. W. (2012). Decolonization is not a metaphor. *Decolonization: Indigeneity, Education & Society, 1*(1), 1–40.

Tudela-Talavera, P., La Torre-Cuadros, M. A., & Native Community of Vencedor. (2016). Cultural importance and use of medicinal plants in the Shipibo-Conibo Native community of Vencedor (Loreto) Peru. *Ethnobotany Research and Applications, 14,* 533–548.

Tupper, K. W., & Labate, B. C. (2014). Ayahuasca, psychedelic studies and health sciences: The politics of knowledge and inquiry into an Amazonian plant brew. *Current Drug Abuse Reviews, 7*(2), 71–80.

Viveiros de Castro, E. (2004). Exchanging perspectives: The transformation of objects into subjects in Amerindian ontologies. *Common Knowledge, 10*(3), 463–484.

Wilson, S. (2008). *Research is ceremony: Indigenous research methods.* Nova Scotia, Canada: Fernwood Publishing.

Chapter 12
Gnosis Potency: DMT Breakthroughs and Paragnosis

Graham St John

Abstract DMT (N,N-dimethyltryptamine) is a powerful tryptamine that has experienced growing appeal in the last decade, independent from ayahuasca, the Amazonian visionary brew in which it is an integral ingredient. Investigating user reports available from literary and online sources, this chapter focuses on the *gnosis potency* associated with the DMT "breakthrough" experience. I explore the parameters of the tryptaminal state and, in particular, the extraordinary *paragnosis* associated with the DMT event, perceived contact with "entities," and the transmission of visual language. As the reports discussed illustrate, for milieus of the disenchanted, among other entheogens, DMT is venerated as a gift that enables connection to a reality (nature, the universe, divinity) from which modern humanity is imagined to have grown alienated. Through an exploration of the legacy of principal actors, including Terence McKenna, Jonathan Ott, Jim DeKorne, and Nick Sand, the chapter navigates the significance of DMT in modern Western esotericism.

Introduction

Known to produce out-of-body states and profound changes in sensory perception, mood, and thought, DMT (N,N-dimethyltryptamine) is a potent short-lasting tryptamine. While DMT has been outlawed in most nations following the UN Convention on Psychotropic Substances of 1971, recent surveys have shown that this relatively harmless tryptamine compound has grown increasingly desirable (Sledge & Grim, 2013; Winstock et al., 2013). Independent from ayahuasca, the Amazonian visionary brew in which DMT is integral, the modern usage of DMT followed the discovery of its psychopharmacological actions in the 1950s. The promotional tours of psychedelic raconteur Terence McKenna in the 1980s and 1990s were integral to its underground appeal, as was the Internet. Users typically participate in an informed networked milieu where knowledge of chemical synthesis, botanical

G. St John (✉)
Social Sciences, University of Fribourg, Fribourg, Switzerland
e-mail: graham.stjohn@unifr.ch

© Springer International Publishing AG, part of Springer Nature 2018   205
B. C. Labate, C. Cavnar (eds.), *Plant Medicines, Healing and Psychedelic Science*,
https://doi.org/10.1007/978-3-319-76720-8_12

identification, extraction techniques, and methods of administration circulate. DMT is today commonly smoked using crystal-vaporizing methods or blended with other herbs, as in "changa" (St John, 2017a). While sociocultural research on this phenomenon remains scarce, a circumstance hampered by criminalization, evidence builds on familiarity with the effects of DMT, as evidenced in clinical research (Strassman, 2001), and through research using interviews (Tramacchi, 2006), surveying (Cott & Roc, 2008), ontology (Luke 2008, 2011) and cultural history (Gallimore & Luke, 2015; St John, 2015).

While dependent on broad variables commonly recognized as "set" (i.e., the mood, expectations, and attentions affecting the individual's state of being) and "setting" (i.e., social and environmental context), as well as source (i.e., botanical or synthetic), technique of administration, and dose, the DMT event typically involves the rapid onset of an out-of-body experience of brief duration (i.e., its effects typically last about 15 min), with a sensation of transit common to the experience. While distortions in space and time, complex geometric patterns, energetic light sources, and veridical encounters with sentient entities are reported features of this visionary space, the experience possesses phenomenological diversity, as found in Strassman's clinical trials (2001). The wide parameters of the DMT "world"—its *hyperliminality*—are to be addressed in a future publication.

Examining user experiences in literary sources, from existing research and in anonymous reports archived on the Internet, including those found on Erowid and DMT-Nexus, this chapter navigates the *gnosis potency* of the DMT event. It therefore addresses the profile of DMT, among other tryptamine sources, within one of three interconnected modalities of use: gnosis, therapeutic, and recreational (St John, 2015, pp. 305–307). While there are diverse "events" shaped by a spectrum of variables, the user reports presented illustrate DMT events are extraordinary "breakthrough" experiences that not uncommonly facilitate outcomes that bear the stamp of gnosis—i.e., access to the truth of one's connectivity with nature—including one's divine self, as well as the natural world, or more generally the cosmos or universe from which humanity is understood to have grown alienated. Not uncommonly received as a gift, experients will act upon such knowledge in various ways. An exploration of the ontology of the DMT breakthrough experience is undertaken in three sections. The first explores the *tryptaminal paragnosis* of DMT *hyperspace*. The second addresses the profile of DMT within the development Wouter Hanegraaff names "entheogenic esotericism" (Hanegraaff, 2013), a profile elevated through the prodigious commitment of Terence McKenna. Drawing largely on the examples of three figures, William Burroughs, Jim DeKorne, and Nick Sand, the third section navigates the wide parameters of *entheogenesis.*

DMT Hyperspace and Tryptaminal Paragnosis

> Ontological warp speed arrived in a startlingly immediate flash as the universe quite literally deconstructed itself in front of my eyes into a complex green and red geometrical grid that artist Alex Grey has rendered as the "Universal Mind Lattice." An impossibly elaborate onrush of candy-colored, chaotically presented patterns of pure visual information then ensued as the intergalactic Wagnerian horn section continued to blow a spectacular fanfare. The emotional content was one of genuine awe, a briefly terrifyingly integration of my neurology into the submolecular fabric of the universe (Gehr, 1992, p. 47).

This comment presents a not untypical example among DMT users in which this compound is recognized to enable a category of immediate knowing commonly designated as *gnosis*. Compared with other forms of knowing, gnosis is associated with the direct experience of the truth, unmediated by doctrine, faith, or reason. It has been established that a mix of hermetic, Neoplatonic, Occult, Kabbalistic, and other traditions have contributed to a dazzling variety of ideas and practices that have been associated with "gnosis" (Hanegraaff, 2006). As has also been recognized, the conditions for gnosis are often altered states of consciousness (ASC), such as ecstatic and trance states (Hanegraaff, 2008a; St John, 2011). The perspective on "gnosis" adopted here approximates what Hanegraaff, in his study of modern esotericism, *New Age Religion and Western Culture*, called the "third option" (beyond "faith" and "reason") in a spectrum of Western knowledge (Hanegraaff, 1998). As knowledge claims harboring discontent with established theologies and scientific rationalism, the idea was provoked by the work of Dutch historian of Christianity and Gnosticism, Gilles Quispel, who traced the history of "a certain type of religious or religiophilosophical thought and practice from antiquity to the present" (Hanegraaff, 2008b, p. 133). The key aspect of what Quispel called the "third component" in the European cultural tradition was "gnosis," a Greek term meaning "knowledge" and, more specifically, "a kind of intuitive, nondiscursive, salvational knowledge of one's own true self and of God" (Hanegraaff, 2008b, p. 133). Developing his own tripartite classification, i.e., faith, reason, and gnosis, Hanegraaff (2008b) was careful to state the classification is analytical and not historical, since they cannot be neatly bounded. It is also important to note that the catalytic role of psychoactive drugs, plant derived or otherwise, has been typically overlooked or ignored in official academic and "state-of-the-art" accounts of gnosis and histories of Western esotericism. For example, while ASC, including those enabled by psychoactive compounds, have been integral to experimental ecstasies and "psychedelic" reveries, there were neither entries on psychoactive drugs nor ASC in *The Dictionary of Gnosis & Western Esotericism.*

As evidenced in a variety of sources, alongside tryptamine analogues and among a host of "teacher" plants and their compounds, DMT holds appeal as a powerful means for gnosis inducement or, more pointedly, *paragnosis* potentiation. The latter term refers to extraordinary and paranormal means of knowledge acquisition. Known to expose users to "worlds" previously hidden from view, encounters with sentient otherworldly "entities," and transmissions of "visual language," the strangely familiar transpersonal DMT state is persistently recognized within the user community as a state of paragnosis. From my reading of user accounts, amid a diversity of experiences, including those of principal figures discussed in this chapter, there remains a persistent feature that the DMT user purportedly arrives at, or approximates, a direct and unmediated awareness of the intrinsic nature of reality (i.e., as it truly is), a reality that had previously been occulted. This awakening not untypically involves (a) the awareness that nebulous and normally unseen forces are the cause of tyranny, oppression, and alienation and (b) that one is intrinsically connected to the divine universe. The first condition is sometimes articulated using a term attributed to Gnosticism, i.e., "archons" (DeKorne 1994). Such revelations typically inspire action in the world. As a transpersonal experience potentiating an awakened identity and altered worldview, such events appear consistent with the transformational status of an "exceptional human experience" (Krippner, 2002).

The faculty of becoming endowed with enhanced visual perception is common during the DMT trance and integral to its paragnosis potency. Experients are not uncommonly feted with a presque vu, an ability to see, or almost see, through a reality filter previously unnoticed. The resulting effects are visions of "hidden" realities and "parallel universes." While launched through alien cities at such a lightning speed that content retention was virtually impossible, smoking DMT at the Chan Kah Hotel, Palenque, gave Daniel Pinchbeck an awareness of the realm "next door." As he wrote in *Breaking Open the Head*, "behind every billowing curtain, hidden inside the dark matter of consciousness, now playing every night in disguised form in our dreams. It is so close to us, adjacent or perpendicular to this reality. It is a soft shadow, a candle flicker, away." It was in this realm that those Pinchbeck called the "cosmic supervisors" repeated: "This is it. Now you know. This is it. Now you know" (Pinchbeck, 2002, p. 242). In collated reports on DMT ventures, science columnist Clifford A. Pickover has commented that most users feel "as if a veil has been lifted, allowing them to view events that have been continuously transpiring in the DMTverse with an existence independent of the psychonaut." Accessing this divine universe where explorers are accessing another reality "mere millimeters away from our own," Pickover refers to the "feeling of enchantment, of sanctity, of beauty, a sense of gaining privileged access to knowledge and intelligence" among travelers in this space, for whom the world "appears to be 'constructed,' composed with care like a work of art or an intricate hand-spun fabric" (Pickover, 2005, p. 91).

Whether explained as travails through parallel universes, odysseys in other dimensions, or journeys to the psychic antipodes, the vicissitudes of *travel* are implicit to DMT hyperspace, the passage through which is often embraced as a breakthrough event. The experience had been widely asseverated via the concept of "hyperspace," a psychoactively induced higher-dimensional space-time championed by T. McKenna, whose exploits in those realms are transmitted via a torrent of oral presentations circulating virally on YouTube. The "space" of the DMT event is commonly reported by users to be above the four dimensions of space-time (i.e., non-Euclidian). Enabling anonymity and modes of communication with some semblance to the virtuality of the experience, the virtual world of cyberspace has been pivotal to communities vested in DMT "hyperspace" (St John, 2017b). The authenticity of the event is connected to the way this virtual "space" and its occupants are received as sources of information "seen," felt, or otherwise sensed noetically as "gifts." Hyperspace is often characterized as a liminal realm of universal knowledge, such as that accessed by D. M. Turner who, in *The Essential Psychedelic Guide*, described "CydelikSpace" as a "storehouse of universal experience" containing "all thoughts which did not occur but could have, and each variation of experience that did not take place" (1994, p. 127).

Travelers of the interdimensional interstices write reports on the parameters of these spaces, which are then passed on, like return gifts, to their own communities. Such include James Oroc who uses quantum physics to explain his access to "all knowledge in the universe, at once" (the "Akashic Field") under the influence of 5-MeO-DMT (Oroc, 2009, p. 197).[1] While the experience is reported to be like receiving the complete encyclopedia of cosmic history, pan-cultural awareness, and total biographical recall within a momentary download, returnees understandably face difficulties retaining the information. As a kind of Ur-space of primary wisdom that is apparent and yet incomprehensible, immediate and yet profoundly other, this space is sometimes described as a "vaulted dome." While returnees chart the multidimensionality of hyperspace, and report on the "dome effect," experience of this space is characterized by ontological variability (St John, 2018).

Among the visceral affects of one's passage through this space is the sensation that experients have undergone an initiation or induction of some kind. This passage is most often characterized by the perception of a newfound and unheralded connectedness. Commentary from musician Devin James Fry illustrates this cosmic initiation while at the same time illuminating DMT's popular appeal. Inspired to write the song "I Touch My Face in Hyperspace Oh Yeah" after a DMT experience, Fry has been reported to state: "It's like seeing the source code of the universe: a river of vibrating mandalas, geometric shapes shifting and moving. That night I became it. There wasn't a separation anymore—I was part of that. I was certain that consciousness is a non-local event … It's more like we're antennas beaming something in for the duration of our time in these bodies" (Curtin, 2015, paras. 7, 9).

The sensation of dissolving boundaries previously separating the user from the universe, divinity, or reality itself, is not uncommon and was succinctly announced by a returnee reporting on Erowid: "I definitely felt I had been closer to the core of the real than ever before and that this mystery is front and center to who we are as humans, who we really are. I felt very connected to my universe, very sensitive and strong and in touch with things" (SFos, 2000, para. 11). "Entities" are a common medium for the transmission of this gnosis. While a veritable "bestiarum" has been identified—from teachers to archons, elves to mantids, and therianthropes to tree spirits, among a wide spectrum of beings (Hanna, 2012; Tramacchi, 2006)—as

---

[1]5-MeO-DMT (5-methoxy-N,N-dimethyltryptamine) is included in this discussion, given reports of its gnostic potency paralleling that of N,N,DMT, both short-acting hallucinogens of the tryptamine family. That is, they are simple indole alkaloids derived biosynthetically from tryptophan, an essential amino acid present in all plants and animals (D. McKenna & Riba, 2015). Despite this similarity, they are different chemicals with distinct strengths and profiles (see Erowid Crew, 2009).

mentioned, accounts typically acknowledge the reception of a "gift." The following offers one example.

> The female being got in my face and communicated to me (not in words) look at whats ON the pedestal! I looked up and saw a diamond shaped object that was made of similar stuff to the walls but infinitely more brilliant, more dazzling, more unspeakably awesome. And as my smile grew and total awe and amazement filled me, this female being began flying around the object at great speed, keeping her eyes fixed on me. She was doing flips and sharp turns and cheering as though she was celebrating the fact that she had the chance to show me. She kept communicating to me, Look at it! Look at it! Isn't this awesome?! This continued, and I kept my eyes on that unbelievable object as the scene began to fade. (Universal Shaman, 2004, para. 10)

The "impossibility" of episodes reputedly defying the five senses and testing the limits of language poses serious challenges for users attempting to transpose their experiences post-event. These challenges are among the reasons why art inspired by DMT (and other compounds), such as work produced by Alex Grey, is appealing to users and why many prefer to adopt media other than written language (e.g., painting, sculpture, film). Otherwise, users may coin neologisms to translate the "unEnglishable," as they have done at the DMT-Nexus, where a list of terms—the "Hyperspace Lexicon"—has been created. The common perception that one can "see" light with all of one's senses is, for instance, posited as "kinesioöptic," referring to a state where "the body can dissolve in the experience and be left with just the sensing of light." Another term, "kalonkinesioöptic," prefixes "kinesioöptic" with "kalon," a Greek term referring to the Platonic idea of transcendental beauty, thereby referring to immersion in astonishing beauty (Hyperspace Lexicon, n.d.)

It cannot be ignored that DMT inaugurates a diverse range of phenomenological experiences, as reported by Tramacchi (2006) in his ethnography of Australian DMT users. While at one extreme, Tramacchi reported a preoccupation with death and dismemberment, in another pattern, interlocutors interacted with "earth spirits or earth energies," communications thought "potentially therapeutic for both the individual and the planet" (2006, p. 73). Consistent with the wide visionary spectrum to which Aldous Huxley (2009 [1955]) was familiar, dramatic variability is native to psychedelics. At one extreme, a palpable atmosphere of decay and senescence is present in user reports and artistic expressions—an enveloping shadowland not unlike that depicted in the screenplay of Gaspar Noé's perverse 2009 epic feature, *Enter the Void*. At the other, outcomes are consistent with the "ecodelic" thesis of Richard Doyle in *Darwin's Pharmacy*, where ayahuasca, DMT, and other substances are inspiring language and evolving consciousness to the benefit of "the *Noösphere*" (Doyle, 2011).

Despite this spectrum of extraordinary experience, one also cannot ignore the common threads, as evidenced by the rhetoric of returnees. A case in point is D. M. Turner, the comparative psychonaut who advised on various combinations like harmala alkaloids with DMT in smoking blends that prolonged the effects by 30–40 min. In this duration, Turner reported: "I often feel that my body and Being are 'embraced' by an ancient earth spirit. And this earth spirit is instructing me to become aware of, and open up, many lines of communication that exist between my mind, body and the external world" (Turner, 1994, p.: 78).

Atomic Age Gnosis

As apparent in such paragnosis, and in invented nomenclature, the revelatory character of the breakthrough event is consistent with the way DMT enables transparencies typically involving a realization of one's prior alienation, e.g., from one's higher self, nature, or the universe. Typically, the experience amounts to liberation from oppression, an emancipation not disconnected from an awareness of the powers—entities, faiths, and dogmas—that sustain it. Enabling awakening, and fueling conspiracies, sometimes with the assistance of sentient intermediaries, DMT is often approached as a sacrament. In this way, it can be likened to the use of psilocybin-containing mushrooms, mescaline, or ayahuasca used in nontraditional contexts, as explained by Wouter Hanegraaff.

> Entheogenic sacraments like ayahuasca are credited with the capacity of breaking mainstream society's spell of mental domination and restoring us from blind and passive consumers unconsciously manipulated by "the system" to our original state of free and autonomous spiritual beings. . . They are seen as providing *gnosis*: a salvational knowledge of the true nature of one's self and of the universe, which liberates the individual from domination by the cosmic system. (Hanegraaff, 2011, p. 88)

As an integral component of ayahuasca, but also as an independent agent, DMT carries this liberating potential and should be recognized within the context of "entheogenic esotericism" (Hanegraaff, 2013), which takes its place, previously neglected, in the history of Western esotericism. In his revisionism, Hanegraaff (2010) names Terence McKenna as the figurehead in this development, pointing out that, as demonstrated in public orations such as the Lectures on Alchemy delivered at Esalen in 1990, McKenna sought in pre-Enlightenment hermeticism "models of a 'magical' and enchanted revival" relevant to the crises of the present (Hanegraaff, 2013, p. 406).

While any such label will likely have been disputed by McKenna himself, "entheogenic esotericism" resonates, especially as it appears to recognize what McKenna called the "Re: Evolution"-ary impact of plant "allies," that they provide the keys for ingestees (i.e., humans) to realize their own divine nature. McKenna had been outspoken on the idea that psychoactive compounds (notably, hallucinogenic mushrooms) were integral to the emergence of human consciousness. He was also a trenchant critic of modern culture, the "ennui" of which, he commented in *The Food of the Gods*, "is the consequence of a disrupted quasi-symbiotic relationship between ourselves and Gaian nature." Among the most appalling symptoms of this disruption, he averred, are the conventions prohibiting plants that are themselves empowering and evolutionary. And perhaps the greatest indictment of all is the fact that, under national and international legal frameworks implemented at the turn of the 1970s that had deemed it to possess no medicinal or therapeutic value, DMT is criminalized.[2] The folly is noteworthy, not least since DMT exists everywhere in nature and occurs naturally in humans. "Only a restoration of this relationship in some form," he continued, "is capable of carrying us into a full appreciation of our birthright and sense of ourselves as complete human beings" (McKenna, 1992, p. 56).

With such a restoration in mind, McKenna advocated an "archaic revival" and a "renewed shamanism" (1992, p. 98). In a 1992 spoken word performance—"Re: Evolution," backed by UK act The Shamen—McKenna stated that, with the "dissolution of boundaries" triggered by tryptamines, especially an "heroic dose" of DMT or psilocybin-containing mushrooms,

> one cannot continue to close one's eyes to the ruination of the earth, the poisoning of the seas, and the consequences of two thousand years of unchallenged dominator culture, based on monotheism, hatred of nature, suppression of the female, and so forth... So, what shamans have to do is act as exemplars, by making this cosmic journey to the domain of the Gaian ideas, and then bringing them back in the form of art in the struggle to save the world. (McKenna, Colin & West, 1992)

McKenna did not advocate these experiments as self-directed therapy. With intention and courage, and with attention to dose and technique, psychedelic tryptamines were to be ingested in feats of world-saving heroism. The following is a crucial insight from a 1995 lecture:

> Everyone of us when we go into the psychedelic state, this is what we should be looking for. It's not for *your* elucidation, it's not part of *your* self-directed psychotherapy; you are an explorer and you represent our species and the greatest good we can do is to bring back a new idea because our world is endangered by the absence of good ideas. Our world is in crisis because of the absence of consciousness. To whatever degree any one of us can bring back a small piece of the picture and contribute it to the building of the new paradigm, then we participate in the redemption of the human spirit. (Burn in Noise, 2008)

The perspective is indebted to the Platonic idea that humans, having fallen from perfection—the world soul—could return to the stars, and many of McKenna's ideas regarding the virtuous use of psychedelics and "alien gnosis" can be read through this lens.

Seized by the "DMT flash" in Berkeley in the fall of 1965/1966 and driven, with brother Dennis, to uncover its source in an epic psychonautical adventure to the

---

[2]With its possession and distribution subject to prohibitions across the United States, beginning in California in 1966, by 1970, DMT and analogues DET (N,N-diethyltryptamine) and bufotenin were included in the Controlled Substances Act of 1970, which was followed closely by the UN Convention on Psychotropic Substances of 1971, putting pressure on foreign governments to follow suit. As a "Schedule I substance" in the United States, DMT has not only been classified together with LSD, mescaline, psilocybin, and other nonaddictive psychedelic compounds; it is typically classed alongside heroin and cocaine as a "dangerous drug" with "no recognized medicinal value." While 5-MeO-DMT and other short-acting entheogenic tryptamines remained legal in the United States, they became subject to classification as illegal DMT analogues under the Controlled Substances Analogue Enforcement Act of 1986. In 2011, 5-MeO-DMT was added to Schedule I.

Amazon in 1971 (McKenna & McKenna, 1993 [1975]), McKenna recognized DMT as "the quintessential hallucinogen" (McKenna, 1994, para. 1). With knowledge of its endogenous status, DMT was championed as nothing short of a human "birthright"—as much, or so he thought, as "our sexuality, our language, our eyesight, our appreciation of music" (McKenna, n.d., para. 5).

Throughout the 1990s, McKenna made a lasting impression speaking at dance festivals and proto-visionary arts gatherings, becoming chief bard to the neo-psychedelic counterculture. The repertoire on "hyperspace" McKenna forged to reckon with the perplexities of the DMT trance state have had a profound impact on countless participants in an emergent research culture whose members build, share, and debate interpretative frameworks to comprehend their experience (St John, 2015).

Within this culture, and with the assistance of the heuristics provided by T. McKenna (who, following his death in 2000, became something of a digitized cult figure), along with the influence of Strassman and Alex Grey, psychedelic trance and visionary arts events, such as Portugal's Boom Festival and Symbiosis Gathering, became the revelatory topography for rediscovering a symbiotic relationship with the Earth. Intentionally "transformational" and participatory festivals celebrated awareness of one's enmeshment in the web of life. Psychoactive compounds, notably DMT, have had a catalytic role in the emergence of psyculture (St John, 2015), with DMT among an assemblage of spiritual technologies, or *spiritechnics* (St John, 2012), championed by expressive expatriates aggrieved by the disastrous effects of monotheism, possessive materialism, and ecological maladaptation. Among the adopted alchemies is the popular experimental DMT smoking mix "changa," sometimes referred to as "smokeable ayahuasca" (St John, 2017a), with transformational experiences interpreted as "psychedelic gnosis" (Gaia, 2016). In a hybridization of the New Age and New Edge movements, with the assistance of sensory technologies from digital electronics to ethnobotanicals, with repertoires from super diets to microdosing, and adopting trance dancing, yoga, and meditation, among a range of human potential maximizing techniques evidencing "entheogenic religion" in the "wide" sense (Hanegraaff, 2013, p. 393), protagonists seek passage from conditions of cosmic alienation.

This broad, and sometimes questionably, "transformational" milieu has inherited an ambience of discontent, an awareness that humanity is in the grip of a crisis in consciousness. For McKenna, and those surfing his wake, the solution to this crisis resided in psychedelic shamanism. Anarchic, experimental, and radically libertarian and empirical, this neo-shamanism would be integral to the evolution of the human condition. Rather than singularly figured to heal the individual self, psychedelic shamanism is ultimately figured to evolve the human spirit. The perspective has deep roots, though immediately indebted to Huxley, who understood that psychedelics like mescaline and LSD could empower the individual user in their knowledge of being. In *The Doors of Perception*, Huxley endorsed psychedelics as means by which to cleanse the "filters" ordinarily protecting humans from the infinite, practices previously the domain of saints, seers, mystics, and prophets. Perhaps more essential than ever in the mid-twentieth century, in the shadow of the mushroom cloud, Huxley, and later psychedelic chemists Bear Owsley and Nick Sand, recognized the urgency of an atomic blast of consciousness in an Atomic Age.

The mounting crisis of the late 1960s demanded that the envelope be blown out on standard consciousness. The times demanded an uncommon courage in the human interfacing with psychoactive compounds. When announcing that "the last best hope for dissolving the steep walls of cultural inflexibility that appear to be channeling us toward true ruin is a renewed shamanism" (McKenna, 1992, p. 98), McKenna wasn't simply backing a shamanic revival; he was propagating gnosis-enabling tools for the modern age. You don't need to go "500 miles up a jungle river and live with primitive peoples and study techniques for 30 years," an eager audience was informed. "If I had a pipe loaded with [DMT] in my hand, each one of you would be thirty seconds away from … this absolutely reality dissolving, category reconstructing, mind boggling possibility" (McKenna, 1998). By virtue of possessing a set of lungs, the secret was only seconds away.

Entheogenesis and Its Polarities

The revisionism that enables such practices to be recognized as legitimate foci for researchers of history, religion, and culture relies on a concept framed specifically in relation to plant products and derivative compounds that, by way of their visionary capacity, are thought to awaken the "divine within": *entheogen* (Ruck et al., 1979). The concept is traced to pioneering natural product chemist Jonathon Ott's (1996 [1993]) assiduous attention to the spiritual potency of a compendium of drugs, including DMT (and 5-MeO-DMT), alongside other tryptamines and psychoactive compounds deriving from plants like *Salvia divinorum*, the San Pedro cactus, and *Tabernanthe iboga*. The product of a long search for appropriate non-ethnocentric terminology, "entheogen," was deemed appropriate for "describing states of shamanic and ecstatic possession induced by ingestion of mind-altering drugs." *Entheos*—literally "god within"—had been used by the Greeks to denote "prophetic seizures, erotic passion and artistic creation" and to refer to "those religious rites in which mystical states were experienced through the ingestion of substances that were transubstantial with the deity" (Ruck et al., 1979, pp. 145–146). By adding the root *gen*—denoting the action of "becoming"—the term evoked a substance that could generate or awaken divinity. The newly minted terminology, then, highlighted the therapeutic and spiritually transformative potential associated with a variety of plants and compounds as they are adopted in nontraditional contexts and where they are typically subject to prohibition.

Among the notable aspects of Ott's work is his millenarian reading of entheogenesis, a position not far removed from McKenna, despite the latter's preference for the word "psychedelic." In this view, a pharmacopeia of botanicals is capable of redeeming "hypermaterialistic humankind" in the otherwise dire conditions of the Anthropocene. The experience conferred by these "wondrous medicaments" could inaugurate, Ott averred, "the start of a new Golden Age," thereby constituting "humankind's brightest hopes for overcoming the ecological crisis with which we threaten the biosphere and jeopardize our own survival" (Ott, 1996, p. 77). In Ott's view, amateur ethnomycologist Robert Gordon Wasson's rediscovery of the shamanic cult of *teonanacatl* (as reported in *Life* [Wasson, 1957]) presaged the modern advent of the entheogen and the revival of ecstatic religion. In this development, "ethnopharmacognostic" agents are adopted in response to the disenchanting conditions of modernity. "When people have direct, personal access to entheogenic, religious experiences," Ott related, "they never conceive of humankind as a separate creation, apart from the rest of the universe" (Ott, 1996, p. 59).[3]

Today, "entheogen" enjoys interdisciplinary cachet, especially among those establishing the therapeutic value of a range of compounds, plants, and concoctions, including psilocybin and ayahuasca (Griffiths et al., 2006; Ellens, 2014). Over the last two decades, and generally within the "narrow" sense outlined by Hanegraaff, entheogenic practices have been explored within widening experimental, therapeutic, and academic circles. Huston Smith was a persistent voice of wisdom, stating that "nonaddictive mind-altering substances that are approached seriously and reverently" can enhance a religious life, even though they do not themselves facilitate a religious life (Smith, 2000, pp. xvi–xvii). While this period saw a growth in studies focusing on the significance of unique compounds and practices, notably the ayahuasca brew and its diasporic proliferation beyond the Amazon (Labate & Cavnar, 2014), studies of the "wider" implications of entheogenesis have moved apace (Fadiman, 2011; Grof, 2009; Roberts, 2013).

Signaling this paradigm shift, the concept of "entheogen" has gained appeal among research scientists and theologians. Staking down a position at a sharp remove from the neo-shamanic millenarianism of McKenna and Ott, psychiatrist William A. Richards encourages the association of entheogens with "the reality that theologians call *grace*" (Richards, 2014, p. 653). While the therapeutic value of "entheogens" has been established, little sociocultural research has been conducted on the contemporary use of psychedelics or entheogens, DMT or otherwise, within healthy user communities (cf. Milhet & Reynaud-Maurupt, 2011). While prohibition has played a role in preventing, obstructing, and discouraging such research, one could imagine research addressing the gnosis potential of the breakthrough experience aided by circulating nomenclature. In reference to its relationship to a near-death experience (NDE), a concept that specifically addresses the DMT event is "necrotogen." Purportedly arising from a conversation between T. McKenna and Rupert Sheldrake, this term references how the DMT event anticipates the death state (Bell, 1999). Strassman's research illuminated this association. Many volunteers were observed to be "embraced by something much greater than themselves, or anything they previously could have imagined: the 'source of all existence.'" Furthermore, those who attain this experience, not unlike those undergoing an

---

[3] As an apparent testament to this proposition in current psychological research, see Forstmann and Sagioglou (2017).

NDE, "emerge with a greater appreciation for life, less fear of death, and a reorientation of their priorities to less material and more spiritual pursuits" (Strassman, 2001, p. 221).

The powerful tryptamine-induced reverie in which one may become reconciled to the inseparability of death and life is figured in the word "ontoseismic." A portmanteau of "ontos" (Greek for "being") and "seismos" (earthquake, from "seiein," meaning "to shake" in Greek), the word refers to the way a breakthrough event may shatter the world image and conditioning of first-time users of DMT. While the "ontoseismic" state may be traumatic and overwhelming, "the cause of the trauma is an Platonic experience of total truth, beauty and love" (Hyperspace Lexicon, n.d.). This concept seems appropriate in relation to some of the more notorious reports on experiments with DMT. Perhaps chief among these are commentaries from William Burroughs when injecting DMT (called "Prestonia") in Tangier at the turn of the 1960s. In a letter to Brion Gysin on April 8, 1961, Burroughs likens the experience to a mental holocaust. "Trip to the ovens like white hot bees through your flesh and bones and everything, but I was only in the ovens for thirty seconds" (Burroughs, 2012, p. 70). And in another letter to Gysin, on April 20, 1961:

> Took again of dim-N and stood in front of the Mirror waiting for the Attack that always comes when the dim-N hits. The attack came from the left side of the mirror—Blue eyed red haired Russians in Tunics and Chinese Partisans among the marchers many women as they advanced towards me to the sound of gongs all chanted "we'll show you something show you something Johnny Come Lately WAR"—Tracer bullets and shells and flame throwers threw me back onto the bed groaning in the torn flesh of a million battle fields. (Harrop, 2010, p. 204)

After months of experimentation, Burroughs turned away from what he had called in his April 8, 1961, letter to Gysin "the nightmare hallucinogen" (Burroughs, 2012, p. 70).

In another example, founding editor of *The Entheogen Review*, Jim DeKorne, described the effect of an early 1990s breakthrough on an extract of *Phalaris arundinacea*, of which the main active alkaloid is 5-MeO-DMT. Using metaphors reminiscent of Burroughs, DeKorne reported an experience "analogous to having a psychic hydrogen bomb go off" in his brain. But, unlike Burroughs, who kept an antidote handy as a virtual sidearm to prevent complete psychic capitulation, DeKorne's attitude was to "resist any impulse to resist: flow with it, breathe with it. Imagine a Zen meditation at Hiroshima ground-zero." While DeKorne was at ground zero consumed by "an atomic fireball at the instant of detonation," his ontoseismic flash receded, allowing him to receive a revelation, related by way of verses from the *Bhagavad Gita* where Krisna gives Arjuna "divine eyes," through which he is able to behold Krisna's "mystic opulence" (DeKorne, 1993, p. 2). In *Psychedelic Shamanism*, DeKorne championed the shaman as rebel, the mind-tinkering outcast who, by way of ethnobotanical experimentation, can heal the "planetary disease caused by human refusal to acknowledge whole systems" (1994, p. 81).

DeKorne described the realm behind "the veils," visible to the psychedelic shaman with "divine eyes" as the pleroma, an unconscious or imaginal realm, transit to which should be undertaken by those suitably equipped for cosmic battle. A Greek word meaning "fullness" or "plenitude," pleroma is a term borrowed from Jung, who took it from the Gnostics, who knew of a hidden kingdom inhabited by gods and demons, among them, the Archons—entities that are "cruel, unfeeling and dictatorial in their relationship with humans" and who are otherwise "dissociated intelligences who feed off of human belief systems the way that we eat hamburger" (DeKorne, 1994, p. 69). For DeKorne, what is at stake is liberation from the coercive power of these invisible rulers. In this view, DMT and other psychoactives enable modern explorers recognition of the otherwise hidden agendas of the gods and, further, to convert their coercive powers into those at one's own disposal.

DeKorne's entheo-millenarian prognostications were announced in an early edition of *The Entheogen Review*. Entheogens, he averred, "may be the only realistic chance we have to make such an unlikely quantum leap of consciousness in the brief time remaining" (DeKorne, 1992, p. 2). Demonstrating a debt to Huxley and McKenna, and searching for a paragnostic weapon that could "transform our world," he set his mind on *Phalaris* as a

> *catalyst* to blast us out of our material myopia. To be effective, this catalyst must be available to the widest possible number of people at little or no cost—something so common that it would be impossible for the entrenched power structure to control or destroy. It must be easy to use, requiring minimal preparation. And it must be potent, even psychologically danger-ous, for nothing less will open our awareness to the encompassing Mystery. (DeKorne, 1992, p. 2)

These views hold correspondence with those of Nick Sand, the first underground chemist on record to synthesize DMT (eventually manufacturing between 20 and 30 kg) (Hanna, Manning & Slattery, 2012). A yogi from the age of 15 and student of anthropology, in the early 1960s, before he manufactured the famed Orange Sun-shine LSD (with Tim Scully), Sand discovered in DMT a powerful compound that triggered a lifelong dedication to manufacturing psychedelics. While it had previ-ously been injected only, in 1964, Sand made the chance discovery that the vapor from DMT could be inhaled. In a biographic description of his life as a devoted alchemist of these sacraments, for which he spent time in 15 jails and prisons, Sand became, as Jon Hanna (2009) related, "a criminal as a matter of principle and as an act of civil disobedience, because he believed he was working for a higher good."

In an article published in *The Entheogen Review* only months after his release from prison, and using a pseudonym, Sand wrote a concise missive on the healing and transformative power of DMT, all dependent upon appropriate set and setting (described at some length) (∞Ayes, 2001, p. 54). A student of world spiritual traditions, including the Kabbalah, Krishna consciousness, Sufism, aikido, t'ai chi, Zen, and tantra, and familiar with the teachings of Krishnamurti, Milarepa, Ramakrishna, and Rajneesh, among others (Hanna, 2009), for Sand, DMT, "the touchstone of the psychedelics," was a powerful spiritual teacher that, under the right conditions and given appropriate support, could facilitate a mystical visionary state of consciousness. "We are not alone; we exist as an integral part of all life, breathing, pulsating, vibrating, giving off plant food, absorbing animal food, in a multi-level fabric of incredibly beautiful designs and patterns. This is what DMT shows us"

(∞Ayes, 2001, p. 51). One might imagine the subject taken up in *Psychedelic Secrets*, the unpublished tome Sand wrote in prison.

> It opens the doorway to the vastness of the soul; this is at once our own personal soul, and its intrinsic connection to the universal soul. When the underlying unity of this fictional duality is seen and felt, one experiences a completeness and interconnection with all things. This experience, when we attain it, is extremely beautiful and good. It is a song that rings and reverberates through the lens of God. Now we know why we were born; to have this intense experience of the sacred, the joyous, the beauty, and the blessing of just being alive in the arms of God. (∞Ayes, 2001, p. 56)

Beyond misguided recreational use, as a mobilizing agent for truth seekers, and ultimately "self-realization," DMT was promoted as a powerful tool in a loose spiritual practice that adopted the language of Gurdjieff and transpersonal psychology. "This quest then, is about re-emerging from the swamp of forgetfulness and distraction in which we live, and being reborn in consciousness" (∞Ayes, 2001, p. 53).

While adopted as a technique among many others for accessing truth or remembering ourselves, as the most respected of all tools, DMT required discipline. "Properly prepared," Sand wrote, "we meet the Gods that live deep within all of us. In that meeting we experience intense recognition of the oneness of all things. We receive true and simple instructions." Enraptured by "the exquisite beauty and truth of this inner knowing" (∞Ayes, 2001, p. 56), he could not have been further removed from Burroughs, whose paranoid struggles with the same substance were influenced by the "psychotomimetic" and "psychotogenetic" paradigms of 1950s psychiatry, in which DMT, among other substances, was thought to cause psychopathologies.

Conclusion: A Passage Beyond Hyperspace

As was also the case for Sand, the "secret" isn't down in the Amazon, as Burroughs believed. It is right here, right now. This allusion to the capacity for humans to access an alternate dimensional space-time with the assistance of a compound known to be endogenous since the 1950s conveys the radical immediacy of an experience involving a rapid plunge across an invisible threshold into dramatically disembodied "worlds." The implication that many advocates of psychedelics—e.g., Huxley, Leary, McKenna, and Sand—have championed is that these passage-like events are a human birthright, sans shamanic, guru, or cultic intermediaries. As a corollary to this neo-gnostic transit, in which individuals are emboldened to potentiate their *selves* with the assistance of plant allies and spirit molecules, any "ritual," as such, is nonprescribed. As Tramacchi documented, the disembodied character of the DMT visions is "ritual-like." He conjectured that there is little conspicuous ritual associated with DMT use "because the visions themselves can possess an intrinsically ritual-like quality" (2006, p. 177).

It's a curious point. What is this "ritual-like" character? Could it be an experiential black hole, at best "liminoidal" or "rituoid," and therefore echoing Victor Turner's (1982) lamentations on the effect of the attenuation of the transformational potency of ritual in modern leisure practices? Might DMT "events" be illegitimate by contrast with the ceremonial practices associated, for example, with ayahuasca shamanisms? Such recreational practices may well be examples of ritual ceasing to be an "effective metalanguage or an agency of collective reflexology" (Turner, 1985, p. 165). But usage occurs on a spectrum, with other uses illustrative of therapy and, as found in this chapter, paragnosis. Technicians of gnosis, amateur botanists, and other members of a worldwide milieu of returnee enthusiasts familiar with the aesthetics of hyperspace are committed to optimize the means of perception, achieved by way of extraction methods, phytochemical and ethnobotanical research, sustainable plant propagation, administration techniques, experimental assaying, environmental augmentation, and safe user guidelines. In addition, they actively translate the experience via artistic media, including visionary art, often present in the contexts of use. These practices combined suggest the intentional augmentation of what is already felt to be a quintessentially liminal experience: the arts and techniques of superliminalization serving to potentiate experimental paragnoses, enable transpersonalism, and facilitate extraordinary experiences on a widening scale.

I have indicated elsewhere the limitations of applying standard sensory transmission in extant models of ritual to synesthetic, transpersonal, and "higher-dimensional" experiences that, nevertheless, possess initiatory and transformational efficacy (St John, 2018). While "travels" in "hyperspace" replete with veridical "entities" present serious challenges for researchers coming to grips with experiential virtuality, specific components are evident. Many telling examples in the literature involve physical travel—e.g., to secluded sites, wilderness areas, or festivals—with hardship, ordeals, and other experiences that are hallmarks of rites of passage. The cases of entheogenesis recounted in this chapter are illustrative of induction into microcommunities of the experienced, whose members may exchange the noetic information ("gifts") received and whose "breakthroughs" may enable reputation and stature.

Moreover, as has been illustrated in this chapter, a range of commentary has been assembled to demonstrate how the DMT event and, in particular, the breakthrough experience, amounts to paragnosis, which is essential to understanding the ritualized proclivities of DMT, the liminality of hyperspace, and the superliminal aesthetics of its protagonists. Reports from key advocates in DMT's modern history of use and promulgation, along with anonymous net-archived commentaries, have been illustrative of "entheogenic esotericism." This association has necessitated a discussion of the gnosis potential of DMT, among other "entheogens," as implicit to entheogenesis. Thoroughgoing analysis of the gnosis of connectedness with which returnees appear to be typically endowed, and how this gift animates efforts to augment the means of perception, awaits future studies.

References

∞Ayes. (2001). Just a wee bit more about DMT. *The Entheogen Review, 10*(2), 51–56.

Bell, A. (1999, April 1). Interview with Terence McKenna, Retrieved from http://www.jacobsm.com/deoxy/deoxy.org/tmab_4-1-99.htm

Burn in Noise. (2008).Transparent. On *Passing Clouds* [CD]. London: Alchemy Records.

Burroughs, W. S. (2012). *Rub out the words: The letters of William S. Burroughs 1959–1974.* New York, NY: Penguin.

Cott, C., & Roc, A. (2008). Phenomenology of N,N-Dimethyltryptamine use: A thematic analysis. *Journal of Scientific Exploration, 22*(3), 359–370.

Curtin, K. (2015, November 25). DMT journeys with Devin James Fry. *The Austin Chronicle.* Retrieved from http://www.austinchronicle.com/daily/music/2015-11-23/dmt-journeys-with-devin-james-fry/

DeKorne, J. (1992). Entheogen: What's in a word? *The Entheogen Review, 1*(2), 2.

DeKorne, J. (1993). Smokable DMT from plants. *The Entheogen Review, 2*(4), 1–3.

DeKorne, J. (1994). *Psychedelic shamanism: The cultivation, preparation, and shamanic use of psychotropic plants.* Port Townsend, WA: Breakout Productions.

Doyle, R. M. (2011). *Darwin's pharmacy: Sex, plants, and the evolution of the noösphere.* Seattle, WA: University of Washington Press.

Ellens, J. H. (2014). *Seeking the sacred with psychoactive substances: Chemical paths to spirituality and to god* (Vol. 1 & 2). Santa Barbara, CA: Praeger.

Erowid Crew. (2009). 5-MeO-DMT is not 'DMT': Differentiation is wise. *Erowid Extracts* Retrieved from www.erowid.org/chemicals/5meo_dmt/5meo_dmt_article1.shtml

Fadiman, J. (2011). *The psychedelic explorer's guide: Safe, therapeutic, and sacred journeys.* Rochester, VT: Park Street Press.

Forstmann, M., & Sagioglou, C. (2017). Lifetime experience with (classic) psychedelics predicts pro-environmental behavior through an increase in nature relatedness. *Journal of Psychopharmacology, 31*(8), 975–988.

Gaia, G. (2016). *Changa's alchemy: Narratives of transformation in psychedelic experiences* (Master's thesis). University of Amsterdam, The Netherlands.

Gallimore, A., & Luke, D. (2015). DMT research from 1956 to the end of time. In D. King, D. Luke, B. Sessa, C. Adams, & A. Tollen (Eds.), *Neurotransmissions: Essays on psychedelics from breaking convention* (pp. 291–316). London: Strange Attractor.

Gehr, R. (1992, May 5). Omega man: It's the end of the world as we know it (and Terence McKenna feels fine). *Village Voice, 37*(18), 47–48.

Griffiths, R. R., Richards, W. A., McCann, U., & Jesse, R. (2006). Psilocybin can occasion mystical-type experiences having substantial and sustained personal meaning and spiritual significance. *Psychopharmacology, 187*(3), 268–283.

Grof, S. (2009 [1975]). *LSD: Doorway to the numinous: The groundbreaking psychedelic research into realms of the human unconscious.* Rochester, VT: Park Street Press.

Hanegraaff, W. J. (1998). *New age religion and Western culture: Esotericism in the mirror of secular thought.* Albany, NY: State University of New York Press.

Hanegraaff, W. J. (2006). Introduction. In W. J. Hanegraaff (Ed.), *The dictionary of gnosis and Western esotericism* (pp. vii–xiii). Leiden, Netherlands: Brill.

Hanegraaff, W. J. (2008a). Reason, faith, and gnosis: Potential and problematics of a typological construct. In P. Meusburger, M. Walker, & E. Wunder (Eds.), *Clashes of knowledge* (pp. 133–144). New York, NY: Springer.

Hanegraaff, W. J. (2008b). Altered states of knowledge: The attainment of gnōsis in the hermetica. *The International Journal of the Platonic Tradition, 2*(2), 128–163.

Hanegraaff, W. J. (2010). "And end history. And go to the stars": Terence McKenna and 2012. In C. M. Cusack & C. Hartney (Eds.), *Religion and retributive logic: Essays in honour of Professor Garry W. Trompf* (pp. 291–312). Leiden, Netherlands: Brill.

Hanegraaff, W. J. (2011). Ayahuasca groups and networks in the Netherlands: A challenge to the study of contemporary religion. In B. C. Labate & H. Jungaberle (Eds.), *The internationalization of ayahuasca* (pp. 85–103). Zürich, Switzerland: Lit Verlag.

Hanegraaff, W. J. (2013). Entheogenic esotericism. In E. Asprem & K. Granholm (Eds.), *Contemporary esotericism (Gnostica)* (pp. 392–409). New York, NY: Routledge.

Hanna, J. (2009). *Erowid character vaults: Nick Sand extended biography.* Erowid.org/culture/characters/sand_nick/sand_nick_biography1.shtml

Hanna, J. (2012). Aliens, insectoids, and elves! Oh, my! *Erowid.org.* Retrieved from http://www.erowid.org/chemicals/dmt/dmt_article3.shtml

Hanna, J., Manning, T & Slattery, D. (2012, May 6). *Interview with Nick Sand* (unreleased). Mind States. Unpublished document in the private collection of John Hanna.

Harrop, J. (2010). *The yagé aesthetic of William Burroughs: The publication and development of his work 1953–1965* (Doctoral dissertation). Queen Mary, University of London, UK.

Huxley, A. (2009 [1955]). *The doors of perception and Heaven and Hell.* New York, NY: Harper Perennial.

Hyperspace Lexicon. (n.d.). *DMT Nexus Wiki.* Retrieved from https://wiki.dmt-nexus.me/Hyper space_lexicon

Krippner, S. (2002). Dancing with the trickster: Notes for a transpersonal autobiography. *International Journal of Transpersonal Studies, 21*(1), 1–18.

Labate, B. C., & Cavnar, C. (Eds.). (2014). *Ayahuasca shamanism in the Amazon and beyond.* New York, NY: Oxford University Press.

Luke, D. (2008). Disembodied eyes revisited: An investigation into the ontology of entheogenic entity encounters. *The Entheogen Review, 17*(1), 1–9. 38–40.

Luke, D. (2011). Discarnate entities and dimethyltryptamine (DMT): Psychopharmacology, phenomenology and ontology. *Journal of the Society for Psychical Research, 75*(1), 26–42.

McKenna, D. J., & Riba, J. (2015). New World tryptamine hallucinogens and the neuroscience of ayahuasca. In M. A. Geyer, B. A. Ellenbroek, C. A. Marsden, T. R. E. Barnes, & S. L. Andersen (Eds.), *Current topics in behavioral neurosciences.* New York, NY: Springer.

McKenna, T. (n.d.). *DMT, mathematical dimensions, syntax and death.* Transcript by E. Petakovic of MckennaCountrCulture (YouTube account) [video]. Uploaded August 28, 2013. Retrieved from http://terencemckenna.wikispaces.com/DMT%2C+Mathematical+Dimensions%2C+and +Death

McKenna, T. (1994, July 19–24). Rap dancing into the 3rd millennium. Presented at Starwood XIV Festival, Brushwood Folklore Center, Sherman, New York.

McKenna, T. (1998, December 13). *Dreaming awake at the end of time.* Talk presented at Fort Mason, San Francisco, California. Transcript by spooky.physics of nndm tube (YouTube account) [video]. Uploaded September 17, 2012. Retrieved from https://terencemckenna. wikispaces.com/Dreaming+Awake+at+the+End+of+Time

McKenna, T. (1992). *Food of the gods: The search for the original tree of knowledge.* New York, NY: Bantam Books.

McKenna, T., Angus, C. & West, R. (1992) Re: Evolution. On Boss Drum [Vinyl record]. London: One Little Indian.

McKenna, T., & McKenna, D. (1993 [1975]). *The invisible landscape: Mind, hallucinogens and the I Ching.* New York, NY: HarperOne.

Milhet, M., & Reynaud-Maurupt, C. (2011). Contemporary use of natural hallucinogens: From techno subcultures to mainstream values. In G. Hunt, H. Bergeron, & M. Milhet (Eds.), *Drugs and culture: Knowledge, consumption and policy* (pp. 149–170). New York, NY: Ashgate.

Oroc, J. (2009). *The tryptamine palace: 5-MeO-DMT and the Sonoran desert toad.* Rochester, VT: Park Street Press.

Ott, J. (1996 [1993]). *Pharmacotheon: Entheogenic drugs, their plant sources and history.* Kennewick, WA: Natural Products Co..

Pickover, C. A. (2005). *Drugs, sex, Einstein and elves: Sushi, psychedelics, parallel universes, and the quest for transcendence.* Petaluma, CA: Smart Publications.

222   G. St John

Pinchbeck, D. (2002). *Breaking open the head: A psychedelic journey into the heart of contemporary shamanism.* New York, NY: Broadway Books.
Richards, W. A. (2014). Here and now: Discovering the sacred with entheogens. *Zygon: Journal of Religion and Science, 49*(3), 652–665.
Roberts, T. B. (2013). *The psychedelic future of the mind: How entheogens are enhancing cognition, boosting intelligence, and raising values.* Rochester, VT: Park Street Press.
Ruck, C. A., Bigwood, J., Staples, D., Ott, J., & Wasson, G. (1979). Entheogens. *Journal of Psychedelic Drugs, 11*(1–2), 145–146.
SFos. (2000, June 14). The elven antics annex: An experience with DMT (ID 1841). *Erowid.org.* Retrieved from: http://erowid.org/exp/1841
Sledge, M., & Grim, R. (2013, December 9). If you haven't heard of DMT yet, you might soon. *Huffington Post.* Retrieved from http://www.huffingtonpost.com/2013/12/09/dmt-use_n_4412633.html
Smith, H. (2000). *Cleansing the doors of perception: The religious significance of entheogenic plants and chemicals.* New York, NY: Tarcher.
St John, G. (2011). Spiritual technologies and altering consciousness in contemporary counterculture. In E. Cardeña & M. Winkelman (Eds.), *Altering consciousness: A multidisciplinary perspective* (Vol. 1, pp. 203–225). Praeger Perspectives: Santa Barbara, CA.
St John, G. (2012). *Global tribe: Technology, spirituality and psytrance.* Sheffield, UK: Equinox.
St John, G. (2015). *Mystery school in hyperspace: A cultural history of DMT.* Berkeley, CA: North Atlantic Books.
St John, G. (2017a). Aussiewaska: A cultural history of changa and ayahuasca analogues in Australia. In B. C. Labate, C. Cavnar, & A. Gearin (Eds.), *The world ayahuasca diaspora: Reinventions and controversies* (pp. 144–162). London: Routledge.
St John, G. (2017b). Hyperespace dans le cyberespace: DMT et méta-ritualisation. *Drogues, santé et société, 16*(2), 76–103.
St John, G. (2018). The breakthrough experience: DMT hyperspace and its liminal aesthetics. *Anthropology of Consciousness, 29*(1), 57–76.
Strassman, R. (2001). *DMT, The spirit molecule.* Rochester, VT: Park Street Press.
Tramacchi, D. (2006). *Vapours and visions: Religious dimensions of DMT use* (Doctoral dissertation), University of Queensland, Australia.
Turner, D. M. (1994). *The essential psychedelic guide.* San Francisco, CA: Panther Press.
Turner, V. (1982). *From ritual to theatre: The human seriousness of play.* New York, NY: Performing Arts Journal Publications.
Turner, V. (1985). Process, system, and symbol: A new anthropological synthesis. In E. Turner (Ed.), *On the edge of the bush: Anthropology as experience* (pp. 151–173). Tucson: University of Arizona Press.
Universal Shaman. (2004). Mother spirit awaits: Experience with DMT (ID 30919). *Erowid.org.* September 28. erowid.org/exp/30919
Wasson, R. G. (1957, May 13). Seeking the magic mushroom. *Life, 49*(19), 100–102, 109–120.
Winstock, A. R., Kaar, S., & Borschmann, R. (2013). Dimethyltryptamine (*DMT*): Prevalence, user characteristics and abuse liability in a large global sample. *Journal of Psychopharmacology, 28*(1), 49–54.

List of Editors and Contributors

Editors

Beatriz Caiuby Labate has a Ph.D. in social anthropology from the State University of Campinas (UNICAMP), Brazil. Her main areas of interest are the study of psychoactive substances, drug policy, shamanism, ritual, and religion. She is Adjunct Faculty at the East-West Psychology Program at the California Institute of Integral Studies (CIIS) in San Francisco and Visiting Professor at the Center for Research and Post Graduate Studies in Social Anthropology (CIESAS) in Guadalajara. She is cofounder of the Drugs, Politics, and Culture Collective in Mexico (http://drogaspoliticacultura.net) and cofounder of the Interdisciplinary Group for Psychoactive Studies (NEIP) in Brazil, as well as editor of NEIP's website (http://www.neip.info). She is also Chief Editor at Chacruna (http://chacruna.net). She is author, coauthor, and coeditor of seventeen books, one special-edition journal, and several peer-reviewed articles (http://bialabate.net).

Clancy Cavnar has a doctorate in clinical psychology (Psy.D.) from John F. Kennedy University in Pleasant Hill, CA. She currently works in private practice in San Francisco and is an associate editor at Chacruna (http://chacruna.net), a venue for publication of high-quality academic short texts on plant medicines. She is also a research associate of the Interdisciplinary Group for Psychoactive Studies (NEIP). She combines an eclectic array of interests and activities as clinical psychologist, artist, and researcher. She has a master of fine arts in painting from the San Francisco Art Institute, a master's in counseling from San Francisco State University, and she completed the Certificate in Psychedelic-Assisted Therapy program at the California Institute of Integral Studies. She is author and coauthor of articles in several peer-reviewed journals and coeditor, with Beatriz Caiuby Labate, of eight books. For more information see: http://neip.info/pesquisadore/clancy-cavnar

© Springer International Publishing AG, part of Springer Nature 2018
B. C. Labate, C. Cavnar (eds.), *Plant Medicines, Healing and Psychedelic Science*,
https://doi.org/10.1007/978-3-319-76720-8

Contributors

Alexander Dawson is a historian of modern Mexico and is associate professor of history at SUNY Albany. He is the author of three books, including *Latin American Since Independence: A History with Primary Sources* (Routledge, 2011, 2014), *First World Dreams: Mexico Since 1989* (Zed Books, 2006), and *Indian and Nation in Revolutionary Mexico* (Arizona, 2004), and has published essays in *Latin American Perspectives*, the *Journal of Latin American Studies*, *The Americas*, and the *Hispanic American Historical Review*. He is currently working on a book titled *The Peyote Effect: Making Race Along the US-Mexican Border* (under contract with the University of California Press), which examines the ways peyote, whiteness, and indianness have been linked over time in Mexico and the USA by indigenous peoples, ecclesiastical authorities, government officials, and others.

Laura Dev is a PhD candidate at the University of California, Berkeley, in the Department of Environmental Science, Policy, and Management, within the Society and Environment division. Her studies are focused on the intersection of political ecology, science studies, and ethnobotany. Using a multispecies ethnography approach to investigating relationships among medicinal plants and humans, her work points to the complex power relations at play as plants become agents in global markets. She conducts her field work following plants, rituals, and knowledge through emergent social networks between the Ucayali Region of Peru and California. In addition to interrogating knowledge-making practices, her research aims to contribute to understanding how indigenous Shipibo communities can retain greater benefits from the commoditization of their plants and rituals. Laura's background is in plant community ecology, and she holds an MS in ecology from Colorado State University.

Erika Dyck is a professor and Canada Research Chair in Medical History. She is the author of *Psychedelic Psychiatry: LSD from Clinic to Campus* (Johns Hopkins, 2008; University of Manitoba Press, 2011); *Facing Eugenics: Reproduction, Sterilization and the Politics of Choice* (University of Toronto, 2013), which was shortlisted for the Governor General's award for Canadian nonfiction; and a forthcoming book *Managing Madness: the Weyburn Mental Hospital and the Transformation of Psychiatric Care in Canada* (University of Manitoba Press, 2017). Her research explores the interaction between patients, doctors, and policy makers as a series of exchanges that help us appreciate the dynamic relationship between scientific expertise and society.

Kevin Feeney has a law degree and a PhD in cultural anthropology. He is currently a lecturer at Central Washington University. Research interests include examining legal and regulatory issues surrounding the religious and cultural use of psychoactive substances, with an emphasis on peyote and ayahuasca, and exploring modern and traditional uses of *Amanita muscaria*, with a specific focus on preparation practices.

His research has been published in the *International Journal of Drug Policy*, *Journal of Psychoactive Drugs*, *Human Organization*, and *Curare*, and he is coauthor, with Richard Glen Boire, of *Medical Marijuana Law* (2007).

Ben Feinberg is a professor of cultural anthropology and chair of the Division of Social Sciences at Warren Wilson College. He received his PhD from the University of Texas at Austin in 1996 and is the author of *The Devil's Book of Culture: History, Mushrooms, and Caves in Southern Mexico* (2003, University of Texas Press). He first visited the Sierra Mazateca in 1987 and has been returning ever since. He is currently researching the history of cave exploration in Oaxaca from both Mazatec and cavers' perspectives and continuing research into American students' narratives of study abroad. He lives in Asheville, North Carolina, with his children and pets.

J. Hamilton Hudson is a lawyer from the USA, born and raised in Hong Kong. He earned his JD with an MS from Tulane University in New Orleans and his BA magna cum laude in anthropology from the University of Colorado, Boulder. Currently, he is research associate at the Interdisciplinary Group for Psychoactive Studies (NEIP), Brazil/USA.

O. Hayden Griffin III is an associate professor of criminal justice at the University of Alabama at Birmingham. He has a PhD in criminology, law, and society from the University of Florida and a JD from the T.C. Williams School of Law at the University of Richmond. His main areas of interests are drug policy, corrections, and law and society. He is the first author (along with Vanessa Woodward and John J. Sloan, III) of *The Money and Politics of Criminal Justice Policy* (Carolina Academic Press, 2016) and second author (with Lior Gideon) of *Correctional Management and the Law: A Penological Approach* (Carolina Academic Press, 2017) and coeditor (with Vanessa Woodward) of *Handbook of Corrections in the United States* (Routledge, 2017). He has more than thirty publications that have appeared in peer-reviewed journals, law journals, and as book chapters.

Katherine Hendy is a visiting assistant professor in the Department of Comparative Studies at the Ohio State University. Her research explores the politics and practices of knowledge making inside of biomedical and scientific settings, as well as the shifting boundaries and meanings surrounding medicinal and recreational substances. Trained as an anthropologist at the University of California at Berkeley, she conducted an ethnographic study of the clinical trials seeking to develop the drug MDMA (Ecstasy) as a prescription pharmaceutical and on the underground psychedelic therapy scene. Prior to her doctoral research, she worked as an ethnographic interviewer and fieldworker on a study of club drug use funded by the National Institutes of Drug Abuse. The Wenner-Gren Foundation has supported her research.

Graham St John, PhD, is an Australian cultural anthropologist specializing in event-cultural movements and entheogens. Among his eight books are *Mystery School in Hyperspace: A Cultural History of DMT* (North Atlantic Books 2015), *Global Tribe:*

Technology, Spirituality and Psytrance (Equinox 2012), and *Technomad: Global Raving Countercultures* (Equinox 2009). He currently works in the Department of Social Science, University of Fribourg, Switzerland, as senior research fellow on the SNSF project Burning Progeny: The European Efflorescence of Burning Man and is adjunct research fellow at Griffith Centre for Social and Cultural Research, Griffith University, Australia. He is executive editor of *Dancecult: Journal of Electronic Dance Music Culture*. His website is: www.edgecentral.net

Beatriz Caiuby Labate has a Ph.D. in social anthropology from the State University of Campinas (UNICAMP), Brazil. Her main areas of interest are the study of psychoactive substances, drug policy, shamanism, ritual, and religion. She is Adjunct Faculty at the East-West Psychology Program at the California Institute of Integral Studies (CIIS) in San Francisco and Visiting Professor at the Center for Research and Post Graduate Studies in Social Anthropology (CIESAS) in Guadalajara. She is cofounder of the Drugs, Politics, and Culture Collective in Mexico (http://drogaspoliticacultura.net) and cofounder of the Interdisciplinary Group for Psychoactive Studies (NEIP) in Brazil, as well as editor of NEIP's website (http://www.neip.info). She is also Chief Editor at Chacruna (http://chacruna.net). She is author, coauthor, and coeditor of seventeen books, one special-edition journal, and several peer-reviewed articles (http://bialabate.net).

Ana Elda Maqueda is an author, clinical psychologist, and a neuroscientist studying the medicinal and psychoactive plant *Salvia divinorum* and the ayahuasca brew at the Human Neuropsychopharmacology Research Group, at the Hospital de Sant Pau in Barcelona, Spain. She is also a fieldwork researcher specializing in *Salvia divinorum* and has spent the last six years exploring the Mazatec Sierra, thoroughly investigating the current uses of this plant. During her fieldwork, she lived with Mazatec families, learning from traditional doctors and healers, and contributed her support to the preservation of their language, habitat, and customs. She is the founder of the nonprofit Xkà, which aims to recuperate the Mazatec knowledge.

Sidarta Ribeiro is full professor of neuroscience and director of the Brain Institute at the Universidade Federal do Rio Grande do Norte. He holds a bachelor's degree in biology from the Universidade de Brasília (1993), a master's degree in biophysics from the Universidade Federal do Rio de Janeiro (1994), and a PhD in animal behavior from the Rockefeller University (2000), with postdoctoral studies in neurophysiology at Duke University (2005). He has experience in neuroethology, molecular neurobiology, and systems neurophysiology, with an interest in the following subjects: memory, sleep, and dreams; neuronal plasticity; vocal communication; symbolic competence in nonhuman animals; drug policy; and neuroeducation. From 2009 to 2011, he served as secretary of the Brazilian Society for Neuroscience and Behavior. From 2011 to 2015, he served as chair of the Brazilian Regional Committee of the Pew Latin American Fellows Program in the Biomedical Sciences. He is a member of the Advisory Board of the Brazilian Platform for Drug Policy and secretary of the Brazilian Society for the Advancement of Science. Sidarta Ribeiro is greatly interested in the study of the neural bases of consciousness and its alteration, including investigation of the ayahuasca experience. He is also involved in the public debate on medicinal uses and the legalization of cannabis in Brazil.

Jordan Sloshower is a fourth-year resident physician in the Department of Psychiatry at Yale University. He was born and raised in Winnipeg, Canada, and completed a master's degree in medical anthropology at the University of Edinburgh prior to entering medical school at Yale. While a medical student, he pursued research and clinical opportunities in India, Nepal, Ecuador, Peru, and South Africa. As a psychiatry resident, Jordan's clinical interests have largely been in community-based mental health, addictions, psychodynamic and mindfulness-based psychotherapy, and integrative psychiatry. His research focuses on the therapeutic application of psychedelic substances and plants, and he is cofounder of the Yale Psychedelic Science Group.

Joanna Steinhardt is a PhD candidate in the Anthropology Department at the University of California Santa Barbara. She is also the recipient of a master's degree in cultural studies from Hebrew University in Jerusalem. Her master's thesis was on an American-Jewish mystical religious revival in Israel/Palestine. She is writing her dissertation on do-it-yourself (DIY) mycology based on field work in the San Francisco Bay Area and the Pacific Northwest. Her interests are in contemporary spirituality, secularity, multispecies ethnography, open source, and DIY science.

Printed by Printforce, the Netherlands